Let Me Heal

Advance Praise for
Let Me Heal

This latest gem from Ken Ludmerer is a monumental treasure trove on the subject of residency education and its relationship to patient care that will be read for decades. More important, it is a must read now for anyone who cares about how we train our future doctors. His descriptions of current problems and prescriptions for change are right on target—essential reading for anyone concerned about the future of health care in this country.
Dr. Timothy Johnson, MD, MPH, Retired Medical Editor, ABC News

Ludmerer's vantage point of physician-historian enables him to unwrap and analyze the residency experience in a unique and penetrating manner. This brilliant work will enlighten the current contentious debate surrounding residency training and demonstrate the inextricable relationship between the quality of residency training and patient care in America. Everyone interested in providing and receiving quality health care is in his debt because of this engaging and powerful book.
Samuel O. Thier, MD, President Emeritus of the Institute of Medicine, Professor of Medicine and Health Care Policy, Emeritus, Harvard Medical School

This thoughtful scholarly treatise on the residency, the most influential learning period for young physicians, is a major contribution to our understanding of how America produces its physician workforce. It notes the educational, scientific, economic, social, legal, ethical, and political influences which produce tensions and conflicts in the training experience.

Dr. Ludmerer provides a platform for examining these influences and he proposes ways for the learning environment to be more flexible, while maintaining high standards and the professionalism we all want to retain in our nation's physicians.

I heartily recommend this superb book to all who are interested in our nation's healthcare system.
Louis W. Sullivan, MD, President Emeritus, Morehouse School of Medicine, U.S. Secretary of Health and Human Services, 1989-1993

In engaging and compelling prose, Kenneth Ludmerer vividly chronicles and insightfully analyzes the medical and social history of the residency phase of American medical education. Based on rich observational and documentary data, he brilliantly evaluates the achievements, tensions, and shortcomings of the residency system. "Let Me Heal," the entreaty that he chose for the book's title, has contemporary as well as historic significance. It is associated with Ludmerer's stirring analysis of how the present-day struggles with patient care and health care delivery in the United States create challenges for good medical education, and of how the residency system can contribute to making medical care better and more affordable.

This landmark book should be read by all who are concerned with medical education and patient care in America.
Renée C. Fox, Annenberg Professor Emerita of the Social Sciences, University of Pennsylvania

In a most readable and engaging way, Ken Ludmerer traces the development of graduate medical education in the United States in parallel with the major developments in the science and practice of medicine over the past century and a half. With his intimate knowledge of and decades of personal experience with medical education, he brings to this work a deep appreciation of the social value and moral purpose of physician training. If you're concerned about the skills and dedication of tomorrow's doctors—and everyone should be—read this insightful and authoritative book.
Jordan Cohen, Immediate Past President, Association of American Medical Colleges

Let Me Heal is as much an entreaty to the profession and the public to solidify the future of graduate medical education in the United States as it is a historical treatise on the evolution of perhaps the greatest and most efficient medical education system in the world. While tracing and interpreting its evolution, Ken Ludmerer points out not only the successes but also the failures of the system, past and present. The inescapable conclusions to the challenges he outlines to the training and professional maturation of physicians are a call-to-arms for those of us engaged in the education of the next generation of doctors and a call for understanding and support from the public, whose future care depends on our success!
Thomas J. Nasca, MD, Professor of Medicine and former Dean, Jefferson Medical College, and Chief Executive Officer of the Accreditation Council for Graduate Medical Education (ACGME)

Let Me Heal

The Opportunity to Preserve Excellence in American Medicine

Kenneth M. Ludmerer

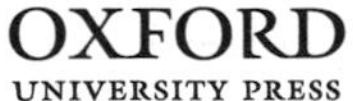

OXFORD
UNIVERSITY PRESS

Oxford University Press is a department of the University of Oxford. It furthers the University's objective of excellence in research, scholarship, and education by publishing worldwide.

Oxford New York
Auckland Cape Town Dar es Salaam Hong Kong Karachi
Kuala Lumpur Madrid Melbourne Mexico City Nairobi
New Delhi Shanghai Taipei Toronto

With offices in
Argentina Austria Brazil Chile Czech Republic France Greece
Guatemala Hungary Italy Japan Poland Portugal Singapore
South Korea Switzerland Thailand Turkey Ukraine Vietnam

Oxford is a registered trademark of Oxford University Press in the UK and certain other countries.

Published in the United States of America by
Oxford University Press
198 Madison Avenue, New York, NY 10016

Library of Congress Cataloging-in-Publication Data
Ludmerer, Kenneth M., author.
Let me heal : the opportunity to preserve excellence in American medicine / Kenneth M. Ludmerer.
p. ; cm.
Includes bibliographical references and index.
ISBN 978-0-19-974454-1 (alk. paper)
I. Title.
[DNLM: 1. Internship and Residency—history—United States. 2. Education, Medical, Graduate—standards—United States. 3. Quality of Health Care—United States. W 20]
R840
610.71′55—dc23
2014004264

3 5 7 9 8 6 4
Printed in the United States of America
on acid-free paper

To the Ideals of the Johns Hopkins Medical School and Hospital

CONTENTS

PREFACE

This book had its immediate beginnings while I served on the Institute of Medicine's "Committee on Optimizing Graduate Medical Trainee (Resident) Hours and Work Schedules to Improve Patient Safety," which published its report in January 2009.[1] However, this book would have been impossible for me to conceptualize or write without my two earlier books on medical education: *Learning to Heal*,[2] which explores the creation of the modern medical school and teaching hospital in America, and *Time to Heal*,[3] which examines the evolution of American medical education from the early twentieth century to the era of managed care. Thus, *Let Me Heal* builds on a lifetime of experience in medical education, both as a professor of medicine who is practicing and teaching on the wards and as a medical educator and historian of medicine who is researching, thinking, and writing about medical education in the United States. It discusses a subject about which I have long been passionate, having for decades witnessed the residency system's achievements and failings as well as its fundamental importance to the health of the nation.

While on the committee, I discovered the great need for an analytic account of the residency system. In the making of a doctor, the residency represents the dominant formative influence. It is during the three to nine years that medical graduates spend as residents and clinical fellows that doctors come of professional age—acquiring the knowledge and skills of their specialties or subspecialties, forming professional identities, and developing habits, behaviors, attitudes, and values that last a professional lifetime. The four years of medical school, in contrast, provide only a general introduction to medical practice. Yet, despite the growing historical literature on medical students and medical schools, no history of the residency system existed.

This book represents an attempt to fill that void. It is intended to provide a contextualized, interpretive account of the development of the residency system in the United States. It is also meant to offer insight into our current dilemmas in residency training and medical care and to offer guidance for improvement. Those who hope to improve the training of doctors and the quality of patient care in America will find much to contemplate in these pages. The book is written for doctors who wish to reconnect with the educational and moral roots of the profession, physicians of tomorrow who aspire to understand the heritage of the profession they will be joining, individuals and scholars of diverse interests who seek to understand the history and meaning of residency training, educational and health care leaders who strive to improve our systems of producing doctors and providing patient care, and patients who desire to understand their own dilemmas in receiving medical care and, perhaps, to work proactively to create a health care system that more effectively focuses on their needs.

The residency system in America had dual roots. It arose in part from the revolution in scientific medicine in the late nineteenth century and the infatuation of American educators of the period with the ideal of the German university. Thus, the residency system represents an important chapter in the history of American higher education. It was no accident that the first formal residency program was introduced at Johns Hopkins, which also established the country's first research university and first scientific medical school. However, the residency system also had roots in medical practice, particularly in the apprenticeship system. Accordingly, it developed many characteristics of an institutionalized apprenticeship. These dual roots of the residency system account for its defining dilemma: the tension between the responsibility of residency training to provide high-level professional education and the desire of sponsoring hospitals to extract as much inexpensive labor from their residents as possible. The "education versus service" tension has shaped the residency system at every moment of its development.

Throughout its history, the residency system was continually influenced by evolving scientific and medical circumstances. These are explored fully in the pages that follow. However, cultural conditions indelibly affected the residency system as well. Changing attitudes toward work and poverty impacted the ways doctors learned and practiced medicine, as did the civil rights movement, feminism, the rise of consumerism, and the evolving health care delivery system. These considerations, too, are included here.

At the core of the residency system are fundamental educational principles: the assumption of responsibility by residents in patient management, and the importance of providing residents sufficient time to reflect and pursue subjects in depth. Also at the core are the moral principles of residency training: thoroughness, attention to detail, and learning that the needs of patients should come first. The subject includes a sociological dimension: Who are the residents? What was it like to be a resident? What were the stresses and rewards? How did the experiences of residents shape their attitudes and behaviors toward patients? How did the experience of being a resident change over time? The topic also involves consideration of the financing, administration, and regulation of graduate medical education as well as the relation of residency training to public goals, such as the quality of doctors produced, the geographical and specialty distributions of physicians, and the ability of doctors to retain a caring, patient-centered focus in an increasingly technological and commercialized health care system. All these perspectives are explored in this book.

As I wrote this book, an emotional public controversy over resident work hours was raging, fueled by the fear that tired house officers pose a threat to patient safety. This is the most intense, divisive controversy in medical education in generations. In one sense this debate is misguided. The evidence is much stronger linking patient safety to the workload of house officers and the quality of supervision than to fatigue from long hours. Indeed, there is growing evidence that the current imposition of rigid, highly inflexible work rules that often do not allow house officers to complete their responsibilities is detrimental to both education and patient care. Yet, as the following account demonstrates, more reasonable work schedules have long been needed to make the residency experience more humane. This book is sympathetic with current efforts to lighten the back-breaking work schedules that residents have traditionally endured, but it makes a strong plea for the provision of much greater flexibility in constructing work schedules than the present system allows.

But that is only part of the story. The danger in the current controversy over resident work hours is that attention will be diverted away from the factors most essential to producing outstanding doctors. From the beginning of the residency system, work hours were but one part of the much larger issue of work conditions. This book examines the evolution of the learning environment for resident training and thus speaks directly to the challenge of establishing and maintaining excellence in residency education. To achieve that goal, attention needs to be paid to the totality of the learning experience. This includes the quality of the house officers and faculty, the characteristics of the teaching, giving residents the opportunity to assume responsibility in patient management, the availability of time to reflect and wonder, the opportunity for residents to establish meaningful personal relationships with faculty, patients, and each other, the provision of manageable patient loads, freeing residents from too many extraneous chores, holding high expectations of residents, and conducting residency training in an atmosphere of professional excitement. All these factors influence the quality of training and the characteristics and capabilities of our country's doctors. It would do well for medical educators to heed this lesson, particularly those who wish to see residency training continue as professional education and not devolve into vocational training.

The most important factor affecting residency training is the quality of patient care that house officers observe. Residents learn their specialty by practicing, under supervision, in the real world of health care delivery. Thus, the quality of residency training ultimately depends on the standards of care maintained in the settings where residents learn and acquire professional values. At the moment, the education of tomorrow's doctors is endangered by our country's commercialized system of health care that, despite lip service to patient-centered care, fails to deliver on that promise. Residents are acquiring habits and approaches to patient care amid a culture of excess in which tests and procedures are often obtained because they are there, not because they are needed. Residents are also learning their specialties in a health care environment that encourages doctors to see as many patients as possible as quickly as possible without necessarily providing the time, caring, thought, and attention to detail that many patients need. Patients are not consistently well served in such a system; neither is medical education. These problems in America's system of health care delivery represent the greatest challenge facing residency training at the present moment.

However, the relationship between residency training and the health care delivery system is reciprocal; the fate of one affects the other. During residency, doctors acquire the habits and approaches that they carry with them throughout their careers. Thus, there is much that good residency training can do to make medical care in America better and more affordable. Medical educators have the opportunity to teach a much more parsimonious approach to patient care—one in which doctors evaluate patients thoughtfully and proceed with only the tests or treatments that are dictated by the patient's particular circumstances. This approach—deemed the method of the "scientific practitioner" by the original medical faculty at Johns Hopkins—has long been the ideal of medical education and practice, if never even closely approximated in reality. As this book points out, closer adherence to this approach would both reduce costs and improve quality, thereby potentially alleviating some of the major stresses in America's system of health care. This reciprocal relationship between residency training and the health care delivery system, and the potential for residency education to contribute to health care renewal, are the most important messages of the book.

With the health care delivery system rapidly changing, the 2010s represent an uncertain time for medical education and practice. Yet there is also much for physicians to embrace. Developments in medical science bring us to the brink of unparalleled opportunity in preventing and treating disease and relieving suffering. The current turmoil in health care delivery offers the profession and public the opportunity to redesign medical education and practice in ways that more fully serve the needs of patients, present and future. The opportunity is there to envision medical education and practice as they should be, not as they are, and to work toward achieving that end. Such opportunities are to be treasured, not feared. The country will always need good doctors, and the medical profession has little to fear in the changes ahead as long as it remembers that it exists to serve, that the needs of patients come before its own, and that it always must be thinking of improving the future as well as caring for the present.

ACKNOWLEDGMENTS

One of the great joys of writing a book is the opportunity to thank those whose ideas, encouragement, and support were so instrumental along the way. Thus, it is a deep pleasure to acknowledge the many friends and colleagues whose contributions have facilitated and enriched this book.

Let Me Heal, like my two earlier books on medical education, *Learning to Heal* and *Time to Heal*, is based on years of extensive research in archival repositories throughout the country. The notes will serve as an index to the staffs that proved so friendly and helpful. For this book, I am particularly indebted to Carol Tomer (Cleveland Clinic), Steven Novak (Columbia University Medical Center), Scott Podolsky (Countway Medical Library, Harvard Medical School), Nancy McCall (The Johns Hopkins Medical Institutions), Jeffrey Mindlin (Massachusetts General Hospital), and Stephen Logsdon (Washington University School of Medicine). I am also grateful to Thomas Nasca and Kevin Weiss for providing me access to the records of the Accreditation Council for Graduate Medical Education and of the American Board of Medical Specialties, respectively. I owe a special thanks to Debra Weinstein for introducing me to the collection of Chief Resident Letters in the department of medicine of the Massachusetts General Hospital and to Jatin Vyas for granting me permission to examine those letters.

Throughout the project I benefited from the encouragement and assistance of many friends who were always available to discuss ideas and provide support. I would particularly like to thank Marcia Angell, Garland Allen, DeWitt Baldwin Jr., Iver Bernstein, Henry Berger, Melvin Blanchard, Timothy Brigham, Douglas Carlson, Ralph Dacey, Thomas De Fer, Bradley Evanoff, Mark Frisse, Lara Goitein, Lee Goldman, Daniel Goodenberger, David Hellmann, Michael Johns, Joel Katz, David Kipnis, David Konig, Alan Kraut, Howard Markel, Thomas Nasca, Ingrid Philibert, Arnold Relman, Walton Schalick, Dale Smith, Murray Weidenbaum, and Sankey Williams. I am also grateful for the insights of those who have written about the history of American medical education before me, especially Thomas Bonner, Gert Brieger, Donald Fleming, and William Rothstein. During the project I benefited greatly from the nurturing environment of Washington University's department of medicine, chaired by Kenneth Polonsky and Victoria Fraser; the department of history, headed by Jean Allman; and the Center for the History of Medicine, led by Thomas Woolsey. Louise Ishibashi and Betsy Presson provided outstanding secretarial assistance.

A number of individuals took the time to offer detailed and helpful comments on an earlier version of the manuscript. I would like to express my gratitude to Mary Ann Dzuback, Daniel M. Fox, Renée C. Fox, David Hellmann, Joseph Kett, Loren Ludmerer, and Rosemary Stevens for their sage insights, constructive suggestions, and helpful advice. I would also like to thank my agent, Glen Hartley, who brought me to Oxford University Press, and my editor, Andrea Seils, who has been an invaluable source of ideas and encouragement. Her insights, good humor, and strong support have made the book immeasurably better. I am grateful to the Spencer Foundation and the Josiah Macy Jr. Foundation for providing grants to write the book. George Thibault, the president of the Macy Foundation, has been a friend of the author and the book from the beginning of the project.

To a few individuals, I would like to express my special appreciation. Daniel M. Fox has been a valued friend throughout my professional career. My outlook that the medical profession has obligations and responsibilities, not just rights and entitlements, owes much to conversations he and I have had over the years. Renée C. Fox has been both a wonderful friend and great source of inspiration. Her brilliant intellect, sociological perspective, and strong value system have had an influence on every page of the book. Mabel Purkerson has been another special friend; she knows how deeply indebted to her I am. Throughout the project, Jordan, Lindsey, and Loren Ludmerer have enriched the book through their presence. Loren has also been a magnificent critic and adviser as well as a continual source of ideas, encouragement, and inspiration. Neither this book nor my trilogy on medical education would have been possible without her.

I have written this book with gratitude for the privilege of being a doctor and with the conviction that despite the present turmoil in health care delivery, there remains much in medicine to embrace and celebrate. The values expressed here—that the medical profession exists to serve, that doctors should never be content with current knowledge and practices, that academic medical centers should have a passion for expanding and not just transmitting knowledge, and that doctors should aspire for perfection and not just excellence in medical care—are values that

I acquired as a student at the Johns Hopkins School of Medicine. These ideals, like most ideals, have never been fully realized, even at Johns Hopkins. However, they are timeless principles that speak to medicine at its best. Medical education and medical practice have much to look forward to in the century ahead, as long as these values remain anchored as the core of the enterprise.

Let Me Heal

CHAPTER 1
Antecedents

It was late one night in 1882 at Episcopal Hospital in Kensington, Pennsylvania, and the staff was worried. Several days before, a young woman had been admitted for a rapidly enlarging abdominal mass, which her surgeon had diagnosed as a "large fibroid tumor." After much hesitation and delay, the surgeon scheduled an operation. This was a huge decision, for in those earliest days of antiseptic surgery, opening the abdomen on the operating table was far from a routine procedure. On arrival the next morning, the surgeon was met at the door by a nurse. "Doctor, there won't be any operation today. The tumor was born last night."[1]

Mistaking pregnancy for an abdominal tumor was hardly unusual in nineteenth-century America, given the prevailing conditions of medical education and practice. Nowhere in the country was training in any medical or surgical specialty available. More striking still, American physicians while in medical school received very little clinical experience of any sort. This was true for all doctors, including the great majority who entered general practice.[2] Accordingly, physicians typically learned from their first patients in practice. This was why many ambitious physicians chose to learn their art after graduation from medical school by practicing on the poor. They received no fees from those patients, but they gained invaluable clinical experience that later made them attractive to paying patients.[3]

These deficiencies of medical education were widely recognized within the medical community. All century long, some ambitious physicians found ways to circumvent the formal educational system by acquiring additional educational experiences after graduating from medical school. These alternative paths of medical education—called nineteenth-century America's system of "professional improvement" by one historian[4]—helped doctors better prepare for practice and a career. Whatever a physician's objectives—obtaining more thorough clinical experience, acquiring training in a medical or surgical specialty, or systematically learning the techniques and methods of medical research—these alternative educational paths provided opportunities that could not be found in American medical schools of the era.

Most physicians who undertook one or more of these alternative educational paths were recent medical school graduates. Nevertheless, these pathways did not represent "graduate medical education" as the term later came to be understood—that is, intensive, multiyear hospital-based training programs in a medical specialty. Indeed, "graduate medical education" did not exist even in name in America for most of the nineteenth century. Instead, medical educators of that time concentrated on the urgent educational challenge of the moment: upgrading "undergraduate" medical education (the instruction of medical students) and thereby improving the standards of medical practice. Medical educators, particularly after the Civil War, saw their work as introducing far more rigorous standards of admission and instruction, providing students the opportunity to do laboratory experiments and work with patients, transforming medical schools into genuine university departments with full-time faculty members committed to investigation and discovery, and persuading hospitals to accept a more active role in medical education and research.[5] However, the institutions they created to serve the needs of undergraduate medical education—the modern medical school and teaching hospital—ultimately provided a home for graduate medical education as well. And the objectives of these nineteenth-century paths of "professional improvement"—clinical experience, specialty education, and research training—ultimately became the objectives of the American residency system, contested and debated as these objectives always were to be.

THE SEARCH FOR CLINICAL EXPERIENCE

Would-be doctors have always sought opportunities for practical clinical experience. In colonial and postrevolutionary America, such experience was provided by the apprenticeship, the dominant method of medical education at that time. In this venerable method of instruction, which dated to ancient times,[6] the student became associated with a practicing physician, who taught the learner the various branches of medicine until the learner was prepared to enter practice on his own.

In the context of eighteenth-century America, the apprenticeship proved a useful learning device. Under a qualified and committed practitioner, called a preceptor, students engaged in supervised work in an active medical practice. Students also had the opportunity to read books from the preceptor's personal library, participate in scientific conversations with their mentor, and ask whatever questions might come to mind. One particularly notable preceptor, famed throughout the colonies for his educational work, was John Redman of Philadelphia.[7]

However, the apprenticeship suffered from major educational deficiencies. Even the finest preceptors could not be knowledgeable in all areas of medicine, nor could they guarantee a full complement of books, equipment, and clinical opportunities. Apprentices derived little stimulation from other students and teachers or from learning medicine in an environment in which new knowledge was being sought. These problems were magnified in the more typical cases where preceptors were less accomplished than Dr. Redman. Many preceptors made little effort to provide systematic instruction, keep up-to-date with recent medical developments, or offer trainees sufficient clinical opportunities. In many cases, apprentices spent more time performing menial household chores for their mentors than learning medicine. Accordingly, in the nineteenth century the apprenticeship fell into disfavor. The American Medical Association declared in 1867: "Private pupilage, as it is now generally conducted, is worse than useless. It is, in fact, simply a waste of time and money, without one solitary compensating advantage."[8]

The limitations of the apprenticeship system were a major factor underlying the proliferation of proprietary medical schools in the early and mid-nineteenth century. As suggested by the name, these were profit-making schools, owned by the professors. They were unaffiliated with universities or any other educational institutions. Medical schools of the era offered lectures, typically four months in duration, in the scientific and clinical branches of medicine. Schools were in session during the winter only since many students worked on farms during the warmer months. To receive an MD degree, students needed to attend two terms of lectures (the second identical to the first) and pass an examination. The objective was to provide a theoretical framework to place the clinical experience of the apprenticeship in context.[9]

Initially, medical schools were intended to supplement the apprenticeship, not replace it. Before accepting a student, medical schools required documentation that the student had already completed an apprenticeship of at least three years in duration. However, by midcentury this requirement had become a formality. A student could purchase a certificate from a preceptor, even if he had not apprenticed with that individual. "The relations of students and preceptors have become merely nominal," one noted medical educator wrote in 1877.[10] In the 1870s, medical schools abandoned the requirement of an apprenticeship as a prerequisite for admission.[11] However, because medical schools of this era made little effort to include practical clinical instruction as part of the curriculum, the typical medical graduate entered practice with no meaningful clinical experience to draw on.

Some students tried to circumvent the deficiencies of their medical education by attending summer sessions at a nondegree-granting extramural private school. A number of such schools appeared after the Civil War, particularly in eastern cities. These schools provided students more practical experience than could be obtained during the winters when medical schools were in session. They specialized in teaching physical diagnosis and the use of new diagnostic instruments such as the ophthalmoscope and otoscope. Some of them provided opportunities for students to learn to bandage wounds and perform minor procedures. Thus, they provided important practical experience that was not available during conventional medical study. However, they offered no real opportunities to take charge of patients, make decisions, or manage cases.[12]

For a fortunate and ambitious few, however, the opportunity to acquire in-depth clinical experience did exist: serving as a "resident" or "house physician" in a general hospital. These positions, the forerunners of the twentieth-century rotating internship, enabled individuals to live in the hospital, assume responsibilities for routine ward work, and round with the various attending physicians and surgeons. Typically, residents served for one year, though the length of service varied from hospital to hospital. Some institutions offered positions for as short as six months; others, for as long as 18 months. The experience at Boston City Hospital, which opened in 1866 with four resident house officers, was representative:

> They [the house officers] shall accompany their superiors in their daily visits, shall make the necessary record of treatment and diet of patients, and shall see that their directions are complied with. They shall, when requested by the physician or surgeon, make autopsies and other pathological examinations; and the House Officer in the Surgical Department shall take charge of the instruments and apparatus. . . . They shall, when requested by the Superintendent or Visiting Committee, investigate the claims of applicants for admission, whether made at the Hospital or from the city. They shall attend to patients on their admission, and give the necessary directions for their comfort, before they are seen by their regular medical attendant, and shall make a daily evening visit to each patient.[13]

Following the example of hospitals in England and Scotland, formal systems of hospital training were instituted in the eighteenth and early nineteenth centuries at a few important American hospitals, such as the Pennsylvania Hospital, New York Hospital, "Old Blockley" (later the Philadelphia General Hospital), Bellevue Hospital, and the Massachusetts General Hospital.[14] The number of hospitals offering such positions grew slowly during the first half of the nineteenth century but accelerated during the Civil War because of the need to treat battle casualties. By 1873, 178 hospitals offered a combined total of 309 hospital positions.[15] The number of positions grew more rapidly in the 1880s and 1890s, as the advent of antiseptic surgery made hospitals busier places and created a greater need for resident physicians to be available to help care for patients.

From an educational perspective, house positions represented the transfer of the apprenticeship from an individual to an institution. Indeed, at the beginning, such positions literally were institutionalized apprenticeships. At the Pennsylvania Hospital, for instance, apprentices were bound by a legal indenture to serve the hospital for five years, in exchange for instruction in the art of medicine. At other hospitals, a resident physician paid $50, $100, or even $250 for that privilege and then agreed to a bond for faithful fulfillment of duties.[16] In the early nineteenth century the formal legal aspects of indentured service were dropped, but the residency continued to display the characteristics of an institutionalized apprenticeship: House officers helped established physicians with their patients, and for that educational opportunity they performed a large number of menial chores for the physicians and the hospital.

Hospital positions went by different names at different places. Variously, the learners were known as "house officers," "house physicians," "residents," "resident physicians," "interns," "strikers," "walkers," or, most famously at the Massachusetts General Hospital, "house pupils." These terms were used interchangeably, and all denoted a similar experience. Most resident physicians were newly minted graduates of medical schools. However, a few hospitals accepted medical students or medical school graduates who had not yet received an MD degree. In these instances conferral of the degree came after the completion of the hospital year.

Competition for house positions was fierce because of both their scarcity and their professional desirability. They were regarded as professional plums because they not only provided educational opportunities but also allowed house officers to become known to a community's medical elite. Such personal contacts frequently proved highly advantageous in jump-starting a young physician's career.[17] Often, hospitals accepted graduates only from a particular local medical school: For instance, Presbyterian

Hospital appointed its house physicians from students at the College of Physicians and Surgeons; Lakeside Hospital, from Western Reserve Medical School; and the Massachusetts General Hospital, from Harvard Medical School. Appointments typically were made by competitive examination. However, nepotism also played a role, particularly at "blue-blooded" institutions such as the Massachusetts General Hospital. There, staff physicians observed that "nepotism exerts such an influence in the choice of candidates at the Hospital, that when a relative of any member of the Staff applies for a position he is sure to obtain it to the exclusion of all others."[18] Reflecting the values of the larger society, almost all house officers were white males. Only certain hospitals would accept Jews; even fewer would consider women, and virtually none would hire African-Americans.

The duties of house officers were similar from one institution to another. Residents evaluated patients for admission to the hospital, performed the initial "workups" of newly admitted patients, checked on hospitalized patients once or twice a day, accompanied the attending physicians on their daily rounds, made certain that the attending physicians' orders were properly executed, kept a record of diet and medications, performed minor procedures, bandaged and dressed patients, and vaccinated patients prior to discharge. Residents also rounded on private patients when the attending physician was unable to do so. Residents also performed many menial tasks, such as washing surgical instruments, ordering food and hospital supplies, stocking supply rooms, and helping the hospital treasurer collect bills from paying patients. For this reason the historian of the Massachusetts General Hospital spoke of how house pupils were financially "exploited as apprentices by [the] institution, profession, and community."[19]

House officers endured a paternalistic existence. They were prohibited from marriage, required to live in the hospital, and could rarely leave the premises, sometimes only with the permission of the hospital matron. Like children, house officers were expected to follow rules and be submissive, thereby helping maintain the order that the nineteenth-century hospital so highly valued.[20] "Every effort is made to preserve absolute quiet," stated the rule book of one important hospital.[21] House officers worked long hours and were no strangers to the loss of sleep. They typically lived in cramped quarters, ate poor-quality food, and suffered from the lack of recreation or exercise. Hospital administrators tended to be unsympathetic toward their plight. At Old Blockley, residents nicknamed the hospital superintendent "the tyrant of Blockley" for his nonchalance regarding their desire for better food and quarters.[22] The daily life of house officers could be grim, particularly on the surgical wards. There, bedsores in patients were common, surgical complications frequent, and hospital-borne infections always lurking. Residents were continually at risk of acquiring a major infection themselves or even of dying from such an infection.[23] How the widespread prevalence of death and suffering and the presence of personal risk affected the attitudes of house officers of the era is not known.

However, the experience of being a house officer was far from bleak. Residents reveled in the knowledge that they were receiving far better clinical training than most of their contemporaries, and they knew they were making invaluable personal connections. One house pupil at the Massachusetts General Hospital in 1888, who described the experience as "absorbingly interesting," spoke of the excitement and personal satisfaction he derived. "The hours were long and the work was hard, but you felt all the time that you were learning something.... The experience was indeed thrilling."[24] In addition, even the sternest hospital matron could not suppress the high spirits of residents, who had, in the words of one house officer, "that buoyancy of disposition common to the American college man."[25] Many were the pranks, parties, and games that took place in house staff quarters. Camaraderie was excellent (often exceptional), and life-long friendships resulted. At the Massachusetts General Hospital, Boston City Hospital, Presbyterian Hospital, and other institutions, thriving associations of former residents appeared, and graduates of these programs reminisced fondly of those days.

Nineteenth-century house officers had but one overriding frustration: They received little responsibility for patient management. Typically, they followed orders and observed procedures; they were not permitted to assume much professional responsibility themselves for patient care. At the Massachusetts General Hospital in the 1860s, it was deemed best to leave the prescribing of pills entirely in the hands of the chief of service and not to delegate this task to house pupils.[26] At Presbyterian Hospital in the 1890s, resident physicians were not permitted to perform vaginal examinations (except in emergencies) or to discuss autopsy results with a patient's family.[27] House officers were present begrudgingly, and if they exceeded their authority, they could expect to be rebuked.

Conditions at the Massachusetts General Hospital, the most prestigious hospital of all, were typical. There, the trustees and medical staff frowned upon allowing house pupils to assume too much responsibility. The trustees felt that "these young men were in the Hospital on sufferance and should be allowed the privilege of performing hospital service only under carefully defined restrictions."[28] In 1874, the medical staff listed the requirements for an appointment as house pupil as, among other things, "Subordination, Capacity for Labor, Conduct."[29] Originally, residents at the hospital were medical graduates known as "house physicians and surgeons." In 1849 the hospital famously changed its policy so that appointments were offered to medical students only, and the trustees adopted the term "house pupils" to help keep them in their place. The reason for this change was that the trustees and medical staff felt that the house physicians and surgeons had been assuming too much authority in the care of patients. As one trustee noted, "What is lost from their [house pupils] having one year's less professional experience will be more than made up by their greater degree of docility & obedience."[30] Only in the 1880s did house officers at the Massachusetts General Hospital and elsewhere begin receiving greater responsibility for patient care.

The nineteenth-century house-staff positions should not be confused with later hospital training positions that went by similar names. These earlier positions represented on-the-job vocational training under an institutionalized apprenticeship system, not a formally directed educational experience. Nevertheless, in their day they played an important educational role. They provided to a lucky few an extensive clinical experience on the standards of the time. They helped create a professional elite, many of whom later participated in the advancement of medical knowledge and the creation of the modern medical school in the United States. And the existence of this system provided an institutional home for the later emergence of graduate medical education in the United States.

Nor should the overriding tension of the system be overlooked: The desire of ambitious house officers to assume as much independence and clinical autonomy as possible clashed with the desire of hospital officials to keep residents in a subordinate position and extract as much menial service from them as possible. This tension would soon resonate throughout graduate medical education in the United States, as the nineteenth-century house positions evolved into the twentieth-century internship and as the modern residency system developed and spread. Indeed, the conflict between the educational needs of house officers and the desire of institutional officials to obtain cheap labor became the system's essential and most enduring tension.

THE QUEST FOR SPECIALTY TRAINING

The nineteenth-century hospital positions served a useful purpose, and American medical education owed much to them. However, as the century progressed, they provided an insufficient educational experience for those desiring an elite career in medicine. All century long, but especially after the Civil War, ambitious doctors increasingly desired a career in a medical specialty (a field of medical activity organized about a focus of interest, such as a body organ, technical procedure, or specific age group). Some nineteenth-century physicians chose to specialize for compelling intellectual reasons, others for the easier hours, higher incomes, and social prestige that specialty practice allowed, and most for a combination of these reasons. However, prior to the 1880s, there were no educational opportunities at all in the United States for those who wished thorough training to be a specialist.

Medical specialization dated to antiquity. However, until the nineteenth century, specialization carried an enormous stigma within the medical profession, in large part owing to its domination by uneducated itinerant practitioners. Peripatetic oculists, stone-cutters, and others perceived as pretenders gave specialization a bad name among physicians. The medical profession viewed specialization as the province of charlatans and quacks, not respectable physicians. Physicians too quick to call themselves specialists risked being ostracized by their professional brethren.[31]

In the nineteenth century traditional professional attitudes toward medical specialization began to change. Contrary to common opinion, much more than the proliferation of knowledge and new technologies played a role, though these certainly were important factors. In the later eighteenth and early nineteenth centuries, an important intellectual precondition for specialization was met. Physicians abandoned belief in the ancient "humoral" system of pathology, and they adopted instead an "oncological" conception of disease—that is, the idea that numerous separate disease types existed, each of which arose from a specific pathology localized in a particular organ or tissue. Changing social conditions played a role: the growth of the population, the congregation of the population into populous urban areas, the development of large urban hospitals where patients with specific diseases could be studied and treated (and where the benefits of specialized practice could be demonstrated), the accumulation of wealth, and the rise of a middle class that demanded and could afford specialized care. After the Civil War, the idea of medical specialization was reinforced by the country's growing infatuation with the division of labor, specialized knowledge, scientific expertise, professional authority, and the idea of progress.

At the core of the forces that gave rise to specialization was the rapid proliferation of medical knowledge. By the 1860s, it was impossible for any individual to keep up with the entirety of medical science. By then doctors were advised to read journals rather than textbooks,[32] and young physicians studying abroad viewed the splitting up of the profession into specialties as inevitable.[33] In 1878 John Shaw Billings, who played a seminal role in planning the Johns Hopkins Medical School and Hospital, wrote that medical specialization could not be avoided "because it is no longer possible for any one man to grasp and retain a knowledge of all the branches of medical science."[34] In 1864, the country's first specialty association, the American Ophthalmological Society, was established. It was followed by the American Otological Society (1867), the American Neurological Association (1875), the American Gynecological Society (1876), the American Dermatological Association (1876), the American Laryngological Association (1879), the American Surgical Association (1880), the Association of American Physicians (1886), the American Pediatric Society (1888), and others before the end of the century.[35]

For most of the nineteenth century, American physicians who sought to learn a medical specialty had but one choice: study in Europe. Before the Civil War, Paris was by far the most popular choice for American students because of the exceptional availability of practical instruction at the bedside and in the dissecting and autopsy rooms. Many Americans fell under the lure of inspiring French clinical teachers, most notably Pierre Louis, but the real attraction was the opportunity to take personalized private courses for a fee with junior instructors or hospital *internes* seeking to enhance their incomes. These instructors provided exceptional opportunities to work with real patients both in general medicine and in the medical specialties. By 1861, nearly 700 Americans had studied medicine in Paris, at least 67 of whom later became medical school professors in the United States. This left an indelible French imprint on American medicine and created the first large group of American physicians to defend the validity of specialization as a model for practice in the United States.[36]

In the 1850s, the pattern of European migration began to change. In 1855, the dean of the Paris medical faculty released an edict that suppressed the teaching by internes of private clinical courses. Around the same time, opportunities for private, bedside instruction with a personal tutor became readily available in Vienna and Berlin.[37] This occurred as the German university was in its ascendance, making the country the undisputed international center of scientific medicine as well as of other scholarly areas, such as the social sciences, philosophy, literary criticism, linguistics, and the natural sciences.[38] As a result, those who desired to study a medical specialty started turning to Germany rather than France. Between 1870 and 1914, approximately 15,000 American physicians undertook some form of serious study in Germany or at German-speaking universities in Austria and Switzerland. The migration peaked in the 1870s and 1880s, remained strong in the 1890s, and continued in smaller numbers until 1914, when the outbreak of World War I destroyed German-American relations and impoverished and demoralized the German universities.

American physicians who studied in Germany tended to be young, male, from the East Coast, and from the upper strata of society. Family affluence was typically a prerequisite for study because of high travel costs and the absence of fellowship support. Many travelers had spent a year as a house officer in an American hospital; some were established physicians who viewed specialty study in Germany as a fine way to spend a long vacation. Most stayed for a few months, though some studied for years and a few remained permanently. On their return to the United States, they often rose to great prominence in the profession, as measured by the frequency with which they were listed in standard biographical guides.[39]

American doctors found Germany an outstanding place in which to study a clinical specialty. All who undertook the journey reveled amid the large hospital clinics, the immense amount of "clinical material," the personalized instruction, the freedom they received to pursue their interests, and the stimulating atmosphere of the German university. Study could be undertaken in dermatology, ophthalmology, obstetrics, gynecology, laryngology, or any other specialty a physician wished. The most popular places of study were Berlin and Vienna, where courses were short (frequently only several weeks in duration) and instruction often provided in English. One young American enthused from Vienna that he was in a "Garden of Plenty every tree of which is laden with ripe fruit."[40]

On their return to the United States, most physicians who had studied in Germany pursued successful careers as consultants or specialists. Few of them aspired to scientific careers. However, they emerged from their German experience with an understanding of the true university spirit, an appreciation of the importance of research, and a recognition of how the scientific branches of medicine could contribute to clinical practice. They also understood that a rigorous system of specialty training was needed at home. Clarence Blake, a pioneering otologist at Harvard Medical School, told his parents while studying in Germany, "A radical change is needed in the American system of medical education and practice, and it devolves upon the young men who have gained broader views by studying on the Continent... to inaugurate this change."[41] As they later assumed important positions in medical schools, hospitals, and professional societies, many found themselves able to lead or support such changes.

As specialization started to take hold in the United States, however, troubling questions arose. How many specialists does the country need? Should specialty training be built on a prior general medical education or should it proceed independently without such a foundation? And some began to wonder whether specialization might not be an unmitigated good. For instance, Billings, though highly supportive of specialization, pointed out that it "is apt to produce narrowness of view, the assigning of undue importance to local affections, and a strong tendency to magnify unduly the branch which the specialist professes."[42] At century's end few medical leaders were troubled by such concerns, so slight was the presence of specialization in the country's medical culture at that time. But as specialization proceeded and a system of residency training was created, such questions proved haunting.

THE PASSION FOR DISCOVERY AND THE BIRTH OF CLINICAL SCIENCE

In the 1860s, as American doctors turned toward Germany for specialized graduate study, America's medical subservience to the Continent was apparent in research as well as in education. Throughout the century few Americans undertook investigative work, and the research that was done tended to be derivative and confirmatory.[43] In this regard, America's indifference to basic research extended to all scientific and scholarly fields. American culture at that time did not encourage contemplative work, and opportunities for original study in all fields were scarce. University positions for investigators did not exist, financial support for research and training programs was not available, professional journals and societies had not been created, and universities had yet to embrace research as part of their mission. Research had not been transformed into a professional enterprise in any academic area.[44]

Of the 15,000 American physicians who made the pilgrimage to Germany, a few went not to learn a clinical specialty but to study the fundamental medical sciences and learn the techniques of experimental medical research. Their influence was far out of proportion to their numbers since they included such luminaries as William Welch, Franklin Mall, John Jacob Abel, Henry Bowditch, Victor Vaughan, and others who acquired faculty positions at the pioneering medical schools of Johns Hopkins, Michigan, Harvard, Pennsylvania, and, later, other institutions. These individuals usually remained in Germany for years, not months, and their favorite places for scientific study were the smaller German universities, particularly those in Leipzig, Strasburg, and Breslau. There they conducted intensive laboratory studies under the careful guidance and warm mentoring of Germany's leading medical scientists. While in Germany, they not only became accomplished scientists but also acquired a new role model: the full-time teacher and investigator. On their return to the United States, they were responsible for establishing America's reputation in medical research and also for creating the modern American medical school.[45]

As American doctors began the pursuit of laboratory medical research, it was assumed that they would not be practicing or teaching clinical medicine. Rather, it was thought that, if successful, they would become "scientific men" pursuing the fundamental sciences of anatomy, physiology, biochemistry, experimental pathology, or pharmacology. To American physicians of the latter nineteenth century, the relevance of the laboratory sciences for clinicians was not apparent. Clinical faculty at medical schools were practitioners, not investigators. They were active medical consultants who taught part-time. They often had an encyclopedic knowledge of clinical medicine, but they pursued little research, and what studies they did publish usually consisted of case reports and literature reviews. They did not have a sufficient background to appreciate what physiology and chemistry might have to offer future developments in medical practice, and they did not believe that laboratory research was something for a clinician to do.

This attitude was illustrated by Clarence John Blake, the aforementioned pioneering otologist at Harvard Medical School and the Massachusetts Eye and Ear Infirmary. Blake studied in Vienna for several years in the late 1860s, and while there he recorded his thoughts about choosing a career in a series of letters to his parents. He found himself intensely interested in biochemistry but was perplexed by its seeming irrelevance to those who wished to practice medicine. "At present in the United States, a Chemist, though he may be an M.D., is a Chemist and not a physician.... If it were possible to unite chemical knowledge with some particular branch of medical investigation and make a remunerative specialty of it I should very much like to do so, but as yet do not clearly see an opening which will lead to the desired end."[46] Since his first love was clinical medicine, he eventually chose to specialize in otology. "I cannot see any opportunity of uniting chemistry with medicine and am every day less and less inclined to practice any other than the medical profession."[47]

Aspiring American medical scientists worked in the German laboratories at that critical time when the fundamental medical sciences were blossoming. New discoveries were being announced "like corn popping in a pan," the neurosurgeon Harvey Cushing later said of that period.[48] However, by the 1870s and 1880s, the fundamental sciences and the clinical disciplines were both rapidly expanding. German clinicians had pioneered the application of chemical and physiological methods to the study of disease and therapeutics. The result was an explosion of information directly pertinent to practitioners' everyday work. Examples included the demystification of gout, diabetes, and other metabolic conditions, the recognition of myxedema as a special type of disease (a recognition that also led to the understanding of the function of the thyroid gland), the development of methods for the examination of urine and the study of kidney function, the understanding of the energy aspects of human metabolism made possible by the quantitative calorimetric method, and the identification of the mechanisms of congestive heart failure enabled by new methods for determining cardiac stroke volume. Early on, this new field was called "physiological medicine," but by the end of the century it was usually known by its contemporary name, "clinical science." Regardless of terminology, its identifying feature was the application of experimental scientific methods to clinical research. The experimental methods employed had been developed chiefly by biochemists and physiologists, but German clinicians quickly adapted them to clinical investigations.[49]

In Germany, leading clinical scientists mentored aspiring American clinical scientists, as the basic scientists mentored Americans seeking proficiency in the fundamental sciences. Perhaps the most notable clinical teacher was Friedrich von Müller, called by Abraham Flexner "a great teacher as well as perhaps the most eminent physician on the Continent."[50] In addition to his extensive clinical training in internal medicine, von Müller had acquired rigorous experience in physiology, metabolism, chemistry, biochemistry, and pharmacology, all of which he studied with great masters, including the renowned chemist Emil Fisher. As a professor of medicine at Marburg, Basel, and Munich, von Müller was sought out by dozens of able young Americans because of his brilliance, encyclopedic knowledge, clinical acumen, pedagogical skill, and gracious nature. Impressionable young Americans studying under his direction absorbed his conception of clinical medicine as an applied science based on chemistry, physiology, and pathology and his belief that a modern clinical professor should dedicate his life to clinical teaching and research. Lewellys Barker, one of von Müller's students and William Osler's successor as Professor of Medicine at Johns Hopkins, said of his teacher:

> In von Müller I found a great clinical teacher—one of the best Germany has ever produced. He exerted a profound influence upon me. An accurate diagnostician and a reliable therapist, he had early recognized the importance of the clinical laboratories in which physical, chemical, and biological methods could be applied to the study of the patients in his wards.[51]

By the last quarter of the nineteenth century, the clinical scientist in Germany had developed a distinct identity. A clinical scientist was versed in both bedside medicine and the application of the knowledge and techniques of the fundamental sciences to the study of human disease. In the words of the eminent internist A. McGehee Harvey, the clinical scientist occupied "the position of middle man in the medical world—a compleat [*sic*] clinician who served to bridge the gap between the practicing physician and the laboratory-based scientist."[52] Because of their interest in the problems of patient care, clinical scientists found the clinical rather than the scientific departments to be their natural abode. As Samuel J. Meltzer, a prominent early clinical scientist in the United States, put it: "The regeneration or rather creation of a science of clinical medicine must come from the innermost of medicine itself. It is true . . . that the men who are to tackle these problems must have a thorough training in the sciences allied to medicine, but the center of their activities must be within clinical medicine itself."[53]

The exposure of American physicians to clinical science in Germany led to intense dissatisfaction with the conditions of clinical teaching in their homeland. Graham Lusk, another eminent early American clinical scientist, was deeply frustrated that in Germany there was a class of "magnificent men whose counterparts do not exist in this country." The development of clinical medicine in America, he argued, "can come only through men who have a knowledge of modern chemistry, physiology, pharmacology and pathology."[54] These physicians deplored the fact that most clinical teachers in the United States were busy consultants who were not able to devote much of their time to teaching and who did not have scientific training in modern medicine. This, according to Meltzer, was American medical education's "greatest evil." Modern clinical teachers "must have an education and training radically different from those which were customary and sufficient in former years."[55]

Where in the United States might clinical science be taught? To this group of American doctors, there was one especially viable potential site: the clinical departments of medical schools. While in Germany, they had been deeply impressed with the organization of the German clinics, which typically had a full-time chief, a number of full-time junior faculty, some talented practitioners working as volunteers, and a cadre of young assistants learning clinical science and preparing for academic careers. William Osler, while visiting various German clinics in 1884, wrote that "the wards are clinical laboratories utilized for the scientific study and treatment of disease, and the assistants, under the direction of the professor, carry on investigations and aid in the instruction. The advanced position of German medicine and the reputation of the schools as teaching centers are largely fruits of this system."[56] Time spent in a laboratory of one of the fundamental sciences was always considered a good idea for an aspiring clinical scientist, but the main home for training in clinical science was thought best to be a clinical department.

The birth of clinical science created new requirements for clinical teaching in the United States. It created a need for medical scientists, not clinical consultants, to lead modern clinical departments. It required that clinical teaching, at least for some, become a full-time activity. It required that clinical medicine, not just the fundamental sciences, be made a genuine part of the university. And it gave clinical departments the obligation of training the next generation of clinical scientists. At the turn of the century, how these forces were to affect clinical education in America was not yet clear. However, one thing was apparent: Clinical education was about to change.

CHAPTER 2
Johns Hopkins and the Creation of the Residency

The central event in American higher education during the latter nineteenth century was the birth of the research university. Sleepy, traditional colleges, whose mission was the preservation of culture, evolved into dynamic universities, charged with the responsibility for the production, not just the transmission, of knowledge. The fledgling research university made possible the realization of the dreams of aspiring scholars in all fields who had been struggling to legitimize the pursuit of research as a career, devote their lives to advanced teaching and research, and bring to an end America's intellectual servitude to England and the Continent.[1] No university more clearly epitomized this movement than Johns Hopkins, which opened in 1876 as America's first research university and established in 1893 the country's first mature scientific medical school.

It was also at Johns Hopkins that the first modern residency program in the United States was established. When the Johns Hopkins Hospital opened in 1889, it had a resident staff in its three clinical departments of medicine, surgery, and gynecology. Soon thereafter residency programs in pathology, obstetrics, pediatrics, and other fields were added. The residencies were analogous to the fellowships established in the scientific departments of the medical school and to the assistantships in the university's graduate school. To the Johns Hopkins faculty, enamored of the German model, the idea that advanced clinical training should be lodged in the university made good sense. This seemed the proper way to ensure that the clinical disciplines would develop along genuine academic lines and that the residency experience would represent true graduate education rather than mere vocational training. Of note, because of financial shortfalls, the opening of the medical school was delayed. The hospital opened four years before the medical school and six years before the first medical students arrived to the wards and clinics. Thus, the residency was the first of this pioneering university's lasting contributions to medical education.

Eventually, the Johns Hopkins residency program became the model for graduate medical education in the United States, much as its medical school did for undergraduate medical education. The spread of the residency system was delayed, so overwhelming was the immediate task of creating the modern American medical school. However, the success of the residency program at Johns Hopkins was undisputable, and many graduates of the program later established residency programs at other institutions based on the model they had experienced at Johns Hopkins. As they did, they carried with them not only an educational concept but also a way of thinking about patients' problems that offered doctors the potential of providing good stewardship of the nation's financial resources available for medical care.

GRADUATE MEDICAL EDUCATION ENTERS THE UNIVERSITY

When the Johns Hopkins Hospital admitted its first patient on May 15, 1889, it already had a resident staff in place. That this happened represented the planning and efforts of William Osler, the chief of medicine; William Halsted, the chief of surgery; Howard Kelly, the chief of gynecology; and Henry Hurd, the hospital superintendent. However, the idea that the Johns Hopkins Hospital should have a resident staff dated to the earliest planning stages of the institution. From the start, those assigned the responsibility of creating the hospital believed that the hospital should be something more than just an institution dedicated to the care of the sick. Rather, they believed that the hospital should be part of the university, guided by the same educational principles that guided the development of the Johns Hopkins University.[2]

Early planning for the hospital fell on the shoulders of Daniel Coit Gilman, the president of the Johns Hopkins University, and John Shaw Billings, Gilman's medical adviser. Gilman, among the most prominent first-generation university presidents, had become familiar with modern concepts of medical education while president of the University of California in the early 1870s. On arriving at Johns Hopkins, he was determined that the hospital, medical school, and university all be guided by academic values.[3] Billings, perhaps the most versatile physician ever in America—he achieved renown as a medical educator, hospital architect, medical bibliographer, statistician, hygienist, civil servant, and administrator—acquired his views of medical education while a "house pupil" in Cincinnati in the 1860s. These views matured during a long trip to the Continent in 1876 to study European systems of medical education. There, he admired aspects of the English and French systems but concluded that the German system offered the most for American medicine.[4] Billings became the chief planner of the hospital. According to Hurd, his importance to the Johns Hopkins Hospital "can never be overestimated," and he was "able to impress his views upon all who came in contact with him," especially Gilman and the hospital trustees.[5]

From the start Billings and Gilman insisted that university principles be adopted in the hospital. Billings told Gilman in 1876, "It is essential that from the very beginning the Hospital organization shall be harmonious with that of the University."[6] He spoke regularly with Gilman about the importance of the hospital having an advanced resident staff to pursue clinical science.[7] Gilman agreed. In his 1878 report to the trustees of the hospital, Gilman wrote, "The plans of the hospital . . . include provision for a certain number of resident graduates or advanced students of medicine, and in other ways have regard to the promotion of medical science and education."[8] With the appointment in 1884 of the German-trained pathologist William Welch as the medical school dean, Billings and Gilman found a resounding supporter. To Welch, "The medical school should be a place where medicine is not only taught but studied."[9]

Thus, Osler, Halsted, Kelly, and Hurd were appointed with the mandate to innovate. Alan Chesney, a former dean of the Johns Hopkins School of Medicine and the historian of its early history, credited Osler for the introduction of the residency system at Hopkins,[10] though the others immediately embraced the idea. The new training system represented a true departure. Before the opening of the hospital, it had been exceedingly rare for a hospital position to last for longer than 18 months. However, residents at Johns Hopkins had already completed internships elsewhere and now planned to live in the hospital for many more years, learning a specialty and investigating clinical problems. Hospital work was facilitated by the administrative departure of having a single chief of service, as in the German clinics, where one individual carried the responsibility of overseeing the department throughout the entire year. This contrasted with the prevailing custom in American hospitals of having a divided service in which different individuals of coordinate rank took charge of a service for short periods of time.[11] The net effect was the creation of a graduate school within the hospital. Welch himself sometimes called residents "graduate students,"[12] and close observers of developments in Baltimore noted, "The Johns Hopkins Hospital is a medical school as well as a hospital."[13]

The Johns Hopkins residency reflected both American and German influences. The program built on the American tradition of hospital appointments for medical graduates, adopting and clarifying some of the old terminology. The faculty chose the term "intern" to designate a medical graduate in the first year of service and "resident" for an advanced graduate engaging in serious scholarly study. It was also understood that the new residency system, like the earlier hospital appointment system, represented an institutional apprenticeship. Halsted sometimes spoke of his residents as serving "an apprenticeship,"[14] and for many decades afterward it was common for former residents to use the term "apprenticeship" when speaking of their experience.[15]

However, the Teutonic model of clinical assistants proved an even stronger influence. This was seen in the cosmopolitan, gregarious, warmhearted Osler, who had spent the least time studying in Germany of any of the original Johns Hopkins faculty members and who was the least scientifically oriented of his colleagues. He used the laboratory mainly for diagnostic, not investigative, purposes, and his classic single-authored textbook, *The Principles and Practice of Medicine*, was notable for its therapeutic nihilism, a contrasting view to the more optimistic hopes regarding therapy that were beginning to permeate medical thinking at that time.[16] However, Osler traveled to Germany on several occasions, becoming friendly with many of the leading medical scientists there. On one trip, he wrote, "The universities of Germany are her chief glory."[17] He described his admiration of the German system to the Johns Hopkins Medical Board, and later he acknowledged one of his great ambitions was "to build up a great clinic on Teutonic lines, not on those previously followed here and in England, but on lines which have proved so successful on the Continent, and which have placed the scientific medicine of Germany in the forefront of the world."[18] He considered the creation of a German-inspired residency system to be his greatest contribution to clinical medicine.[19]

The Teutonic influence was also apparent in Osler's colleagues. No American surgeon admitted his debt to German medicine more readily than Halsted. This brilliant, taciturn, aloof surgeon—perhaps America's most productive cocaine addict—introduced German methods of strict asepsis, the careful handling of tissues, and absolute hemostasis into American surgery, and he pioneered the study of surgical problems in the physiological laboratory.[20] He, too, greatly admired the German system of clinical training, and he designed his surgical residency program "to adopt as closely as feasible the German plan."[21] Kelly, a brilliant operator and devout Christian who prayed before every operation (which made him an anomaly at the secular Johns Hopkins University, which famously had broken with tradition by not having a prayer at its 1876 opening ceremony), made four trips to Germany in the 1880s—the first three to study and the fourth to get married.[22] He also was enamored with the German system of clinical assistants and based his gynecological residency on that model.[23]

The Johns Hopkins residency was designed to be an intensive academic experience for mature scholars who desired to continue their hospital training to study a specific field of medicine. Initially, the selection of individuals to the resident staff was limited to physicians who had already completed a hospital internship or period of study in Europe. As Billings said at the hospital's opening ceremony, "It is intended that these places shall be open only to those who have had a thorough previous training, and who have shown themselves to be fitted to undertake this important part of their studies."[24] After the medical school graduated its first class in 1897, appointments to the house staff were limited to high-ranking, unmarried graduates of the Johns Hopkins Medical School.[25] As Welch explained, "We do not in general accept a year spent in another medical school as equivalent of a year spent here."[26] In the early years, 12 interns were appointed annually, with additional appointments as "externs" available as a consolation prize. Externs lived outside the hospital, worked in the outpatient clinics, received opportunities for scientific investigation, and could be called on to substitute for interns in the case of illness or other unforeseen eventualities.[27]

The Johns Hopkins residency program consisted of three classes of "house officer," now the generic term for any member of the resident staff. At the lowest level were the interns, appointed directly out of medical school, who each served for a 12-month term, assuming responsibility for the moment-by-moment management of patients. Initially an intern spent four months on each of the clinical services, but soon the position changed to a "straight" internship of 12 months in one clinical department. Some interns were selected to stay on as assistant residents. Appointments as assistant residents were also for 12 months, but these appointments were renewable for an indefinite period. Most assistant residents were chosen from the Hopkins interns, but to prevent inbreeding, some were taken from other hospitals. Assistant residents supervised the clinical work of interns and less experienced assistant residents, and they received abundant opportunities for scientific work. A lucky few—"picked men,"[28] as the faculty viewed them—were selected from the assistant residents to serve as chief residents, the crown jewel of the system. Chief residents served indefinite periods as assistants to the department chairs. They oversaw the activities of the interns and assistant residents, taught students and house officers, and pursued clinical research. They remained in this position, gaining experience and reputation, until a suitable opportunity, usually a senior faculty appointment at another medical school, became available. Typically, chief residents served two years, but some stayed much longer. For instance, William S. Thayer served as chief resident in medicine for seven years, and William G. MacCallum was chief resident in pathology for nine years.[29]

Thus, in the German fashion, the Johns Hopkins residency blended the work of the clinic with the study of the fundamental sciences in a several-year training period. Four essential elements of the program were new to American medicine. The first was that the resident staff was given full responsibility, under the guidance of faculty, for the diagnosis and treatment of seriously ill patients. The second was the attitude of inquiry and investigation. Indeed, in the early years a considerable portion of the scientific reputation of the Johns Hopkins Hospital derived from the publications of the resident staff.[30] The third was the participation of house officers in the teaching of students, nurses, assistants, and each other. The fourth was the extended duration of study. The result was a system that steered many who went through it into careers in academic medicine.

Unlike graduate students at the university or in the medical school's scientific departments, residents also acquired practical clinical training. However, the Johns Hopkins faculty considered the clinical experience to be a by-product of residency. Their primary goal was to prepare young physicians for careers in clinical investigation. As Billings put it, clinical training was "the secondary and not the primary object" of residency. The central objective was to "fit its students to increase knowledge."[31] In this regard the creation of the residency played a critical role in the domestication of clinical science in the United States. For the first time, those who wished to become academic leaders in medicine and to pursue careers in teaching and research did not have to study in Europe in order to obtain the proper preparation.

At this time a residency position at Johns Hopkins was only for a few. Even students at the Johns Hopkins Medical School could not be assured of receiving an appointment to the hospital house staff. A residency position, Osler declared, was only for "a superior man who also wishes to do scientific work."[32] However, the exclusivity of the residency at Johns Hopkins made a powerful statement: Graduate medical education, if it were to be done, should be conducted in the most ideal way possible. The faculty should consist of clinical scientists and academic leaders, not just any local practitioners who might be available. Those accepted into a residency should represent the best in terms of academic background, ability, integrity, discipline, and dedication. Clinical learning should be conducted in an atmosphere of inquiry, and the diagnosis and treatment of disease should go hand-in-hand with their study in the laboratory. In short, the hospital should be a graduate school, and the training of residents should reflect the values of the university. This was the contribution of Johns Hopkins to graduate medical education in the United States.

THE SCIENTIFIC PRACTITIONER AND THE PROMISE FOR THE NATION

With the opening of the Johns Hopkins Hospital, a new critical attitude entered American medical education. At first this attitude pervaded the Johns Hopkins residency programs, soon thereafter the Johns Hopkins Medical School, and ultimately all of medical education in the United States, undergraduate as well as graduate. The central elements of this new viewpoint consisted of an emphasis on the acquisition and assessment of information, a decided distrust of authority, and the recognition that the "scientific method" represents a way of thinking that is independent of the subject matter or particular facts being studied. The result was a blurring of the distinction between medical science and practice and also the emergence of a way to practice medicine that was more deeply "scientific" than before.

The origin of these changes lay in the response of medical educators to the evolving information explosion that was transforming medical science and practice in the latter nineteenth century. Not only was knowledge in all areas growing at an unprecedented rate, but there was a concomitant sense of nearly drowning in information. Books were being replaced by journals as the most important vehicle for communicating medical findings, the number of journals was increasing exponentially, and new technologies in communication, such as the telegraph and telephone, were accelerating the speed with which information spread. "The time has gone by when one mind can encompass all which has been ascertained in the medical sciences," Welch wrote in 1886.[33]

As medical knowledge grew, it also changed. Facts and theories were continually being overturned by new observations. A physician could not take comfort in what he thought he knew, for new research might disprove old beliefs. "Your new text books will be antiquated in five years," Billings told a class of medical students.[34] This led to an insight of revolutionary importance: the recognition that knowledge is not fixed, but rather, that it grows and evolves. Among medical educators, an evolutionary view of knowledge replaced the traditional catechistic view—a metaphor that was not lost on them in the wake of the pronouncement of the theory of evolution. In the 1870s and 1880s these ideas began to appear among faculties at a few medical schools, most notably Harvard, the University of Pennsylvania, and the University of Michigan. However, nowhere in American medical education was this evolutionary view of knowledge expressed earlier, more fully, or more forcefully than at Johns Hopkins, where this attitude molded medical education from the earliest stages of the planning period in the mid-1870s.[35]

This evolutionary view of knowledge shaped the educational philosophy of the Johns Hopkins medical faculty in three ways. First and most conspicuously, the faculty recast medical education to have a procedural rather than a substantive emphasis. They encouraged residents and students to learn how to acquire and evaluate information themselves rather than merely to memorize facts. Knowledge obtained or verified with one's senses was deemed much more reliable than that provided by textbooks and lectures. Since the amount of information was beyond anyone's capacity to master, and much of what was considered true or important today would inevitably be regarded differently tomorrow, it was considered more important to understand biological principles and formulate sound judgments than to recite specifics. In short, at Johns Hopkins, medicine was more learned than taught, and what needed to be learned was less the facts about every disease than the techniques for studying disease. This approach seemed the one viable way to manage the challenge imposed by the burgeoning amount of medical information.

This emphasis of the Johns Hopkins faculty on "self education," "learning by doing," and developing sound "habits of thought" could have been borrowed from the educational writings of John Dewey, whose name famously is associated with the ideas of "progressive education." Without knowing it, the Johns Hopkins faculty made their methods and ideas of medical teaching conform largely to the methods of progressive education. It remained for the noted educational reformer Abraham Flexner to show that the Johns Hopkins faculty used the same educational concepts as Dewey.[36] The association between medical education and progressive education has been explored in detail.[37]

Second, aware that medical knowledge was proliferating rapidly and that many traditional "truths" were being overturned, the Johns Hopkins faculty developed an intense disdain toward traditional medical authority. What mattered to them was not what an eminent authority wrote or said but rather the empirically derived proof that could be adduced to document an assertion. As Kelly put it, "We can, however, readily recall the day when the weight of one man's authority was everything, when years of experience and gray hairs were the only capital of value.... Happily for us these *ipse dixit* days are passing away."[38] Or, as William Thayer, an early chief resident in internal medicine and later chair of the department, wrote, "The method of authority has given way to the method of observation and inquiry."[39]

The faculty projected this attitude in all their teaching. They emphasized that the merits of an idea should be subjected to scrutiny quite aside from its source and that true critical thinking involved the willingness to make disturbing modifications, admit errors, and subject reasoning to open criticism. The result was a less authoritarian, more democratic learning environment, where the professor could be wrong and the views of house officers and students mattered. Lectures might summarize what was known, or thought to be known, but conferences, seminars, and rounds provided opportunities to discuss what was not known, to evaluate the evidence behind a certain assertion or clinical strategy, or to make sense of a situation when experts disagreed. Here was yet another way that residency training was conceptualized and practiced as graduate education, not vocational training.

Of note, this distrust of authority and embrace of empirically verifiable information were pervading many other areas of scholarship at this time. Morton White called this the "revolt against formalism" in American intellectual life, and in this way he related the ideas of such diverse thinkers as Thorstein Veblen in economics, Oliver Wendell Holmes Jr. in law, Charles A. Beard in history, and John Dewey in education.[40] All these scholars, in response to the rapid proliferation of information in their respective fields, became cultists of experience, rejecting traditional authority and textbook learning for a radical empiricism and an evolutionary concept of knowledge. As the Johns Hopkins medical faculty were "revolting against formalism" in a fashion analogous to thinkers in other fields, they made a powerful implicit statement that graduate medical education (and undergraduate medical education as well) genuinely belonged in the university.

Third, like John Dewey and other thinkers influenced by the evolutionary view of knowledge, the Johns Hopkins medical faculty viewed the essence of science as its method of inquiry rather than any particular content. "Science," Dewey wrote, "has been taught too much as an accumulation of ready-made material, with which students are to be made familiar, not enough as a method of thinking, an attitude of mind, after the pattern of which mental habits are to be transformed."[41] The Hopkins faculty heartily concurred with this view. By "scientific method," they meant the testing of ideas by well-planned experiments in which accurate facts were carefully obtained. They viewed this method of thinking as applicable equally to the laboratory and the bedside. The clinician's diagnosis was equivalent to the scientist's hypothesis; both diagnosis and hypothesis needed to be submitted to the test of an experiment. In the clinician's case, the experiment might be the results of a laboratory test or the response to a particular treatment. Thus, wrote Lewellys F. Barker, Osler's successor as chief of medicine, Johns Hopkins has been misunderstood as "making scientists, not practitioners." In fact, the institution's goal was to turn out "scientific practitioners"—that is, clinicians who could reason scientifically in the care of patients.[42] Thayer echoed this sentiment: "The training which best fits a man for a professorship differs in no way from that which best qualifies him for the career of a practitioner or consultant."[43]

The concept of the scientific practitioner was endorsed and explained to the American public by Abraham Flexner in his famous report on medical education in 1910. He, too, viewed the essence of science as its method of testing hypotheses with experiments and carefully observing the results. The scientific character of an activity, he explained, "depends not on where or by what means facts are procured, but altogether on the degree of caution and thoroughness with which observations are made, inferences drawn, and results heeded."[44] Thus, clinical practice, when properly done, was like laboratory research, because properly trained clinicians employed the same methods of reasoning as scientists in the laboratory did. Flexner elaborated:

> And just as it makes no difference to science whether usable data be obtained from a slide beneath a microscope or from a sick man stretched out on a cot, so the precise nature of the act or experiment is immaterial: it matters not in the slightest, from the standpoint of scientific logic, whether the step take the form of administering a dose of calomel, operating for appendicitis, or stimulating a particular convolution of a frog's brain with an electric current. The logical position is in all three cases identical. In each a supposition—whether expressed or implied, whether called theory or diagnosis—based on supposedly adequate observation submits itself to the test of an experiment. If proper weight has been given to correct and sufficient facts, the experiment wins, otherwise not, and a second effort, profiting by previous failure, is demanded. The practicing physician and the "theoretical" scientist are thus engaged in doing the same sort of thing, even while one is seeking to correct Mr. Smith's digestive aberration and the other to localize the cerebral functions of the frog.[45]

In the view of the Johns Hopkins faculty, scientific practitioners, like all scientists, were at the core problem solvers. Problem-solving capability was essential to the modern practice of medicine since every clinical situation involved a problem that needed to be figured out. A doctor had to come up with the proper diagnosis, decide what treatment to pursue, or even consider whether to pursue a treatment at all and instead let nature pursue its course. "Every case presents a problem to be solved," declared John Finney, a noted surgeon at Johns Hopkins.[46] This could be done only if clinicians approached their patients with an inquisitive spirit, did a careful and thorough history and physical examination, and subjected their clinical impressions to adequate testing and critical control. In this way the practitioner could most efficiently determine which one of the scores of possibilities could be accounting for a patient's chest pain, or recognize that a patient's abdominal pain might be coming from the heart, or that a patient might in fact have a serious heart problem with no chest discomfort at all. Similarly, the master surgeon was identifiable by the head even more than the hand—knowing not just how to operate but on whom to operate, when to operate, and on whom not to operate, thereby saving many patients from unnecessary surgery.

In the context of later developments in American health care, what was particularly notable about the scientific practitioner's approach to patient care was that it was efficient and cost-effective. The scientific practitioner sought to solve a patient's problem as directly as possible, using the fewest possible tests and procedures, endeavoring to produce the least disturbance, discomfort, and upset. A careful evaluation of the patient, coupled with intelligent reflection on the findings, would suggest precisely which tests, if any, needed to be performed. This reflected a thoughtful, parsimonious way of thinking that guided the scientific practitioner to do what needed to be done in a patient's particular situation. It stood in contrast with the easier but intellectually flabby approach of obtaining every test possible, needed or not, the results of which would be sifted through later. Problem-solving medicine, in short, contained powerful implications for containing medical costs as well as for implementing the most effective and efficient treatment plans. Indiscriminate testing or treatment made no medical or economic sense.

This, then, was the great promise of scientific medicine for the health of the nation. Scientific physicians not only would treat individual patients well, but they also would practice in a mindful, parsimonious fashion that would conserve money and resources. Scientific physicians had the capacity to serve the larger good. They could be stewards for the nation's resources as well as outstanding doctors for their individual patients. How well medical education and practice in the future would make use of this powerful tool, of course, remained to be determined.

WORK AS PLAY

The residency programs at the Johns Hopkins Hospital were a success from the beginning. The delay in the opening of the medical school proved, if anything, a benefit because the faculty could concentrate on graduate medical education without the distraction of having an undergraduate medical curriculum to prepare at the same time. Soon, other residency programs appeared. Within a decade of the hospital's opening, residency programs in pathology and obstetrics were operating. With the opening of the Harriet Lane Home in 1912 and the Henry Phipps Clinic in 1913, important residency programs in pediatrics and psychiatry, respectively, were also initiated.

It was also during the early years of the Johns Hopkins Hospital that formal subspecialty training began, particularly in the surgical fields. William Halsted, the chair of surgery, possessed an uncanny ability to identify the unusually gifted among his surgical assistants, and he directed many of them into their subsequent careers—in some cases by gentle suggestion (which the recipients dared not ignore), in others by overt command. Thus, he guided Hugh Young into urology, Samuel J. Crowe into otolaryngology, William S. Baer into orthopedic surgery, Frederick Baetjer into radiology, Harvey Cushing and Walter Dandy into neurosurgery, and Joseph Bloodgood into surgical pathology. Halsted selected four of these men (Young, Crowe, Baer, and Baetjer) to become division chiefs for their subspecialties in the department of surgery, with full responsibility for organizing and directing those fields, while they were still residents. Young later recalled the informal and surprising way that Halsted made him Johns Hopkins's first chief of urology. In October 1897 Young was running through the corridors of the hospital when he literally ran into Halsted, knocking his chief over, luckily catching Halsted just before his head hit the floor. While Young was profusely apologizing, Halsted interrupted: "Don't apologize, Young. I was looking for you, to tell you we want you to take charge of the Department of Genito-Urinary Surgery." Young said, "This is a great surprise. I know nothing about genitourinary surgery." Whereupon Halsted replied, "Welch and I said you didn't know anything about it, but we believe you could learn."[47]

House officers knew they were lucky to be at the Johns Hopkins Hospital. Selection to the resident staff required a high class standing at the Johns Hopkins Medical School. However, high grades alone were insufficient. The faculty also looked for evidence of scientific aptitude: They were "far more impressed by the student who answered questions intelligently or made an observation that indicated imagination or originality, than... by the usual criterion of his marks in the Dean's office."[48] In addition, the faculty favored students they liked personally. As Osler explained, "These young men come in contact with us at all hours and it is absolutely essential that they should be persons with whom we can work pleasantly and congenially."[49]

The residency programs were academically strong, for the faculty created an environment that allowed their educational principles to be realized. In medicine, Osler emphasized thoroughness, attention to detail, and careful reasoning. Interns and residents in his department quickly realized that the teachers were themselves students, merely a bit further along in the process, anxious to help their juniors. Osler continually emphasized that knowledge can be acquired but is never given and that there is joy in the quest.[50] In surgery, Halsted was equally careful and thorough in his examination of patients, and he stressed the importance of accurate diagnosis so patients would not undergo needless operations. On attending rounds, his residents saw his keen mind at work, for any finding with a patient that suggested a new idea to Halsted prompted him to begin discussing possible laboratory experiments or clinical studies. Many publications by Halsted or his students originated in this way.[51] This spirit of inquiry and investigation, which permeated all the clinical services, was facilitated by the fact that most of the teachers were themselves investigators. As Barker put it, only the "investigating teacher" can help learners "make progress in independent work or in independent thought" as opposed to merely acquiring "large stores of information."[52]

The experience of the Johns Hopkins residency was enhanced by the personal presence of the faculty. The faculty's professional work, whether teaching, investigation, or patient care, was conducted within the hospital, where they accordingly spent much more time than attending physicians at other hospitals customarily spent.[53] Not only were the faculty visible but they cared deeply about their residents, and the residents knew it. On the occasional holiday, Kelly took his residents bicycling through the eastern shore of Maryland or wherever fancy dictated, and he insisted that his house officers receive full credit for any original research they might do. The effusively warm and gracious Osler, with the aid of his wife, held lavish dinners at home, provided the latch key to his house and library to a select few, and praised his house officers generously and unstintingly. Halsted temperamentally was nearly the polar opposite of Osler—taciturn, aloof, sparing in giving praise, and possessing few intimate friends and little social life. However, he was a superb research mentor, cared deeply about his residents' future careers, had a great thirst for knowledge, demonstrated an equal disdain for humbug, and inspired fierce loyalty from members of his resident staff.[54]

The hospital administration also cared deeply about the well-being of its house officers. Superintendent Henry Hurd, called affectionately by the residents "Uncle Hank" (and his daughters, "the Hurdlets"), was a staunch house staff advocate, someone residents could rely on and go to when there was a problem. Uncle Hank could be moody, which was thought to be related to the state of his digestion. Fortunately, the residents learned to read him, and they knew just when to approach him for favors. When his digestion was working well, he was likely to grant any reasonable request.[55]

The duties of a house officer depended on the individual's level of training. Interns in all departments were entrusted with the immediate responsibility for the care of patients in the wards. Junior assistant residents would oversee the interns and assume major roles in the teaching of both interns and medical students. More senior residents would oversee and teach their juniors as well as engage in original laboratory or clinical studies of their own. The amount of research accomplished by the house officers at this time was astonishing. One writer mentioned that she possessed 12 bound volumes consisting of 500 papers published by Hopkins residents or students during the first eight years of the school's existence.[56]

The details of a house officer's day-to-day work also depended on the particular field. In ear, nose, and throat, for example, an assistant resident's typical morning was spent assisting in operations, taking histories and performing physical examinations on new patients, and caring for patients already in the hospital. During some afternoons the resident worked in the outpatient otolaryngology clinic, where he saw patients of his own and provided instruction to medical students. Other afternoons he engaged in experimental work in the laboratory. Periodically there were also rounds, conferences, and opportunities to receive instruction in the use of various instruments.[57] In surgery, a junior assistant resident might spend mornings administering anesthesia in the operating room, early afternoons working in the outpatient surgical clinic, and late afternoons performing experiments in the laboratory.[58] And, of course, evenings were also busy, either caring for patients if on call, or reading, studying, or pursuing a project if not on call.

What was striking on every clinical service was the degree of responsibility residents received. In surgery, for example, the bulk of patient care and medical student teaching was provided by the resident staff. Over time, Halsted entrusted more and more of the actual operating to the residents. By the end of Halsted's period as chief, the chief resident in surgery and senior surgical residents were doing most of the surgery on ward patients and much of the surgery on Halsted's private patients.[59] In every department, clinical responsibility was provided in a graded form, with the more experienced and mature residents receiving greater responsibility. House officers reveled in the independence they received.

At first glance, it might seem that the house officers did not have a heavy workload. In 1898, for instance, the 23 members of the resident staff each averaged between 10 and 11 patients at a time. Each house officer admitted and discharged approximately 150 patients that year, with the average length of stay about 20 days.[60] From a contemporary perspective, accustomed to larger numbers of admissions per day and much shorter lengths of hospital stay, this might seem like a leisurely pace. However, these statistics mask the extraordinary thoroughness with which the house officers cared for their patients. Interns and residents did *complete* histories and physical examinations on their patients and knew *every* detail of *every* patient. They carefully evaluated the progress and status of patients on each subsequent hospital day as well. The house staff also performed many of the standard laboratory studies, such as examining the urine or blood. Thus, they typically felt there were not enough hours in the day.

This concern for thoroughness and attention to detail was emphasized explicitly and implicitly by the faculty. Osler, for instance, regularly preached the importance of what he called the "quality of thoroughness,"[61] and he exemplified thoroughness in his own clinical work. During a typical afternoon in his office, he saw five patients, averaging a half hour per patient. "A case cannot be satisfactorily examined in less than half an hour," he explained. "A sick man likes to have plenty of time spent over him, and he gets no satisfaction in a hurried, ten or twelve minute examination."[62] He was also famous for the care and detail he brought to teaching. He typically devoted his two-hour rounds with house officers and students to two or three patients, rarely to four, to allow enough time to explore all the issues of each patient.[63] House officers on every service dared be careless at their own risk.

Esprit de corps among the house officers was strong. Everyone knew everyone else, even in other departments. All house officers were unmarried and lived in the hospital. Strong friendships were formed, jealousies and rivalries were few, and successes and pleasures were freely shared. Mealtimes were rife with banter and good conversation, and pranks were common. Heightening the good times was the fact that Osler and Halsted, while still bachelors, also lived in the hospital, as did the Hurds and a number of other members of the hospital staff. Osler wrote his famed textbook of medicine in his living quarters in the Johns Hopkins Hospital.

One must resist the tendency to romanticize the past, for the past was never perfect. Such was the case at the Johns Hopkins Hospital. Residents there were no strangers to sleep deprivation, exhaustion, stress, and self-doubts. Tensions among the house officers sometimes arose. The famed neurosurgeon Harvey Cushing, Halsted's chief resident in surgery from 1897 to 1900, could be extremely harsh on his underlings, and his sharp criticisms almost precipitated fistfights on more than one occasion.[64] House officers were often frustrated by the inability of the best care of the period to help their patients, and, from the perspective of the present, the treatment of the charity patients on the ward services sometimes left much to be desired. The faculty members were hardly without their personal idiosyncrasies—Welch's disorganization, Halsted's aloofness, Kelly's religious fervor.

However, on balance, spirits among the house officers remained high. Most residents felt a strong bond with each other and with the institution, a bond intensified by the sense of common purpose. Many lifetime friendships were formed. In later years, many former Johns Hopkins house officers of the period described their residency as an invigorating and delightful experience, referring in large part to the uplifting stimulation of association they derived from their teachers and each other.[65]

However, there was something more than esprit de corps at the early Johns Hopkins Hospital. There was what one chief resident in pathology called "a wonderful happiness in work."[66] Residents experienced the exhilarating thrill of being on the outer boundary of knowledge, a sense of collective pride that they were not only learning medicine but also making medicine, the joy of intellectual effervescence at being part of something new and important. This "contagion of happiness," as Donald Fleming called it, began with the faculty but enveloped the house staff. In Fleming's words, it was "the general sense of happiness in their work that bound members of the Hopkins community together."[67]

From this perspective, the hospital was not so much an institution as a lifestyle, one that was dominated by the ever-present search for new knowledge.[68] As one former resident put it, "Finally, life succeeded in being fun, for most work was not a hardship but rather life itself."[69] Reginald Fitz, a noted Harvard surgeon, once spent a few days at Johns Hopkins, after which he said that the hospital was a happy monastery with the unusual feature that the monks cared nothing about the future.[70] Fleming agreed, discovering many commonalities between the residents and medical staff at the early Johns Hopkins Hospital and monks in a happy monastery. Both had an undistracted devotion to their calling, strong fellowship, and the conviction that pursuit of their individual interests would contribute to the larger good. According to Fleming, the men of Hopkins, like monks, "had this same sense that if they only did well what they would wish to do as individuals they would contribute to the happiness of everyone else."[71]

Insight into the atmosphere at Johns Hopkins is provided by the findings of the psychologist Howard Gardner. From Gardner's perspective, residents at Johns Hopkins were engaged in doing "good work." To Gardner, "good work" is work of expert quality that benefits the broader society. One conspicuous quality of good work is that it "*feels* good." With good work, individuals have "flow experiences," whereby they "feel totally involved, lost in a seemingly effortless performance. Paradoxically, [they] feel 100 percent alive when [they] are so committed to the task at hand that [they] lose track of time, or [their] interests—even of [their] own existence."[72] Of note, Gardner found that "good work" is more likely to occur at work than anywhere else. Judged by the reactions of those who went through it, the pioneering residency program at Johns Hopkins allowed participants the opportunity to engage in "good work." It thus provided an inspiring model of what graduate medical education could be.

DIASPORA

Johns Hopkins clearly represented a departure in graduate medical education in America, as it did in medical student education. However, the faculty did not want its residency program to remain unique. Rather, it wished to see similar programs put into place elsewhere. The overriding goal of the faculty was to inspire emulation at other institutions—to "teach the teachers" who could export the Hopkins vision to other hospitals and medical schools. This was all part of a broader desire of leading medical scientists in America, like leading scholars in all fields, to "professionalize" their disciplines and bring to an end America's intellectual subservience to the Continent.[73]

Over time the dream of the Hopkins faculty to "teach the teachers" came to fruition. The clinical chiefs possessed an exceptional flair for selecting outstanding individuals for positions on the house staff—individuals with keen intellects, bounding curiosity, a passion for discovery, a love of their profession, a commitment to serving the patient, and unusual dedication and discipline. During the first quarter-century of the Johns Hopkins Hospital, over 350 physicians served on the house staff, and over 1,100 Hopkins medical students received their clinical training there.[74] This created a substantial nucleus of extremely capable, well-trained physicians who could—and did—serve as emissaries of the Hopkins residency at other medical schools and hospitals.

This process was well illustrated by events in surgical education. During his years as chief of surgery, Halsted had 17 chief residents, 11 of whom subsequently established surgical residency programs at other medical schools modeled after the one at Johns Hopkins. A "multiplication effect" occurred in the next generation. These 11 surgical centers produced 166 chief residents, of whom 85 became teachers in university medical schools. Halsted also had 55 assistant resident surgeons, who each spent between one and three years with him. Of this group, 41 assumed important positions in academic surgery at various medical schools; only 14 became private practitioners.[75] And one need not have trained with Halsted to view himself as a disciple. For instance, Allen O. Whipple, the Valentine Mott Professor of Surgery at the College of Physicians and Surgeons of Columbia University, did not work under Halsted, but he was fascinated by Halsted, championed Halsted's principles of surgical training, and credited Halsted as his inspiration when he introduced the surgical residency to Presbyterian Hospital.[76]

A similar process occurred in the surgical subspecialties. For instance, Hugh Young modeled his urology residency on Halsted's surgical residency—except, in Young's words, he went "even further" by allowing his urology residents even greater freedom to operate independently on patients in the public wards.[77] Young's program immediately became an incubation center for the development of urology. Men trained by Young subsequently became heads of urology programs at Yale, Harvard, Cornell, the University of Pennsylvania, the University of Rochester, Georgetown, the University of Virginia, Emory, Tulane, Washington University, and the University of California, among others. Three of these individuals went directly from the residency to the chairmanship. Another group of individuals served as assistant residents in urology under Young without finishing the program. Of this group, nearly two dozen became professors or heads of urology at important medical schools.[78] It was difficult to find a leader in urology before World War II who had not trained with Young.

The nonsurgical fields also became fountainheads for the subsequent diffusion of the residency. Pediatrics provided a typical example. The department was headed by John Howland, a charismatic leader who helped modernize pediatric training and practice in the United States. Curiously, as with many other leading physicians, his college friends might not have predicted such a career. At Yale he was an expert oarsman, intercollegiate tennis champion (and one of the top-ranked players in the country), editor of the *Yale News*, member of the sought-after Skull and Bones society, and one of the most popular individuals on campus; however, he was an unremarkable student. In medical school he found his calling, and his abundant energy turned to medicine, then to pediatrics. A brilliant clinical scientist, he pioneered the use of chemical methods to study problems of pediatric illness, and he introduced the residency system to the training of pediatricians. His ideas took root with the talented young physicians who worked with him. From his program went forth one resident after another to head other departments or assume positions of responsibility elsewhere. Among these were James L. Gamble (Harvard), Kenneth D. Blackfan (Cincinnati, then Harvard), Stanley G. Ross (McGill), Frederick Tisdall (Toronto), W. McKim Marriott (Washington University), Horton R. Casparis (Vanderbilt), Harold L. Higgins and A. Ashley Weech (Cincinnati), Benjamin Kramer (Long Island), Grover F. Powers and Alfred T. Shohl (Yale), Edwards A. Park (Yale, then Johns Hopkins), and Wilburt C. Davison (Duke). As with other members of the Hopkins faculty, much of Howland's influence on his residents was implicit. One former resident said, "He was a remarkable example of the unconscious teacher, the teacher... who does not know that he is teaching. He made us all try to be like him."[79]

The Hopkins faculty took great pride in the residency system. For example, consider Halsted. His contributions to surgical practice were legendary: his championship of aseptic surgery; the invention of rubber gloves; the development of important operations for breast cancer, thyroid goiter, inguinal hernia, and many other conditions. An even greater contribution was his general attitude toward surgery. He emphasized the importance of searching scientific study of the underlying pathological condition, and he pioneered the "safety in surgery" school by his painstaking devotion to the gentle handling of injured tissues. However, to Halsted these contributions were less notable than his introduction of the residency system to surgical education. He regularly told his friend and colleague, William Welch, that his "greatest satisfaction" in life came from "the training of surgeons."[80]

The residency system did not immediately spread to other institutions. It took time for this novel form of training to demonstrate its benefits, arouse interest elsewhere, and inspire imitation. In addition, medical educators of the 1890s and 1900s were preoccupied with more urgent problems: upgrading standards in undergraduate medical education and creating the modern medical school and teaching hospital. Hence, it was not until the eve of World War I that the residency began to appear at other places.

However, as momentum for adopting the residency system started to grow, a troubling question arose: To what degree could it be successfully exported? The residency succeeded at Johns Hopkins, where it was led by a gifted faculty and where positions were offered only to unusually talented individuals. Yet to be determined was whether other programs could re-create those same conditions. It seemed likely that certain leading hospitals might succeed, the Massachusetts General Hospital being a prime example. But what about lesser teaching hospitals, public hospitals, or community hospitals? The residency system worked when all residents were "picked men," whether they ultimately entered academic medicine or private practice. But would the residency system succeed if positions were given to more average medical students, as inherently must be done if the system were to grow and spread? The answers to these questions lay in the future.

CHAPTER 3

The Growth of Graduate Medical Education

A central characteristic of an educational system is implicit in its name: It is a *system*. The various components interrelate with each other, and the lower levels of the system articulate with the higher. Thus, in America, the elementary schools feed the high schools; the high schools, the colleges; and the colleges, the graduate and professional schools. The same principle extends to graduate medical education: It depends on the strength of the medical schools and on the number and quality of medical graduates. During the first two decades following the introduction of the residency system at the Johns Hopkins Hospital, the deficiencies of American medical schools diverted attention away from graduate medical education. Medical educators understandably focused on building the scientific medical school, establishing entrance requirements, and articulating medical education with the underlying educational system. They gave little attention at the time to graduate medical education.

In the second decade of the twentieth century, a codified system of "graduate medical education"—that is, formal medical study after the receipt of the MD degree—began to appear. This system consisted of two parts. The first was the "internship"—a period of clinical work for newly minted MDs. The internship provided more responsibility with patients than medical students received, thereby offering a rounding-out experience for general practice. It also provided a foundation on which graduates could continue formal medical study toward a specialty. The second component of the system was the "residency." Modeled after the program introduced at the Johns Hopkins Hospital, the residency provided an intensive, multiyear hospital experience in a particular clinical field following the completion of an internship. It was designed for those physicians wishing to enter specialty practice or pursue an academic career. In this new, two-part system of graduate medical education, the desires of earlier generations of American physicians to acquire clinical experience, study for a specialty, or prepare for a career in research could all be met—without having to leave their homeland to do so.

The growth of graduate medical education into an industry during the past half century should not obscure the fluidity and instability of the system prior to World War II. The emerging system was notable for its lack of uniform standards and the inconsistency of quality and experience from one program to the next. In addition, the residency at this time represented only one of several paths to specialized clinical practice. Many physicians followed alternative paths to specialization, such as courses at a postgraduate medical school, study in Europe, or serving as an assistant to an established specialist. Through the 1930s, it was not clear which of these paths would become dominant. The development of graduate medical education in the United States represented a highly contingent process.

However, as the internship and residency developed, one characteristic was especially noteworthy: These programs were located in hospitals, not in universities. Thus, graduate medical education was unique in American higher education. It was the only branch of graduate or professional training to be situated in an institution in which service rather than education was the primary mission. There were powerful reasons for this, such as the abundance of patients and marvelous facilities for the study and investigation of disease. However, over time the location of graduate medical education in hospitals was to account for many of its most frustrating dilemmas as well.

COMPLETING THE INFRASTRUCTURE

Before World War I, most medical educators scarcely thought about graduate medical education. There was simply too much work directly ahead to improve undergraduate medical education in America. With the exception of a few schools, entrance requirements were lax, laboratories inadequate, clinical facilities scarce, and financial resources meager. On top of this, a scientific spirit had not fully diffused into the methods of teaching.[1] Abraham Flexner, in his famous muckraking report on medical education in 1910, did not mention the internship or residency.[2] In 1916, the faculty of one medical school stated the dominant view: "The urgent questions now being solved in regard to the course for the degree of M.D. must be decided before any attempt is made to develop graduate work of a high grade."[3]

In the early twentieth century, a number of developments occurred that paved the way for the spread of graduate medical education in the United States. Some of these developments benefited both undergraduate and graduate medical education; others uniquely served graduate medical education. Together, they created an infrastructure on which a strong system of graduate medical education could grow.

The first development was the maturation of clinical science into an intellectually important, clinically relevant discipline. Medical discovery no longer depended so completely on basic scientists making discoveries in the laboratory that could be translated to clinical practice (for example, the chemist Louis Pasteur developing a vaccine for rabies). Rather, more and more medical discoveries were the work of clinical scientists—clinically active physicians using the tools of chemistry, physiology, immunology, and other laboratory disciplines to study disease and therapeutics in live patients.

A turning point in the maturation of clinical science occurred during the first decade of the twentieth century. At that time, a new feeling for the value of chemistry in medicine became much more widespread. This change was symbolized by the appointment of Lewellys F. Barker to the chair of internal medicine at Johns Hopkins in 1905. Barker's predecessor, William Osler, had been the apostle of the microscope, the pathology laboratory, and careful clinical observation in the study of disease. Osler introduced clinical laboratories at the Johns Hopkins Hospital to facilitate diagnosis, not to develop new knowledge. Barker, on the other hand, was a first-rate clinical scientist. He understood that the study of disease and therapeutics could benefit greatly from the application of biological and chemical methods.[4]

The importance of clinical science lay in part in its utility as a tool to advance medical knowledge. However, equally important was its transforming effect on the practice of medicine. The growing understanding of abnormal metabolism, blood changes, and chemical derangements within the diseased body did much to aid physicians in diagnosing disease, interpreting illness, and treating those disturbances. One medical school dean noted in 1916: "I have seen the taking of blood pressure transformed from a laboratory fad to a clinical routine; I have noted embryology influencing surgical procedure; I have seen the action current become the basis of electrocardiography; I have seen the theoretical chemistry of the proteins become the cornerstone of dietetics; I have seen... clinicians attempting to measure and understand hydrogen ion concentration."[5] It was now inconceivable that a physician could be an outstanding clinician without a firm grasp of fundamental scientific facts and principles.

The most subtle, but perhaps the most significant, indication of how clinical science began transforming the practice of medicine lay in the way scientific concepts began influencing the thought processes of practicing physicians. Often unconsciously, the "clinical mind" began using the concepts and theories derived from the fundamental sciences in analyzing the clinical circumstances of patients. Elias P. Lyon, a noted physiologist and dean of the University of Minnesota Medical School, observed this phenomenon when he decided to shadow some of the school's noted clinicians.

> So I followed a master of diagnosis in his day's work. I saw him percuss and auscultate; I saw him count corpuscles and analyze excreta; I saw him elicit reflexes and measure temperature; I heard him speak of valves and pressure and enzymes and neurons and calories. I said: "That man is not practicing medicine. He is practicing physiology." I watched a therapeutist at the bedside and found that he was not practicing medicine but pharmacology. I saw a surgeon earning a thousand dollars. I discovered that he was not practicing surgery but anatomy, pathology, physiology—and high finance! Finally, the relation I was seeking came suddenly into mental view. Anatomy and physiology and pharmacology and bacteriology and chemistry and the rest are not the children of medicine; they are not the branches of an evolutionary tree; they are not handmaids; they are not stepping stones or preparatory stages. They are it. They are medicine itself.[6]

As Lyon put it, concepts derived from the fundamental sciences had become "the invisible warp" of the clinician's mind.[7]

A second development was the maturation of clinical science as a profession, not just as a scientific discipline. That is, by World War I a critical mass of clinical scientists had arisen who were carrying on productive research in their home country, publishing their work in American journals, and training the next generation of academic leaders at American medical schools and teaching hospitals. An important sign of the professionalization of clinical science in the United States was the organization of the American Society for Clinical Investigation in 1908. By World War I, a substantial cadre of clinical investigators was at work, most of whom found homes in clinical departments of medical schools. Indeed, appointment to a major clinical position at a medical school now depended mainly on a person's national reputation as a scholar, not on one's local reputation as a clinical consultant. This represented another sign that medicine had entered the university.

The presence of a rapidly growing number of clinical investigators revolutionized the culture of most medical schools. Basic scientists at many schools began to fear their departments might be eclipsed by the clinical departments in terms of size, resources, and influence within the school.[8] Private practitioners, the traditional clinical teachers at medical schools, increasingly found themselves powerless in school governance and policy formation, even as they continued to participate actively in clinical teaching at most medical schools.[9] Despite pushback, however, the growing importance and influence of clinical scientists at medical schools could not be stopped. More and more clinical departments came to be led by scientifically trained individuals who used the laboratory to study clinical problems.[10]

A third development involved the emergence of a new interest among many hospitals in promoting medical education and research. Prior to 1910, the attitude of most hospitals toward doing so had been decidedly chilly, a fact that caused no small amount of consternation among medical educators. Samuel Lambert, the dean of the College of Physicians and Surgeons, spoke for many in 1911 when he deplored "the antagonism that has been felt between hospitals and medical education."[11] With few exceptions, hospitals regarded medical education and research solely as the responsibilities of medical schools. Hospitals consistently refused to allow medical students to work in the wards as clinical clerks, regularly denied medical faculties the opportunity to appoint the hospital staffs, and often exhibited only lukewarm support of clinical research. Even the venerable Massachusetts General Hospital was remarkably cool toward medical education, denying medical students the opportunity to work there as clinical clerks until 1913.[12] Abraham Flexner used his 1910 report to make "one more plea for an understanding between existing hospitals and deserving medical schools."[13]

In the 1910s this situation rapidly changed. The Johns Hopkins Hospital had become a national model, clinical research was succeeding, and hospitals that cooperated with medical schools began to achieve significant advantages in attracting the finest physicians to their staffs. These events inspired the creation of new partnerships between medical schools and their affiliated hospitals, and many leading hospitals quickly became teaching laboratories for their respective medical schools. In this new environment excellence in patient care no longer determined leadership among hospitals. Rather, leadership came to depend on setting new standards for patient care—on helping patients of the future as well as patients of the present. "The reputation of a hospital depends more upon the quality of its publications than upon any other element," an officer of the Peter Bent

Brigham Hospital observed in 1917.[14] By 1920, the "teaching hospital" had become firmly entrenched in American medicine, a remarkable transition considering the intensity of the resistance to the idea only a short time before. Acceptance by hospitals of an expanded teaching mission was clearly to benefit both undergraduate and graduate medical education.[15]

A final development was the maturation of the modern American medical school in the years following the Flexner report of 1910. This allowed the production of large numbers of medical graduates sufficiently prepared to take advantage of the opportunities and benefits of a strong system of graduate medical education. As elementary schools created a pipeline for high schools, high schools for colleges, and colleges for professional and graduate schools, so did the modern medical school create a pipeline for graduate medical education. As one indication of the importance of this development, in the early 1910s the Johns Hopkins Hospital, which previously had accepted only graduates of the Johns Hopkins Medical School for internship positions, began making places available for graduates from other schools.[16]

In short, during the generation that followed the opening of the Johns Hopkins Hospital, several developments critical to the growth of graduate medical education in the United States occurred. These included a rapidly growing body of clinically relevant knowledge (and objective methods for acquiring that knowledge), a rising number of clinical scientists on medical school faculties, a much greater receptivity to teaching and research within hospitals, and the appearance of large numbers of medical graduates properly prepared to take advantage of these opportunities. Before World War I, the impact of these developments on graduate medical education was scarcely felt. However, they provided an infrastructure on which the development of graduate medical education in the United States would soon occur.

THE MATURATION OF THE INTERNSHIP

To some early twentieth-century medical educators, the idea that doctors needed formal instruction after the completion of medical school might have come as a shock. For decades, medical knowledge and practice had been growing and changing, but so had the American medical school. Since the Civil War, the traditional 16-week term of instruction had given way to 32-week or 36-week terms, and the course of study had increased from two years to four. Entrance requirements to medical school had been established, the scientific subjects had been added, laboratory instruction had been introduced, new physical facilities had been constructed, fundamental and clinical research had begun to thrive, and medical education was in the process of becoming a genuine branch of the university. After 1910 the clinical clerkship spread rapidly, a development made possible by the new interest of many important hospitals in partnering with medical schools. The clerkship allowed third- and fourth-year medical students to participate, under supervision, in actual patient care. Accordingly, to some, the need for rank-and-file physicians entering general practice to engage in formal study after medical school seemed small.

However, such confidence in the expansible properties of medical schools was short-lived. The onslaught of new knowledge was too relentless to accommodate even in a four-year course of study. There was too much information to learn, too many principles to understand, and too many diagnostic and therapeutic procedures to master. More and more, medical school faculties became aware that even the university medical school was not sufficiently preparing students for the practice of medicine. In their view, a rounding-out experience had become necessary for all physicians, for general practitioners as well as future specialists.

To some medical educators, the best way to complete the education of physicians was to do more of the same: create a fifth year of medical school. Such an approach offered many advantages. It would allow medical teaching to be distributed in a less concentrated manner, providing students more time for study, reflection, and healthy living. It would also permit more and better clinical opportunities to be provided. In the early 1900s, this idea had prominent advocates, most notably at Columbia University's College of Physicians and Surgeons. However, the idea failed to gain traction. Few medical schools had the physical, human, or financial resources to extend the required course of instruction. The Columbia faculty soon abandoned the idea because "of the impossibility of securing similar action by other important schools within any reasonable period of time."[17] The trajectory of the American medical school toward expanding its length of instruction ground to a halt, and the four-year curriculum triumphed as the standard model.

Instead, medical educators increasingly favored the idea of using hospitals for graduate training after medical school. In this, they were inspired by the hospital positions for medical graduates that had dotted the landscape of American medicine in the nineteenth century. Since the 1880s these positions had become more numerous and visible, and their educational quality had improved. For instance, the number of house officers at Mount Sinai Hospital (New York) grew from one in 1856 to nine in 1893; at Lakeside Hospital, from one in 1872 to nine in 1898; and at the

Massachusetts General Hospital, from six in 1871 to 20 in 1902.[18] Since the 1880s the educational quality of many of these positions had also improved. Speaking in 1911 of the value of an internship in a good hospital—one that was rich in patients, facilities, and scientific opportunities, and where there was actual responsibility for patient care—one medical educator declared: "No one who has had the advantage of such a training doubts its value; no one who has not had it but regrets his inability to secure it."[19]

The growing role of house positions in American medicine in the 1880s and 1890s was not by accident. Hospitals had become much busier places, particularly after the introduction of aseptic techniques in surgery in 1884. The acuity of illness had increased, and the length of stay had dramatically dropped. For instance, at the Massachusetts General Hospital, the average length of stay fell from 81 days in 1855 to 19 days in 1899.[20] There was also much more to do in the day-to-day management of patients. There were new chemical, blood, and urine tests to perform, and more careful monitoring of patients was required, particularly after surgery. Social factors also contributed to the increasing role of the hospital in serious illness. Gas heat, electric lights, telephones, improved roads, faster and more reliable transportation, and urban crowding all led to a growing demand for hospital services or an improved capability of hospitals to respond to that demand.[21] Accordingly, hospitals developed a much greater need for house officers than before. As one observer noted, hospitals had discovered "that it is impossible to get along satisfactorily without these assistants."[22]

In the early 1900s, the nineteenth-century system of house appointments evolved into the internship system. The term "internship" came to connote a hospital-based educational experience for medical graduates that rounded out the medical school course, with particular emphasis on the practical application of knowledge. The goal was for interns to acquire independence, confidence, critical acumen, and judgment by assuming enlarged clinical responsibilities, under supervision, for patient care. The internship was considered part of the basic preparation for general practice; it was also regarded as an essential prerequisite for training in a specialty. As the system came to be codified, the hodge-podge of names previously used for graduate hospital positions was abandoned, and the term "intern" came into universal use. At the Massachusetts General Hospital, for instance, the term "intern" replaced the venerable name "house pupil" in 1922.[23] The adoption of the term "intern" over competing terms probably reflected the earlier decision of the Johns Hopkins Hospital to use this title.

In the early 1900s, there were still relatively few internships, and most were located at large teaching hospitals. Competition among medical students to win a position was fierce. As late as 1914, internships were available for only one-half of that year's medical school graduates.[24] However, as the pace and complexity of hospital care continued to grow, as the amount of patient-related chores such as blood drawing and laboratory work continued to increase, and as graduates of the modern medical school demonstrated their maturity and capability, the demand from hospitals for house officers grew rapidly. By 1923, the number of available internships for the first time became large enough to accommodate all medical school graduates.[25] In the 1930s, virtually all medical graduates were availing themselves of the opportunity to do an internship.[26] By the end of World War II, approximately 1,300 hospitals, or roughly one-third of the nation's total, were approved for internships, and there were 8,500 openings for 5,000 medical graduates.[27] Some of this growth resulted from the expansion of opportunities at teaching hospitals, but most of the growth resulted from the spread of internships to community hospitals, which also began to desire such services.

Nineteenth-century hospital positions, even at their best, represented an apprenticelike experience, offering on-the-job practical training but little exposure to broad principles or organizing concepts. At the Massachusetts General Hospital, as late as 1897 it was deemed inappropriate for house pupils to check out books and journals from the hospital library, so unconcerned were hospital authorities for the educational aspects of the experience.[28] The twentieth-century internship represented the conversion of that system to a formally organized program that was designed to be educational in the university sense of the term. The rich educational features of a well-constructed internship, according to the American Medical Association, "definitely stamp this as 'education', not 'on-the-job' training comparable to that of an apprentice garage mechanic."[29]

Surprisingly, perhaps, clinical research represented only a small part of the experience. Scholarly pursuits were encouraged, but given the heavy time demands of assuming the moment-by-moment responsibility for the care of patients, clinical research was pursued only by rare, exceptionally motivated interns. What made good internships so educational was that clinical care was conducted in a scholarly environment, where there was a thirst for knowledge, an atmosphere of inquiry, and insistence that clinical decisions be documented by the best available evidence. In addition, the practical experience gained by patient care was enhanced by conferences, seminars, rounds, lectures, and other types of instruction, which at some programs were held at night as well as during the day.[30] Much of the best learning occurred informally—the conversations interns had with an attending physician in the hallway, or with each other at mealtimes or at a work station. And, for interns at hospitals affiliated with a medical school, the presence of medical students provided an opportunity to teach as well as to learn, which itself was a valuable learning experience.

Internships came in three varieties. The most common was the "rotating" internship, in which interns rotated through all the clinical specialties. A second variety, the "straight" internship, allowed interns the opportunity to spend their entire time in a particular field, such as internal medicine or surgery. The third variety, the "mixed" internship, represented a cross between the rotating and straight internships. "Mixed" internships provided greater concentration in internal medicine and surgery but less time in the other specialties and subspecialties than rotating internships. Rotating and mixed internships were found primarily in community hospitals; straight internships, mainly in teaching hospitals. In 1939, there were 6,301 rotating internships, 1,013 mixed internships, and 518 straight internships offered.[31]

Which type of internship provided the richest educational experience? A contentious debate raged around that question. The American Medical Association (AMA), whose constituency consisted mainly of general practitioners, favored the rotating internship because of the diversity of experiences it provided, and it viewed the straight service as "unsound."[32] Medical school faculties, on the other hand, deplored the rotating internship because of the perceived superficiality of the experiences it provided. The distinguished surgeon Evarts Graham of Washington University called rotating internships "practically valueless."[33] Heated arguments erupted between the AMA and various medical schools on this issue, thereby revealing the major fault line in the profession between practicing and academic physicians.[34] World War II began with the issue unresolved, though wise words were offered by one medical school dean, Willard C. Rappleye of Columbia University, who wrote, "The type of service is not nearly as important as the opportunities which are provided for the right kind of training."[35]

Extraordinary fluidity and a conspicuous lack of standardization characterized internship programs during the period between the world wars. Programs varied considerably in their length of service. Most commonly, an internship lasted one year, but a rare program was shorter, and many were longer, some for as long as three years. In 1938–39 there were 4,975 12-month internship positions offered, 383 18-month positions, 47 21-month positions, 2,211 24-month positions, 50 27-month positions, 67 30-month positions, and 99 36-month positions.[36] Some hospitals offered internships of different lengths. For instance, Mount Sinai Hospital, one of the few teaching hospitals to offer a rotating internship, provided both a one and a two-and-one-half-year internship. It also went back and forth in the length of its longer internship—some years it was 24 months, but most years it was 30 months.[37] It was also common for there to be staggered starting dates within an internship program: Johns Hopkins, for example, July 1 and September 1; Babies Hospital (New York), January 1, April 1, July 1, and October 1; and the three prominent Boston teaching hospitals (Boston City Hospital, Peter Bent Brigham Hospital, and Massachusetts General Hospital), at three- or four-month intervals throughout the year.[38]

During the interwar years, medical educators debated whether the internship represented the culmination of undergraduate medical education or the first stage of graduate medical education. To some, the keen interest in the internship from the Association of American Medical Colleges and the AMA, which had been so instrumental in medical school reform, gave credence to the idea that the internship represented the completion of undergraduate medical education. In 1915 the University of Minnesota Medical School established its "fifth-year program" in which it deferred conferring the MD degree until the graduate had successfully completed an internship.[39] This action gave further support to the idea that the internship was part of undergraduate medical education.

However, support for the idea was not strong. Most medical schools opposed it, largely because they felt they could not guarantee the educational standards of an internship at any hospital other than their own.[40] Medical students tended to dislike the plan. For instance, when the Georgetown University School of Medicine considered the idea, the Georgetown medical students protested. They pointed out many problems with the plan, including the possibility that an idiosyncratic doctor or hospital could deny a student a degree.[41] By 1939, only 13 schools delayed conferring the MD degree until after the completion of an internship, indicating that most schools considered it a phase of graduate medical education.[42] During World War II the "fifth-year program" disappeared from American medical education, never to return, indicating universal acceptance of the internship as the beginning of graduate medical education.

As the internship grew in importance, so did its regulation. With the acquiescence of the profession, this responsibility fell to the Council on Medical Education of the AMA. In the 1910s the Council began inspecting hospitals to accredit them for internships, as it already had been inspecting medical schools for accreditation. In 1919 the Council published its first "Essentials for Approved Internships," and in 1920 it changed its name to the Council on Medical Education and Hospitals to reflect its enlarged role. Hospitals that violated the Council's educational guidelines would not be accredited and would be removed from the approved list.[43]

State licensing boards played a peculiar role in the regulation of the internship. In 1939, 21 state licensing boards required an internship for licensure, a prelude to the post–World War II era when this requirement became universal.[44] What infuriated many medical educators was that some states went far beyond requiring an internship for a license to specifying the types of service and even the number of hours on each service that were required. Medical educators deplored this intrusion of government into purely educational affairs, but at the time many states considered this their prerogative.[45] After World War II this micromanagement of the internship by state licensing boards ended.

Before World War II, the internship remained the weakest part of graduate medical education. One report called it "the most unsatisfactory and uneven portion of the educational scheme of medicine at the present time."[46] Many internship programs, of course, offered outstanding experiences. However, the bottom was low and the gap in quality between the best and the worst programs was extremely wide. Many approved internship programs offered too little clinical responsibility, too many chores, and too little teaching to allow trainees to accomplish much in the way of professional development. One medical educator observed, in many hospitals "the intern does little more than give an anesthetic, dress and take the blame for the pus cases, and occasionally examine the urine or sputum. No histories or none worthy the name, no laboratory tests, no thorough examination of a patient."[47]

Most of the deficient internships were at community hospitals, and the smaller the hospital, the more likely it was that there were educational problems. This was because the smaller hospitals had greater difficulty providing diverse clinical experiences, stimulating formal and informal educational opportunities, and sufficient support from the clinical laboratories, radiology department, and pathology services. The greatest problems were found at community hospitals with between 25 and 100 beds.[48] These programs provided so much work and so little teaching that they were facetiously called "the self-teaching types of internship."[49] The Council on Medical Education and Hospitals took its responsibility of approving hospitals for internships seriously. However, it was also sensitive to the desire of community hospitals to have an intern staff, and as a result the Council proved much more lenient in approving hospitals than it did in approving medical schools.

Although the Council's sensitivity to the desires of its constituency helps explain its decisions, there may be another factor as well. Guiding the Council's activities was its energetic and devoted secretary, N. P. Colwell.

A sophisticated educational leader, Colwell considered medical research "the very soul of medical education."[50] Earlier, he had played a major role in the efforts to eliminate proprietary medical schools and elevate standards at university medical schools. He understood the characteristics of a strong learning environment. However, he had a tendency to romanticize the educational opportunities small hospitals provided. He spoke of the "undiscovered talents" that might emerge and be utilized for educational purposes in unexpected places. "Most excellent courses for graduate study are found sometimes in small hospitals or hospitals in outlying districts in which a few physicians or even a single physician or surgeon has demonstrated a remarkable teaching ability.... There is an educational opportunity in every hospital regardless of its size and location."[51] In this, Colwell was reminiscent of individuals like Henry Ford and Thomas Edison—innovators who never gave up their infatuation with America's agrarian past, even as they pioneered technological changes that helped give rise to an industrial future.[52]

THE SPREAD OF THE RESIDENCY

In 1916, William Welch of Johns Hopkins, now a senior statesman in American medicine, spoke to the Harvey Society about the extraordinary contribution to American medicine that the Johns Hopkins faculty had made with its introduction of the residency system 27 years before. He described the great advantages of an educational program that allowed residents a prolonged period of advanced training in a medical specialty. Only one thing surprised him: the fact that so few other hospitals had adopted the residency system. He confessed, "I have often wondered that this system has not been more widely adopted in this country."[53]

Yet, even as Welch was speaking, the intellectual and social infrastructure for the residency system was rapidly falling into place. Clinical science had developed to a point where no one doubted its value in helping solve many important medical problems. A young, energetic cohort of clinical scientists had assumed leadership roles in clinical teaching. Medical and surgical practice had become more complex, leading hospitals to look more favorably on the idea of acquiring a resident staff. Medical students were increasingly drawn to specialty practice—in part for intellectual excitement, in part for the accompanying social prestige and economic rewards. And as George Rosen, a noted historian of medicine, demonstrated, the growth of specialization was reinforced by many cultural trends, such as the rapid growth of urban areas with high concentrations of disease, the country's accumulation of wealth, and the public's growing infatuation with specialized knowledge, expertise, and the division of labor—all of which made medical specialization seem inevitable and desirable.[54]

The first major breakthrough in the spread of the residency system occurred in Boston. Curiously, this did not occur at the venerable Massachusetts General Hospital but at the new Peter Bent Brigham Hospital, which was located immediately next to the Harvard Medical School. Until the appointment of David Linn Edsall as chief of the medical service in 1912, the Massachusetts General Hospital had been remarkably conservative in all matters of medical education and research. According to one writer, the atmosphere in the hospital had lacked "a critical scientific fragrance" prior to his arrival.[55] Edsall, a prominent clinical scientist of the new school, led the hospital's development over the next several years into a major center of advanced clinical study. However, Edsall was following the example of the Peter Bent Brigham Hospital, which in its planning stage had announced its intention to allow Harvard medical students to work as clinical clerks, permit the medical school to make its staff appointments, develop a large program of clinical research, and establish a residency program. In Boston, the Massachusetts General Hospital was the follower in medical education, and the Peter Bent Brigham Hospital, the leader.

When the Peter Bent Brigham Hospital accepted its first patient on January 27, 1913, it had in place a residency program in internal medicine and surgery. At the base of the program were 16 "straight" interns, 8 in medicine and 8 in surgery, appointed for a 16-month period. The interns carried the bulk of the responsibility for the moment-to-moment care of patients. Above them were three assistant residents in each department, appointed for renewable one-year terms. The residents supervised the clinical care of the interns and pursued independent investigations on subjects of their choosing. Each service was headed by a chief resident, who was appointed for an indefinite period. The chief resident supervised the entire service, assumed major responsibility for teaching medical students and house officers, and engaged in scholarly studies. As at the Johns Hopkins Hospital, the chief residents were mature, scientifically gifted individuals with academic aspirations. The first chief resident in internal medicine, Francis Peabody, famous for his essay on the doctor-patient relationship, served in that position for three years before embarking on a brief but glorious career in clinical research, first at the Boston City Hospital, then at the Peter Bent Brigham Hospital.[56] The first chief resident in surgery, Emil Goetsch, also served in the position for three years before becoming associate professor of surgery at Johns Hopkins and, later, surgeon-in-chief at the Long Island College Hospital.

Officials of the Peter Bent Brigham Hospital patterned their residency program after the one in place at Johns Hopkins. Henry A. Christian, the physician-in-chief, had been a medical student at Johns Hopkins, where he became enamored of William Osler. Later in life, Christian became editor of Osler's *Principles and Practices of Medicine*. Cushing, the founder of neurosurgery, spent many years as William Halsted's chief resident in surgery at Johns Hopkins, where he imbibed all that was Halstedian and absorbed the spirit and values of the medical school. When the opportunity arrived for Christian and Cushing to lead the Peter Bent Brigham Hospital, they did not have to look far for an educational model. As Cushing put it, "The residential system we have adopted is patterned after that which in the past has proved so effective at the Johns Hopkins Hospital."[57] The diaspora from Johns Hopkins had begun to take roots.

The clinical chiefs at "the Brigham" intended to provide residents a superior clinical experience. However, as at Johns Hopkins, the primary goal of their residency was to support the development of clinical investigation in the United States and thereby help America establish its scientific independence from the Old World. For instance, Christian, who in 1908 had helped found the American Society for Clinical Investigation, expressed this viewpoint in an unpublished memorandum written around the time the hospital opened. "Clinical medicine in America ha[s] failed to keep pace with that in Germany," he wrote. However, "The time has come to take the next step in medical education in America, if we are to gain our proper place in medicine." This involved the promotion of clinical science by developing the residency system to train clinical investigators and creating more job opportunities for clinical scientists at medical schools.[58] Throughout his tenure as chief of medicine, Christian spoke of the clinical work done by the residents as their "routine work," in distinction to their more important "investigative work."[59] In recruiting residents, he looked for individuals with experience and aptitude in chemistry, physiology, and pharmacology, knowing that such individuals would have an easier time drawing the link between clinical care and the fundamental sciences.[60] He recruited the distinguished chemist Otto Folin to the staff as "hospital chemist" and the legendary physiologist Walter Cannon as "hospital physiologist" so that outstanding basic scientists would be present on the clinical team. Cushing, who viewed the extension of knowledge as "the highest function of a hospital," concurred with his colleague in medicine.[61]

From the start the residency programs at the Peter Bent Brigham Hospital were successful. It quickly became apparent that they provided superb clinical training. However, it also became apparent that they succeeded brilliantly in promoting clinical research. Soon the hospital was another germinal center for the production of academic leaders. In surgery, 26 former interns or residents had attained professorial rank in US medical schools by 1929.[62] In internal medicine, 26 former house officers had achieved professorial rank by 1938, as well as 3 as clinical professors, 17 as associate professors, and 20 as assistant professors.[63] In pathology, a smaller program, there were 17 former residents with important academic appointments in 1946, including 11 who were full professors.[64] (Among these were Sidney Farber, for whom the Dana-Farber Cancer Institute is named, and Ernest W. Goodpasture of "Goodpasture's syndrome," a disease in which the body's immune system attacks the lungs and kidneys.)

During the 1920s and 1930s the residency system took root. Under Edsall's leadership, the Massachusetts General Hospital soon created a residency system, becoming a third germinal center (along with the Johns Hopkins Hospital and the Peter Bent Brigham Hospital) for the production of academic leaders. By 1925, 29 hospitals offered residency programs; by 1930, 338 hospitals; and by 1939, 518 hospitals.[65] In the early 1900s, only the Johns Hopkins Hospital had a fully developed residency in surgery. By 1941 there were 30 residencies patterned after it; by 1951, 130 such programs.[66] Most of the early growth occurred at teaching hospitals, but by the 1930s many community hospitals had introduced residency programs as well.

Much of the spread of the residency was led by former residents at the Johns Hopkins Hospital. For instance, George J. Heuer, one of Halsted's chief residents, introduced surgical residencies modeled after the Johns Hopkins program at the Cincinnati General Hospital (the teaching hospital for the University of Cincinnati) and, later, at the New York Hospital (the teaching hospital for Cornell). The success of the program in Cincinnati demonstrated that the residency model was exportable to municipal hospitals, not just private hospitals. At Vanderbilt, G. Canby Robinson, a "first-generation Oslerian" (trained directly by Osler), and C. Sidney Burwell and Hugh Jackson Morgan, two "second-generation Oslerians" (trained by Osler's students), introduced a Hopkins-inspired residency in internal medicine, while Barney Brooks, who had been an intern and assistant resident under Halsted, did the same in surgery.[67] At Stanford, residency programs were started by Arthur Bloomfield in internal medicine and Emile Holman in surgery, both graduates of the Johns Hopkins Medical School and former residents at the Johns Hopkins Hospital, who brought the teaching methods they had learned at Johns Hopkins to the West Coast.

The spread of the residency was also facilitated by the cross-fertilization of ideas that continually occurred within the medical profession. In 1913, Christian established the first "visiting professorship" at an American hospital. Under this program, leading clinical scholars from other institutions were brought to the hospital, spending several days with the house staff and faculty, with abundant opportunity to discuss scientific ideas and educational developments.[68] The "visiting professorship" grew to become an important activity in all departments at virtually all medical centers. Traveling societies, such as the Interurban Clinical Club, the Association of American Physicians, the American Clinical and Climatological Association, the American Surgical Association, the Halsted Club, the Society of Clinical Surgery, and the Clinical Society of Genito-Urinary Surgeons, where camaraderie was high, friendships strong, and information about professional matters freely flowing, provided another venue to discuss ideas about residency training. The residency was also discussed at specialty society meetings, meetings of the Association of American Medical Colleges and Council on Medical Education and Hospitals, and at other educational conferences. Medical educators communicated regularly with each other by letter and telephone, and newly appointed department chairs commonly visited other institutions prior to beginning work at home. Department chairs often published descriptions of their programs in scientific journals, alumni magazines, hospital reports, and other publications.

As the residency spread, it retained its emphasis on combining clinical investigation with bedside work in a particular specialty. The goal, as at the Johns Hopkins Hospital, was to produce physicians capable of scholarly leadership at the highest levels in the various specialty fields. No one anticipated that all residents would pursue investigative careers, but it was believed that investigation was important to the professional development of all specialists. Accordingly, research became a standard part of residency programs. For this reason, some institutions called their residents "fellows," "graduate fellows," or "graduate students,"[69] and leading residency programs continued to be referred to occasionally as "graduate" or "postgraduate schools."[70] It became part of the Essentials for an Approved Residency that residents in all fields should be encouraged to engage in "some investigative work."[71] All residency programs were expected to include work in the basic sciences relevant to the particular specialty; hospitals not part of an academic medical center were instructed to make arrangements with a medical school whereby instruction for their residents in the basic sciences could be given.[72] Residents frequently worked for an advanced degree during their residency. At Presbyterian Hospital, for example, between 1933 and 1941, 113 residents received the Doctor of Medical Science degree from Columbia University.[73] This practice was especially common in the surgical fields, where a graduate degree (DSc, MA, or PhD) was either optional or required at 40 percent of residency programs in 1940.[74]

An excellent example of how residency programs continued to combine clinical research with clinical training was found at Presbyterian Hospital, the teaching hospital of the Columbia University College of Physicians and Surgeons. Presbyterian Hospital had inaugurated graded residency training during World War I, but in the 1920s, under the leadership of Walter W. Palmer in internal medicine (who had come to Presbyterian Hospital from Johns Hopkins in 1922, bringing several notable assistants from Johns Hopkins with him),[75] Allen O. Whipple in surgery (who, as noted earlier, greatly admired Halsted's residency system), and outstanding leaders in the other clinical departments, the hospital emerged as a magnificent center for patient care, graduate medical education, and clinical research, nipping at the heels of Johns Hopkins, "the Brigham," and "the General" for leadership of American medicine. Residents in all fields received instruction in the fundamental sciences and were encouraged to undertake research. For example, in the hospital's three-year ophthalmology residency, one of its strongest programs, there were six resident physicians. Each resident was expected to make a special study of some subject in ophthalmology, write a thesis, and become a candidate for the degree of Doctor of Science from Columbia University.[76] The Columbia-Presbyterian Medical Center also provided scientific instruction for house officers at New York City hospitals that were not affiliated with a medical school. In 1940, 194 resident physicians from 16 hospitals participated in Columbia's graduate program, of whom 52 were registered for the DSc degree.[77]

As in the case of the internship, the residency system in the 1920s and 1930s was conspicuous for its fluidity and the lack of standardization. Different terms for "resident" were used, programs varied in starting dates and duration, and some programs accepted new residents at multiple points during the same academic year or offered residencies of different lengths of time. Structural details invariably varied. In internal medicine, for instance, the University of Chicago and the University of California at San Francisco had specialty wards (that is, they sent patients with heart problems to one area, cancer to another, etc.); the Peter Bent Brigham Hospital admitted patients with any internal medicine problem to the same ward.[78] The level of clinical responsibility delegated to residents varied significantly among programs, as did the scientific sophistication of the work. Residents at teaching hospitals often undertook original experimental studies, while residents at community hospitals usually performed literature reviews or statistical analyses of patient records. Each program had its unique personality and temperament, reflective of local traditions and culture. In addition, since residency programs were departmentally based, not hospital based, there were often notable differences in culture among the programs within the same hospital. In an understatement, a report on graduate medical education in 1940 said of residency programs, "No two are exactly alike."[79]

As the residency system spread, there was a great diversity among the programs. At the top, in terms of prestige, were Johns Hopkins, the Peter Bent Brigham Hospital, and the Massachusetts General Hospital, with Presbyterian Hospital close behind. These were national programs that attracted medical students from schools around the country and whose graduates dispersed widely after leaving the residency.[80] Next came a number of outstanding university programs, such as Pennsylvania, Michigan, Rochester, and Barnes Hospital. All the major university programs at this time were in the Midwest or East, as West Coast schools were handicapped by their geographical remoteness.[81] Some hospitals were considered top-tier in particular areas. A prominent example was the University of Minnesota (which, not coincidentally, had a Graduate School of Medicine and vigorously encouraged its residents to pursue a graduate degree), which developed world-class programs in surgery, pediatrics, and radiology, producing unusually large numbers of academic leaders from those three departments.[82] Also outstanding were programs at a number of municipal hospitals. Most notable were Boston City Hospital, Bellevue Hospital, and Philadelphia General Hospital, which all enjoyed strong relationships with local medical schools. The "average" university hospital and some large community hospitals were also well respected. Among the latter, the Mayo Clinic and Cleveland Clinic became particularly important training sites. The Mayo Clinic, despite its isolated location in Rochester, Minnesota, ultimately became the largest site of graduate medical education in the world.[83] Small community hospitals generally ranked lower. Not to be forgotten were many "niche" programs: the Hospital of the Woman's Medical College of Pennsylvania, providing opportunities for woman; several black hospitals, most notably the hospital of Howard University, offering residency positions to African-Americans; a number of strong Jewish and Catholic hospitals, some affiliated with medical schools, catering to individuals of those respective faiths; and the highly regarded 60-bed program at the Hospital of the Rockefeller Institute for Medical Research, serving a small but exceptionally important group of future physician-scientists with particular interests in infectious diseases.[84]

In residency education, as in undergraduate medical education, a small number of programs set the standards. But of the "big three" teaching hospitals of the period—the Johns Hopkins Hospital, the Peter Bent Brigham Hospital, and the Massachusetts General Hospital—which was the best?

Each claimed that position for itself. Johns Hopkins had the strongest medical tradition, and during the second generation of its existence it continued to lead. However, the university was new, and the two Boston hospitals had the advantage of drawing on the prestige of Harvard University. Thus, at the Peter Bent Brigham Hospital Christian told others that "the facilities and opportunities for work at the Brigham are going to be very distinctly superior to those that exist at the Hopkins, or in any other hospital in this country."[85] A notion of superiority developed quickly within the institution. When one staff member discovered that the Mayo Clinic had a better system of recordkeeping, he reported his finding in the following way: "I realize that the records of the Peter Bent Brigham Hospital are remarkably perfect. I believe, however, that they might be made more perfect if they could be centralized according to the general plan of the Mayo Clinic."[86] A conceit arose among the two Harvard programs that became well recognized throughout the rest of the country. Thus, a former Harvard medical student, now a surgical resident at Johns Hopkins, wrote to one of his mentors at the Peter Bent Brigham Hospital:

> Then, too (as they did repeatedly during my interne year) you'd be surprised how many times a lesson, or a trick, or a point would come back to me from your ward rounds. . . . And I'd have to smile, as I caught myself saying, often with more than a touch of élan, "When I was up in Boston, I saw – "etc."[87]

This élan was thought to be especially conspicuous at the Massachusetts General Hospital. Partly with facetiousness, partly with envy, others in the medical world began to refer to the MGH as "Man's Greatest Hospital."

Unlike the internship, which became available to all medical graduates, residency positions before World War II remained relatively few. Medical educators, who regularly distinguished between the unusually gifted and the ordinary medical student, believed that residency training should be for the former only. As late as 1940 entry-level residency positions were available only for one-quarter to one-third of interns. Competition for a residency position was keen. Obtaining a position required ambition, scientific aptitude, a strong academic record, the ability to forego an income, and often a bit of luck. Acceptance into a program as a junior or assistant resident provided no guarantee that one would complete the program. Programs were organized as so-called pyramids—that is, each year some residents were eliminated from the program, with one final survivor ultimately being designated "chief resident." The exact size and shape of the pyramid varied among specialties and from one hospital to another. However, the principle was everywhere the same: Starting a residency provided no guarantee of completion. The major exception at this time was the Mayo Clinic, which early on organized its residency programs as "rectangles" rather than "pyramids," thereby allowing residents who performed well to complete the program.[88]

The presence of the pyramid system created considerable motion among residents, as they often divided their training among different hospitals. Frequently a resident cut from a prestigious program would find another position at a less prestigious institution. Most hospitals, including excellent university hospitals, could find room for a "Hopkins man" or a "Brigham man" who did not make it through those highly competitive programs. Thus, the chair of internal medicine at the College of Medicine of Wayne University customarily chose three of his five first-year residents from his own intern staff and two from outside, anticipating he would attract outstanding individuals from other programs for those two positions.[89]

Fortunately, those who progressed far enough up the pyramid were considered specialists in the field, even if they did not make it to the top. Thus, being cut from a program was not necessarily a personal professional disaster. A distinguished professor of urology at Jefferson who lived through the period observed:

> To drop out of a pyramidal residency before reaching its peak was no disgrace, since all who started in the competition were especially chosen, superior individuals. I have known many so dropping, and while some were no doubt deeply disappointed, I can recall no one of them who did not go on to a successful career in teaching, research, or practice.[90]

Indeed, some of the greatest academic leaders in the country had suffered major career disappointments while in training. Barney Brooks, a notable surgical leader and department chair at Vanderbilt, finished fifth in his class at Johns Hopkins. He had hoped to study internal medicine under Osler. However, so did the first four students in the class, so Brooks ended up entering the surgery program under Halsted. There he was cut once again, which forced him to finish his surgical residency at Barnes Hospital.[91] Alfred Blalock, chair of the department of surgery at Johns Hopkins and famed throughout the world for developing the "blue baby operation" (to correct the tetralogy of Fallot, a deadly congenital heart condition), had been devastated as a fourth-year medical student when he failed to obtain a surgical residency under Halsted.[92] William MacCallum, the most eminent pathologist of his era and the author of the standard textbook in the field, became a pathologist by virtue of his failure to receive the residency he desired in internal medicine under Osler.[93] And Henry

Christian himself had left Baltimore for graduate training because he had been unable to secure a residency under Osler. He wrote a "courteous" letter to his Johns Hopkins classmate Dorothy Reed (of the "Reed-Sternberg cell" of Hodgkin's lymphoma), inquiring if she might surrender her position with Osler to him. The indignant Reed—who as a medical student had pulled out an unloaded six-shooter to thwart an intruder in her apartment attempting to rape her—was accustomed to handling pressure and simply told Christian to scurry off.[94]

As the residency system became implanted in American medicine, the amount of time a typical resident devoted to clinical research diminished. This was illustrated by the evolution of the residency program at the Peter Bent Brigham Hospital. When Christian became chief of medicine in 1912, he intended for the interns to do the bulk of the "routine" clinical work so that the chief resident and residents would be able "to devote practically their entire time to investigation."[95] Within a decade, as the number of admissions soared, the average length of stay decreased, and the complexity of care increased, the residents found themselves with much less time for research than Christian had originally anticipated. During the 1920s and 1930s this problem became more severe. The house staff grew in size during this period but not fast enough to keep up with the clinical work. Cushing observed that residents in any department who were accomplishing anything in research were doing so with "stolen" hours.[96] It became increasingly difficult for the average resident to find the required time and uninterrupted composure for serious research, even at the Brigham. Accordingly, Christian maintained that "our product of graduate house-officers is no longer as good as it was."[97] When Christian retired, he was understandably proud of what many of his residents had accomplished in research, but he felt there were "more . . . laggards in this aspect of the work than in any other."[98]

Thus, by World War II, the focus of the residency system had changed. The residency had begun at Johns Hopkins as a way to produce academic leaders. But as the system spread, the majority of those who went through it became practicing specialists rather than clinical investigators. Even at the Brigham, that veritable factory for producing clinical scientists, only around 15 percent of the residents during its first quarter-century chose academic careers.[99] At less prominent teaching hospitals, the percentage of residents pursuing academic careers was far less, and at community hospitals, even lower still. The residency remained invaluable for the training of clinical scientists, but most residents did not choose that career.

In these developments, medical specialization in the United States followed the international pattern. As the historian of medicine George Weisz has shown, medical specialization in the nineteenth century in the United States, Germany, France, and Great Britain was understood as a function of medical research and teaching. The roots of specialization were in knowledge production, and specialization was closely identified with academic medicine. At the beginning, according to Weisz, medical specialization was also "part of the much wider change that gradually produced 'professional' scientific and disciplinary communities in many different fields of knowledge." In the twentieth century, medical specialization entered a second stage, one in which it became the dominant form of medical practice. The earlier view of medical specialization as synonymous with research disappeared, and a practice-oriented perspective developed instead. Medical specialization always retained its close association with medical science, but ultimately it became more closely identified with domains of medical and surgical practice rather than with clinical research.[100]

Although the amount of time residents devoted to clinical research was less in 1940 than it had been a generation before, the investigative component continued to be indispensable to the system's success. Medical educators all along believed that the advanced training provided by a residency should fit the learner to solve his own problems rather than merely supply him with information. Medical educators also believed that research helped in the acquisition of problem-solving abilities by making learners more critical and discerning. Accordingly, they considered exposure to research important for all residents, regardless of whether an individual was contemplating full-time practice or academic medicine. Christian himself made this point. "Investigation trains the man conducting it to become careful, patient, persistent, and intelligently critical and so is helpful in whatever work that is undertaken subsequently." The main value of research for residents, he continued, "is rather what it gives in training than what it adds to medical knowledge."[101]

The value of a scholarly dimension in residency training was illustrated when Eugene Stead was recruited from the Peter Bent Brigham Hospital to chair the department of medicine at Emory University in 1942. When Stead arrived, he found that residents at Emory's teaching hospital, Grady Hospital, were knowledgeable and extremely well read but that their reading was uncritical. As Stead described it, "They believed everything they read and were puzzled by the fact that one paper said one thing and a second just the opposite."[102] Stead attributed this to the fact that they never had had a hand in the creation of knowledge and hence were "not aware of the pits into which all authors at one time or another fall."[103] Stead, who brought with him some exceptional colleagues such as Paul Beeson and James Warren, adopted a different approach. He intentionally exposed his residents to controversy at seminars, conferences, and other venues where vigorous discussions could occur. Such discussions quickly dispelled false premises, fallacious arguments, and personal conceit. He encouraged residents to become involved with faculty members in preparing case reports and conducting clinical trials. (As they did, the quality of hospital notes recorded by the residents immediately became more thorough, detailed, and precise.) There was much more discussion with the residents about pathophysiology (mechanisms of disease), leading to a greater understanding of *why* things might be done a certain way. Very quickly a palpable new critical attitude suffused the training program. As one intern, a former medical student at Emory, told a new faculty member, "It's just magical the way this place has changed since Dr. Stead and you people have come to Grady."[104]

In short, medical educators in the 1920s and 1930s saw research as essential for ensuring that residency training would provide university-level graduate education and not vocational training, even as the clinical dimension of the experience increased in importance. As at the Johns Hopkins Hospital, the concern was not for producing "scientists" or "practitioners" but rather "scientific practitioners." The educational objective was for all residents to develop critical intellectual qualities—a spirit of inquiry, dissatisfaction with present methods, rigorous intellectual honesty, and a healthy distrust of authority—regardless of ultimate career goals. Long before the term "evidence-based medicine" became trendy, residents and their teachers were devouring the medical journals, staying up with the literature, seeking evidence to justify or refute a particular clinical strategy or to evaluate whether the claims of a particular author might be warranted by his data. Thus one physician in private practice told Christian why his experience as a house officer at "the Brigham" meant so much to him: He now understood the need for a "careful thorough search for evidence in regard to a case, a sane logical judgment based on that evidence, rational therapy, and a healthy scepticism [*sic*] toward new and improved ideas."[105]

In the 1920s and 1930s, as in the generation before World War I, the scientific practitioner held great promise for the nation. This promise resided not only in the possession of knowledge or technical skill but also in the wisdom and critical judgment to know when to do something and when to refrain. Surgical teachers repeatedly emphasized the importance of proper diagnosis, avoidance of unnecessary operations, good postoperative care, and the adaptability to handle an unexpected occurrence in the operating room. Harvey Cushing once said, "I would like to see the day when somebody would be appointed surgeon somewhere who had no hands, for the operative part is the least of the work."[106] Educators in many specialties pointed out that physicians who understood scientific methods "lean less heavily on the laboratory for diagnosis and rely more on their own observations and capacity for deductive and inductive reasoning."[107] The scientific practitioner, whether in academic medicine or in practice, had the intellectual capacity to practice a judicious medicine in which things were done for a legitimate reason, thereby consuming fewer resources and producing less inadvertent harm.

IN SEARCH OF A SYSTEM

The internship and residency systems spread rapidly between the world wars. Even the challenges of medical preparedness for World War I could not slow down their momentum.[108] For medical schools, this was a transforming event. In 1910, except for Johns Hopkins, the education of undergraduate medical students dominated the time and attention of medical faculties. By 1940, graduate medical education had grown to become a conspicuous activity of every medical faculty. Medical educators rejoiced as they saw a university spirit permeate graduate medical education, and they fully understood that the residency system was a major factor in America's rapid ascendance to international prominence in medicine.

For hospitals, too, particularly those with strong residency programs, the development of graduate medical education was transformational. With their close relationships with medical schools, the teaching hospitals now stood out as America's elite institutions for patient care. Teaching hospitals had accepted the notion that a university hospital cannot justify its existence unless it is setting new standards for patient care, and their participation in medical education and clinical research allowed them to do this. Thus, at Lakeside Hospital, investigations by residents and faculty into the metabolic effects of surgery immediately allowed a reduction in death rates of patients operated on at the hospital for rectal cancer by one-half and for appendicitis, exophthalmic goiter, and gastric procedures to close to zero.[109] At the Massachusetts General Hospital, investigations by Joseph Aub, Walter Bauer, Fuller Albright, Oliver Cope, and others led to the identification of a parathyroid adenoma (a nonmalignant but metabolically deadly tumor of the parathyroid gland) as an important cause of hyperparathyroidism (overactivity of the parathyroid gland), and soon the hospital became the leading clinic for the diagnosis and treatment of parathyroid conditions in the world.[110] As the director of the Massachusetts General Hospital observed, patients come to the hospital "for the sake of receiving treatment which they know it is simply impossible to get elsewhere."[111] Or as the director of Lakeside Hospital put it, "It is generally conceded that a University Hospital is a better institution than a non-teaching one."[112]

As the internship and residency spread, individual programs were in perpetual motion. Programs grew in size and were continually examined and reexamined in their every detail, trying to improve the experience from one year to the next. No feature was too small or too large to escape scrutiny: the amount of time to be spent on this service or that, the distribution of time between inpatient and outpatient work, the size of a house officer's patient load, the appropriate level of clinical responsibility, the expectations for patient-related chores, the number of interns for each resident, or the quality of rounds and conferences. Even the effectiveness of teaching was examined, in the effort to reward the better teachers and weed out the laggards. Thus, at the request of Soma Weiss, Christian's successor as chief of medicine at the Peter Bent Brigham Hospital, the young Paul Beeson graded 27 members of the attending staff in internal medicine from "A" to "F" for their work on ward rounds.[113] (He gave "A's" to Joseph Aub, Sidney Burwell, Charles Janeway, and Eugene Stead.) Without calling it such, "continuous quality improvement" was encoded in graduate medical education from the beginning.

Through the 1930s, it was not clear who controlled graduate medical education. Given the success of medical school faculties in leading the reform of undergraduate medical education, it was a natural response among the profession to look to the medical faculties once again to take charge of graduate medical education. The American College of Physicians, the American College of Surgeons, and other specialty organizations called repeatedly for academic medicine to assume control of residency training. However, medical school faculties, traditionally conservative, concentrated on the programs within their own teaching hospitals. They had no desire to assume responsibility for training at community hospitals or set standards for the nation at large. As a result, no one was in charge.

There was also considerable confusion surrounding the term "graduate medical education" itself. Particularly before 1920, the term connoted to some the "undergraduate repair work" that was provided by many schools for physicians who had graduated from medical school before the Flexnerian reforms had been completed. Older physicians in practice, aware of their deficiencies, often turned to these courses, which sometimes lasted for months, to learn belatedly what younger physicians were learning in medical school. The term "graduate medical education" was also frequently confused with what later came to be called "continuing medical education"—refresher courses of varying lengths and detail for physicians in practice trying to stay up-to-date with their fields.

Most confusing of all, through the late 1930s residency training remained only one of several pathways to specialty practice. There were other educational alternatives for aspiring specialists. One was study in Europe, which resumed after World War I, though at much lower levels than during its peak years. Here, the quality varied, depending on where a physician studied and for how long. This route was taken primarily by physicians unable to obtain residency positions in the United States.

Another common route to specialization was through working in an outpatient specialty clinic at a large urban hospital. There, a young physician might work in a pediatrics, otolaryngology, or dermatology clinic, thereby gaining expertise and peer recognition. Or a young physician might work as a junior assistant to an established specialist, acquiring competence in a field through an apprenticeship approach. The eminent New York pediatrician L. Emmett Holt, who was to pediatrics what Osler was to internal medicine, regularly employed such assistants, many of whom went on to distinguished careers in pediatrics.[114]

A more formal approach involved taking university graduate work in a medical specialty, complete with a dissertation, that led to a PhD or DSc degree. This strategy appealed to Abraham Flexner, who viewed specialty training as "but the upper story of a university department of medicine."[115] In the 1920s and 1930s, a number of universities experimented with this approach. One of the most notable examples was Columbia University. When the Columbia-Presbyterian Medical Center was built in the mid-1920s, there was no single pathway of graduate medical education. Accordingly, the medical school sponsored both a university-based graduate program and a residency program at Presbyterian Hospital.

Many physicians started as general practitioners and then became specialists after a while by concentrating on a particular area. Thus one radiologist "gradually drifted" into the field while in a general medical practice. He described how he had "been doing more and more of this type of work and less and less general medicine until now I am confining myself almost exclusively to this latter field." He was ultimately made a Fellow of the American College of Radiology.[116] Or another specialist, this one in ophthalmology, related his journey from general practice into ophthalmology. "It so happens that I am in general practice, but the eye is my specialty, and a given portion of my time, and all of my Post Graduate study has been given to this particular subject." After extensive course work at the New York Post-Graduate Medical School, he was ultimately placed in charge of the eye clinic at a community hospital in Newark, New Jersey, where he performed a considerable number of eye surgeries.[117]

The most popular alternative route to specialization practice was that of taking a course in the subject at a postgraduate medical school. Perhaps the most prominent was the New York Post-Graduate Medical School, a nonprofit institution that had its own hospital and, from 1931 to 1947, an affiliation with Columbia University. This school offered lengthy courses in the various specialties and provided instruction in the basic sciences as well, in addition to offering continuing education courses for physicians in practice.[118] However, most postgraduate medical schools were highly commercial, for-profit proprietary ventures, more concerned with profits than education. Here, a general practitioner could take a two-week course in any specialty, operate on a few dogs or cadavers, and call himself a urologist or orthopedist or anything else he might wish.

Through the late 1930s, there was no consensus on the proper route to specialized medical practice. As one authority acknowledged, physicians could be "bonafide specialists" even though they "did not learn their specialty in a residency."[119] The most prestigious pathway, the residency system, represented the apprenticeship and university traditions in medical education. The popular short courses at proprietary postgraduate medical schools represented the commercial tradition in American medical education. In the 1930s it was not clear which direction specialty training would follow. The multiplicity of pathways to specialty practice, the fluidity and lack of standardization of the residency system, and the popularity of the short courses at proprietary schools all made graduate medical education seem reminiscent of undergraduate medical education a generation before. In 1931, the dean of the Columbia University College of Physicians and Surgeons considered "this whole problem of postgraduate medical education" to be "the most important single problem before the medical profession of the country at the present time."[120]

Nevertheless, by the 1930s the residency system was in ascendance. More and more, residency training was seen to offer a superior educational experience to any of the alternative pathways, and the residency system was increasingly credited for America's rising reputation in medicine worldwide. What form or shape graduate medical education in the United States would ultimately take was still unclear. However, one thing was certain: The residency system would be at the core.

CHAPTER 4
The American Residency

If any single concept dominated the thinking of medical educators since the late nineteenth century, it was the idea that medical education cannot be separated from the problems of general education. This notion guided their approach to graduate as well as undergraduate medical education. Accordingly, they articulated a group of educational principles to guide the training of interns and residents, and they spoke to the moral basis of graduate medical education and practice as well. These principles had been followed in the original residency programs at the Johns Hopkins Hospital, but it was during the generation between World Wars I and II that these principles became codified.

As educators, medical faculties understood that the environment in which learning occurred was as essential to the development of doctors as the formal educational program itself. Accordingly, medical educators worked with hospital leaders to create a learning environment that reinforced and validated the principles that educators were trying to impart. A well-constructed learning environment allowed house officers to acquire knowledge, techniques, judgment, and independence with maximum efficiency. Equally important, the learning environment proved indispensable for shaping the values, attitudes, and behaviors of young physicians during this highly formative part of their medical training.

It also became clear during the period between the world wars that graduate medical education was shaped by the values and influences of American culture at large, not just by the internal environment of the academic medical center. Cultural attitudes concerning work, delayed gratification, and the balance between professional and personal life played critical roles in shaping the American residency, as did attitudes toward the poor and the role of the consumer in American society. Ultimately, and not surprisingly, the American residency reflected the culture in which it was conducted and not just medical or educational principles alone.

EDUCATIONAL PRINCIPLES

The founding Johns Hopkins medical faculty based their educational philosophy on the assumption that medical knowledge would continue to grow and evolve at an increasingly more-rapid rate. Subsequent developments proved this assumption to be correct. In 1889, surgery was in its infancy, and a tone of therapeutic nihilism still pervaded the medical fields. By World War I, the old fear of the surgeon's knife had been overcome, a much greater confidence in therapeutics had developed, and new fields, such as radiology, pediatrics, and psychiatry, had appeared. A generation later, the capacity of medicine had become more impressive still. Aided by advances in anesthesiology, blood transfusion, intravenous fluid replacement, and oxygen tents, general surgery had spawned many subspecialties, such as thoracic surgery, neurosurgery, urological surgery, and orthopedic surgery. Clinical science had produced an extensive understanding of disease mechanisms, and many new effective therapeutic agents had been discovered. A review in 1943 listed more than 35 important, specific therapeutic agents (including liver extract, heparin, insulin, thyroxin, progesterone, androgenic and estrogenic hormones, pitressin, thiouracil, sulfonamides, penicillin, and various vitamins) compared with only six such agents 30 years before.[1] Some conditions nearly disappeared. For instance, until the early 1920s, syphilis was the leading cause of stillborn babies. After the development of the Wasserman test (a serological test for syphilis that allowed screening for the disease), stillbirths from syphilis nearly vanished.[2] The disease spectrum in America also changed. By the 1930s, chronic diseases had replaced infectious diseases as the leading causes of mortality, a consequence of greater longevity.[3] As the Peter Bent Brigham Hospital's Henry A. Christian noted, "Medicine is ever changing; the problem of the present may not be the problem of the next decade; the problem of the future may not be even remotely related to the problem of today."[4]

Accordingly, the objectives of medical education continued to be those originally articulated at Johns Hopkins. The modern doctor needed to be a thinker, not a parrot. Doctors needed to understand scientific methods and principles, not merely regurgitate facts. Physicians needed to be able to acquire and assimilate new information, to think critically, and always to be skeptical of authority and traditional teachings. They also needed to understand that patients came to them not with diagnoses in hand but with problems to be solved. Hence, doctors needed to develop problem-solving ability and clinical judgment. Such skills were pertinent to making a difficult diagnosis, determining the most judicious course of treatment when there were dangers to standard therapy, deciding when to obtain a test, institute a treatment, or proceed to the operating room, or recognizing and managing an unforeseeable problem or complication. Medical practice was rife with risk and uncertainty, and physicians in every field needed the skill and wisdom to manage the perplexing uncertainties they would inevitably face.

How best to prepare physicians with these qualities? Medical educators agreed that learners should be put to work. In other words, after an appropriate scientific preparation, learners needed to jump into the clinical setting and begin caring for patients themselves. However, this was considered true of medical students and house officers alike, both of whom participated actively in patient care. There, however, the similarity ended. Of necessity medical students during their clinical clerkships remained closely supervised; they did not have the authority to write orders, decide management, or perform procedures on their own. Interns and residents did. It was axiomatic in medicine that an individual was not a mature physician until he had learned to care for patients independently. The assumption of responsibility, then, became the defining principle of graduate medical education.

To develop independence, house officers received major responsibilities for the care of their patients. They typically were the first to evaluate the patient on admission, spoke with the patients on rounds, made all the decisions, wrote the orders and progress notes, performed the procedures, and were the first to be called should a problem arise with one of their patients. As the Johns Hopkins faculty observed of its residency program, "The most distinctive factor is that the resident has full responsibility for the diagnosis and treatment of seriously ill patients."[5] Such responsibility allowed house officers not only to develop independence but also to acquire ownership of their patients—the sense that the patients were *theirs*, that *they* were the ones responsible for their patients' medical outcomes and well-being. The objective of promoting independence applied throughout graduate medical education—to rotating internships, serving the needs of future general practitioners, and to residencies, of future specialists. Medical educators repeatedly described the assumption of responsibility as the factor that transformed physicians-in-training into capable practitioners.[6]

Responsibility in care was not something house officers were cavalierly given. Rather, it was earned by residents who showed themselves to be mature and capable. Responsibility was provided in "graded" fashion—that is, junior house officers had much more circumscribed responsibilities, while more experienced house officers who had accomplished their earlier tasks well were advanced to positions of greater responsibility. Advancement occurred relatively quickly in cognitive fields like neurology, pediatrics, and internal medicine. There, assistant residents in their second or third year received decision-making authority even for very sick individuals. Among these fields, house officers in pediatrics were generally monitored more closely because of the fragility of the patients, particularly babies and toddlers. Advancement occurred more slowly in procedural fields such as general surgery, obstetrics and gynecology, and the surgical subspecialties. In these fields, technical proficiency was so important that residents had to wait many years, sometimes until they were chief resident, to perform certain major operations.[7] Residents in fields like pathology and radiology, where there was little direct contact with patients, also received increasing responsibility over time. For instance, more advanced residents in these fields were permitted to provide interpretations of slides or radiographs without immediate supervision.

There were notable variations in the amount of responsibility allowed. The degree of independence varied from one program to another, reflecting local culture. Thus, surgical residents at the Cleveland Clinic received considerable opportunity to operate; at the Mayo Clinic, much less.[8] The type of hospital also was a factor. At community hospitals, where private physicians were in charge of their own private patients, house officers often received little responsibility. At municipal and county hospitals, where charity patients predominated and attending staffs were often small, house officers could easily receive too much.

The assumption of responsibility did not mean there was no supervision. House officers were accountable to the chief of service, there was regular contact with attending physicians, and chief residents kept an extremely close eye on the resident service. Moreover, someone more senior was typically present or, if not physically present, immediately available. Thus, interns were closely watched by junior residents, junior residents by senior residents, and senior residents by the chief resident. One generation taught and supervised the next, though these generations were separated by only a year or two. Backup and support were available for all residents from attending physicians, consultants, and the chiefs of service. The gravest moral offense a house officer could commit was not to call for help.

The beneficial results of having house officers assume responsibility for patient care were readily apparent. In all specialties, house officers were found to develop more confidence, wisdom, and judgment when granted responsibility in a progressive, graded fashion. At the Cleveland Clinic, for instance, the faculty decided to provide the residents greater independence. The next year they noted "how much the Fellows [the clinic's term for residents] had grown and how much more valuable their opinions were now than a year ago."[9] Nowhere were the educational results of assuming responsibility more apparent than in surgery, where surgical teachers pointed out that surgeons who had received adequate responsibility as residents developed greater diagnostic skill, judgment, confidence, and the ability to deal with the unexpected. Edward Churchill, chief of surgery at the Massachusetts General Hospital, considered the assumption of responsibility the key to the development of "a calm and competent operating surgeon who was ready to meet any situation with equanimity."[10]

House officers understood that the assumption of responsibility was the most important educational feature of internship and residency. Hence, the most prized positions were at voluntary or municipal teaching hospitals with large ward (charity) services, where house officers were given much greater responsibility than at community hospitals with predominantly private patients. House officers at these programs reveled in the responsibility they received. Competition for patients, not always friendly, often broke out. Would the intern or assistant resident manage the patient's diabetic ketoacidosis? Would the hernia repair be "given away" to a junior surgical resident, or would the senior resident or even a staff member keep the case for himself? Even in pathology, where house officers did not manage patients directly, house officers fought for opportunities and defended their turf. Thus, in Stanford's program, the pathology interns usually performed the autopsies, and they regarded the staff breaking in with the same indignation as "surgical residents would the staff men's doing all the appendices, circumcisions, and hemorrhoids."[11]

The assumption of responsibility proved a remarkably effective educational device. It was in keeping with the widely held tenet of progressive education that skill in any practical art is not acquired by being told things but by learning to do things. By itself, however, the assumption of responsibility represented the tradition of the apprenticeship. Graduate medical education could reach a university level only if suffused with the ideals and standards of scholarship and scientific inquiry. This meant imparting scientific knowledge and understanding, not mere tidbits of scientific facts; conveying principles and concepts, not simply procedural techniques or standardized protocols; and promoting intellectual inquiry, not merely providing job training. To accomplish this, medical leaders defined a second educational principle of graduate medical education: the importance of studying problems in depth.

No one articulated this notion more consistently than teachers at Harvard Medical School. Francis W. Peabody, chief of medicine of the Harvard Service at the Boston City Hospital, told his house officers, "One case carefully studied and recorded is worth many cases observed superficially."[12] Henry A. Christian, chief of medicine at the Peter Bent Brigham Hospital, declared, "A thorough study of fewer things is regarded as a better educational method than acquiring meager knowledge of many things."[13] He regularly pointed out that the patient load of house officers should not be too high so that they could have sufficient time for reading, study, reflection, and research.[14] Christian's successor, Soma Weiss, felt the same way. When Weiss met with his interns and residents, he told them, "It is not the number of cases observed, but how well they are observed that count. One case may be more instructive than one hundred."[15]

Patients were not assigned to house officers in any preset fashion prescribing which diseases and conditions they should see, and in what order. Rather, house officers admitted patients by what might be termed the "laissez faire method of learning." Interns and residents received patients randomly, depending on who was in line for the next admission. Medical educators presumed that, over time, on a large and active teaching service, house officers would be exposed to a sufficient volume and variety of patients to emerge as experienced clinicians. Medical educators did not fret over the fact that no house officer saw everything while in training. Educators knew that medical practice was replete with rare conditions, unusual presentations, unexpected complications, difficult diagnostic or therapeutic problems, and other puzzling dilemmas. They anticipated that with proper training, house officers would acquire the problem-solving abilities to handle the unknowns and uncertainties that inevitably occurred in medical practice.

How did house officers explore patients' problems in depth? The work began with careful study of the patient through a detailed medical history and physical examination followed by the pertinent laboratory and radiographic studies. After assembling the information, a house officer devised a differential diagnosis and plan of management, to be discussed with others of greater seniority. The house officer then proceeded to follow the patient carefully throughout the hospitalization, thereby observing the unfolding of disease and the response to the treatment plan, making further diagnostic or therapeutic decisions if needed, and monitoring the results of those decisions as well.

House officers would also try to read as extensively as possible about their patients' condition, focusing on journals for the most recent information, not just on textbooks as was typically done by medical students. Reading was done to build knowledge or deepen understanding, not just to ascertain some immediately relevant fact. House officers (and students) were advised to read mostly about the problems of their patients at hand, on the grounds that such reading brought the topics to life and that the understanding derived would stick with them more readily. At the Peter Bent Brigham Hospital they were told:

> There is no better time to read up a particular medical subject than when you are in charge of a patient manifesting that disease. The information you obtain from reading a review, for instance, of peptic ulcer such as is found in any of the good systems of medicine, when you yourself are taking care of a patient suffering from peptic ulcer, will be more profitable and will become a more permanent part of your knowledge than when done at any other time.[16]

House officers were also encouraged to read critically. That meant evaluating the evidence by which an author might make a claim, making a judgment regarding the applicability of the paper to clinical practice, and not neglecting to read classic articles that had changed medical or surgical practice so they might experience important or lasting scientific work.[17] They were expected to reflect on these matters, relating the problems of the patient at hand to those of other patients or other conditions, and asking themselves where the border of current knowledge might end and what type of investigation might expand that border. All this thinking and reflection would be the stuff of the upcoming conference or seminar with peers and faculty the next day or the day after that.

From the house officers' point of view, the most interesting patients were generally the most challenging ones. This was particularly true of the more capable house officers. Virtually every intern and resident experienced stunning cases that taught them important lessons that they never forgot. As one intern at the Massachusetts General Hospital remarked, "The fun in internal medicine is not dealing with the usual but with the unusual."[18] Faculty members valued this attitude in their house staff, for they sought out individuals with initiative, curiosity, keen intellects, and spirit. Christian commented, "If the work of the resident staff should ever become such a dull routine it is almost inevitable that the men seeking such jobs will be correspondingly dull and stupid."[19]

A busy schedule of conferences and rounds indicated that learning was a communal activity. One popular conference was the weekly "grand rounds" held by each clinical department, where disease problems were thoroughly discussed from every perspective. Discussions were highly clinically relevant (indeed, patients typically were present for questions and examination when their cases were presented), and conferences were conducted with a characteristic formality and protocol. Even more popular was "morning report," where residents met several times a week with the chief resident and senior faculty, including the department chair, to discuss patients admitted to the service the day before. These discussions focused on diagnosis and treatment, particularly of the more difficult or sicker patients. House officers learned from patients others had seen, not just their own patients, and they reflected on those problems as well.

The greatest value of the various conferences and group discussions was that they were interactive. Controversy was welcome, opinions were challenged, and friendly but fierce arguments frequently ensued. One former internal medicine resident at the Peter Bent Brigham Hospital described "the wonderful 'arguments' that so often came up" at the conferences in his department.[20] In these discussions, data and logic mattered, not seniority. House officers learned that the professor might be wrong and that the merits of an idea should be subjected to scrutiny quite aside from its source. House officers learned to submit their reasoning to open criticism, admit errors, and modify their views and opinions. Such discussions promoted judgment, humility, critical reasoning, and the recognition that more medical care was not necessarily better medical care. One surgical resident at the Massachusetts General Hospital later described to his chief what the residency had meant to him: "the opportunity of acquiring a greater objectivity, a more open mind, a more humble evaluation of my knowledge and skill, but a sense of confidence in my independent thought."[21]

In-depth study included learning the scientific foundations of the specialty, not just the clinical issues involved with diagnosis and treatment. Disease was now seen as a dynamic process, and understanding the underlying biological disturbances was the key to developing and using effective diagnostic and therapeutic strategies. Medical educators wanted house officers to learn not only the transitory knowledge of the moment but also the means by which such knowledge was obtained and the ways of questioning and testing it. This way, house officers could become engaged with the underlying science and develop a genuine biological understanding of their field. To medical educators, no other activity was considered more essential to the goal of producing broadly educated physicians and surgeons rather than medical and surgical technicians.

For some house officers, particularly residents, the study of an individual patient led to a project of original investigation. This was especially true at teaching hospitals, and the stronger the hospital, the more often this happened. Depending on the project, the resident, and the program, this work was done while engaged in patient care or in lengthy blocks of time set aside for research, typically from six months to two years. Some residents produced work of outstanding quality and lasting importance. A. McGehee Harvey pointed out that the extraordinary contributions to medicine made at Johns Hopkins "were not made by professors alone, but by residents, interns, students, and technicians as well" who were imbued with the "keen sense of inquiry" fostered by the institution.[22]

If the assumption of responsibility and the emphasis on studying problems in depth represented two core principles of graduate medical education, the recognition that learning occurred informally as well as formally was the third. Medical educators understood that faculty taught implicitly as well as explicitly—by their behavior and actions, not just by their precepts. In some cases informal learning was a force for good. Thus, declared one internal medicine intern at the Massachusetts General Hospital, "I secretly aspire to attaining the lucidity of thought and intellectual honesty of a W. B. Castle."[23] (Castle, one of the most notable figures in the history of Harvard Medical School, discovered that the failure of the lining of the stomach to produce "intrinsic factor" accounted for the inability of the body to absorb vitamin B_{12} in pernicious anemia, and he was a gifted and caring teacher and clinician as well.) In other cases the opposite effect occurred. A report on graduate medical education noted, "One cannot expect a resident to bring a thoughtful approach to the problems of a patient under his care, if the staff physician . . . treats the patient in a superficial or unsympathetic manner."[24] In either case, medical educators understood that values, attitudes, and behaviors were absorbed, not merely taught, and that in these areas the unconscious power of faculty examples mattered more than any words they might utter.

In short, as the internship and residency disseminated widely during the period between the world wars, a mature philosophy of graduate medical education emerged. What medical educators of the time called "the assumption of responsibility" anticipated later discussions of the five stages of learning, from novice to master, delineated by Stuart and Hubert Dreyfus. The emphasis on studying problems in depth anticipated subsequent educational ideas about the importance of "reflection" and "mindfulness" to learning. The importance medical educators placed on directing reading toward issues raised by the patient at hand was later validated by theories of "adult learning," which held that adults learn best when they have a reason to do so. The recognition of medical educators that learning occurred implicitly as well as explicitly, particularly in the internalization of attitudes and behaviors, anticipated later conversations about "the hidden curriculum." Although the terms used to describe these concepts changed with time, by World War II these educational principles had already become the basis of graduate medical education in the United States, and their importance was to endure.

THE MORAL DIMENSION OF GRADUATE MEDICAL EDUCATION

At its core, the practice of medicine represents a profoundly moral activity. Patients are fully served only when their welfare is the foremost concern of the doctor, when the physician practices with thoroughness and attention to detail, and when every effort to ensure maximum safety is provided. As medical leaders created graduate medical education in the United States, they understood the moral dimension of medical work. Accordingly, they sought to help house officers develop a professional identity with an ethical core of service and responsibility. These ethical precepts were taught both explicitly and implicitly. The objective was for physicians in training to internalize a moral responsibility for the welfare of their patients.

How was this ethical dimension to be developed? One way was for training programs to make clear that the doctor existed for the patient and not the patient for the doctor. In their teachings, medical educators continually emphasized that the patient came first. As the surgeon Charles W. Mayo, a grandson of the Mayo Clinic's founder and the last member of the Mayo family to run the clinic, put it, "The secret of the great professional is that he gives service above self."[25] Contemporary writers have correctly portrayed physicians of the era as sometimes paternalistic, but even so, patients were their masters, and doctors in training typically learned that they existed to serve.

Statements such as Mayo's are hardly rare in the history of American medicine. Alone, such words to a cynic could be considered meaningless platitudes. What is notable about graduate medical education before World War II is that medical teachers regularly exemplified the primacy of the patient by their actions, not just their words. From the opening of the Johns Hopkins Hospital, Osler, Kelly, and the others gained the admiration of house officers and students for their deep commitment to the welfare of patients. Thereafter, medical teachers throughout the country typically demonstrated a similar behavior of putting the interests of patients first. House officers quickly learned that illness is no respecter of the time of day or day of the week and accordingly that physicians can never be sure of their time. They were taught that they had a twenty-four-hour responsibility to patients. They were held accountable to this standard, for their teachers expected nothing less of themselves.

No physicians had a greater around-the-clock commitment to their patients' welfare than surgeons, whose dedication to work became legendary. For instance, the neurosurgeon Harvey Cushing, who operated for 24 hours without stop if he thought a patient might be saved, taught his residents that "no one has any right to undertake the care of any patient unless he is willing to give that patient all of the time and thought that is necessary, and of which he is capable."[26] Mayo felt the same way. He described his life as "filled with surgery, which tends to shrink the real world until it consists only of hospitals and patients and shoptalk."[27] To Mayo, "A surgeon was not worth a damn if he could leave his sense of obligation when he left the operating room," and the principal quality he looked for in selecting residents for the Mayo Clinic was "commitment to the patient's welfare."[28] To the surgeon John Finney of Johns Hopkins, it was "surgery first, and everything else secondary."[29] Such devotion to duty, as shall be discussed shortly, did not come without a price, particularly for many family members of physicians and house officers of the era. However, patients could take comfort knowing that their doctors were available. House officers learned that medicine is a calling, that altruism is central to being a true medical professional, and that the ideal practitioner placed the welfare of his patients above all else.

A second moral teaching of residency was the importance of thoroughness. No amount of commitment to the patient could ensure good results if the quality of care was not high. To medical educators, thoroughness was the sine qua non of clinical excellence, and they emphasized the importance of thoroughness to their house officers with the same fervor that they insisted that the patient should come first. As Henry A. Christian put it, "All great clinicians study their patients with the most detailed thoroughness, missing not the smallest departure from normal function." No successful doctor, he continued, "can have any other method than infinite thoroughness in his work."[30]

Thoroughness in doctors was easily misunderstood. It did not mean doing every test or procedure available. Christian cautioned that tests should be minimized "so as to cause as little discomfort and pain as is possible."[31] Rather, thoroughness meant careful, systematic study of the patient, attention to detail, and not cutting corners. It began with a detailed history of the patient's condition. One surgical resident described how he had been taught "to get a thorough medical history, starting with the top of the head and working down to the feet. The questioning of the patient [involved] . . . every detail of his health."[32] It proceeded to an equally careful, systematic physical examination, as house officers put patients on their hands and knees to detect a "puddle sign" for ascites (fluid in the abdomen), carefully percussed the heart to define its size and shape, and scrutinized the nail beds for subtle indications of disease. It concluded with ordering pertinent tests or treatments suggested by the clinical findings and close monitoring of the patient's condition thereafter.

The principle of thoroughness applied to residencies in radiology and pathology, not just those specialties with direct patient-care responsibilities. Thus, in radiology, residents learned to examine X-rays systematically and to identify and explain every marking. One leading radiology chairman instructed his residents to undertake a "more careful scrutiny and more thorough study of the individual patient, rather than a hastier and necessarily more superficial analysis of a . . . larger number of patients."[33] Similarly, pathology residents learned to examine macroscopic and microscopic specimens with exquisite attention to detail. One pathology chairman explained "that the very thorough histological studies that we made were in large part for the benefit of the men we were training and that I simply would not put any limit to their curiosity."[34]

Thoroughness was exceedingly important to good care. It allowed every reasonable step to be taken to diagnose the cause of a patient's problem. Often it was the subtle findings that provided the clue to a diagnosis. In addition, thoroughness facilitated the detection of problems unrelated to a patient's immediate complaint. A careful examination of the skin of a patient with abdominal pain might reveal an early, treatable skin malignancy, or a rectal examination in someone with joint stiffness might uncover a potentially curable rectal cancer. Thoroughness also allowed physicians to arrive at a comprehensive, multidimensional diagnosis. As Lewellys F. Barker of Johns Hopkins explained, "A psychoneurotic may need more than merely mental treatment, for psychotherapy alone will often fail to cure if the patient, in addition to his neurosis, has, for example, two abscessed teeth and is forty pounds under normal weight."[35]

To medical educators, thoroughness was demanded because of the overriding importance of making the correct diagnosis. For instance, appendicitis and pancreatitis, both described by the Harvard surgeon Reginald Fitz, each typically presented as an abdominal emergency. However, appendicitis required immediate surgery, whereas pancreatitis demanded supportive medical care, for surgery in those patients usually led to death. Given the relative scarcity of specific cures at this time, the last thing any physician wanted to do was to overlook a treatable diagnosis.

Given the relative simplicity of laboratory and radiological testing prior to World War II, the history and physical examination provided doctors their most valuable tools for making a diagnosis. It was a "golden era" of physical examination, as clinicians in every specialty perfected the art of detecting findings to a degree scarcely imaginable to today's physicians. Of one internist at the Massachusetts General Hospital, it was said that he seemingly "could make a diagnosis merely by walking up to the patient's bed."[36] House officers everywhere reveled in their mastery of techniques to elicit subtle physical findings, which they then taught to students and other house officers.[37] If they missed a physical finding, house officers, particularly the better ones, often felt embarrassed, sometimes ashamed.

The third component of the moral dimension of residency was its explicit emphasis on patient safety. Safety was a special concern to medical faculties because they oversaw the transformation of inexperienced physicians into mature doctors. Medical educators not only needed to produce a finished product capable of practicing safely and wisely but also needed to protect the safety of patients seen by interns and residents during the process of learning.

From the beginning, medical educators recognized that sparing patients from being seen by inexperienced physicians was not a viable option. Every physician needed to gain clinical experience, and every physician faced a day of reckoning when he practiced medicine independently for the first time—that is, without anyone looking over his shoulder or immediately available for help. The only choice medical educators had was to control the circumstances where this would happen. Should house officers gain experience and develop independence within the structured confines of a teaching hospital, where help could readily be obtained, or must this occur afterward in practice at the potential expense of the first patients who presented themselves?

To maximize patient safety, medical educators employed a system that provided oversight and support as house officers developed independence and maturity. Supervision, particularly at the better hospitals, was regularly provided, if only by someone a year or two more experienced. Chief residents, attending faculty, and the clinical chiefs were available for help, and these more senior physicians reviewed the progress of cases at frequent intervals. Interns and residents were expected to practice within their level of competence and to seek help if they were uncertain. In this fashion medical educators attempted to reconcile patient safety with educational needs—and the needs of the present generation with those of the future.

At most training programs, particularly those sponsored by teaching hospitals, an additional factor promoted patient safety: the multiplicity of individuals examining a patient and participating in that patient's care. For example, on the internal medicine service of the Peter Bent Brigham Hospital, each patient was seen by Christian, another senior faculty member, the chief resident, and the assistant resident, in addition to the intern and sometimes a student—all of whom wrote independent notes in the chart and participated in the discussion of diagnosis and therapy.[38] The multiplicity of examiners promoted not only learning but also safe patient care, as one team member challenged another, sometimes a more junior individual questioning someone more senior. Thus, at Barnes Hospital, a surgical intern saved a patient's life by discovering a pelvic abscess following an appendectomy that had been missed by the patient's private doctor.[39] This was far from a rare occurrence on teaching services everywhere.

Indeed, it was the presence of graduate medical education that helped to make the quality of patient care at teaching hospitals so admired. Sick patients were continually monitored. House staff teams rounded on their patients at least daily, often twice a day,[40] and they were immediately available for problems or complications. The multiplicity of physicians involved in a patient's care made it unlikely that a critical finding would be overlooked or that a management plan would be implemented without sound justification. House officers were known for zealously guarding the welfare of patients under their care, and faculty often commented that patients cared for by residents received better care than private patients.

To the middle and upper classes at that time, the chief disadvantage to being a patient on the resident service was concern not for safety but for personal comfort. Most private patients preferred not to be so frequently poked and prodded, nor did they wish to be among the riff-raff charity patients who made up the bulk of the resident services. Private patients also preferred the greater privacy, better food, and more liberal visiting hours they received. Thus, Henry Christian, while praising the work of his resident staff, spoke of the importance of "reducing to a minimum any inconvenience incident to this."[41] This concern for the disruptive influence of medical education on the tranquility of the hospital and the experience of being a patient was an old one.[42]

Of course, despite safeguarding, errors did occur, as did unfortunate adverse events unassociated with error. This was true of patients cared for by faculty members and private physicians as well as by house officers. When complications happened, it was the desire of medical educators that everyone learn from them. Typically, this was done through regular "morbidity and mortality" conferences, where every detail of the management was scrutinized by an audience of faculty, residents, and students, regardless of whether error was involved or not. Such public give-and-take could be bruising for the individuals who had been involved in the patient's care. However, the goal of these conferences was not personal recrimination but to allow for an extended discussion of management issues so that everyone could learn from the event. The honest recognition of mistakes or bad outcomes, and the careful analysis of these events, helped breed humility and lessened the likelihood of repetition. The discussions also helped create an appreciation of the importance of safety among house officers that they took later with them into practice.[43]

When patients died, even in the great majority of cases when an error was not suspected, vigorous efforts were made to obtain an autopsy. At the Massachusetts General Hospital, house officers were told, "It is the desire of the Hospital to secure post mortem examinations in all cases of death."[44] Autopsies provided a valuable check on a physician's work, and it was believed that every autopsy had something to teach, no matter how common the condition or how well the symptoms were apparently explained during life. Teaching hospitals of the period achieved autopsy rates ranging from 40 to 80 percent.[45] Some surgeons went so far as to publish case reports, including the postmortem findings, when a patient died, in the hope that the lessons learned might be disseminated widely.

In discussions of error, and in all discussions of patient care, total honesty was expected of every physician. Anything less constituted another grave moral offense. It was acceptable, if sometimes embarrassing, for a house officer or an attending physician not to know something. What was not acceptable was for a physician to speak beyond his knowledge, to feign understanding, or to act beyond his competence. Even worse was to be untruthful. One early surgical resident at Johns Hopkins discovered this when William Halsted asked him about the condition of a patient. The embarrassed resident, who had not seen the patient, informed Halsted that the patient was doing well. Later that day, Halsted visited the patient, who in fact was extremely ill, forcing the resident to admit that he in fact had not seen her. The resident was summarily dismissed from the program—not for failing to visit the patient but for saying he had.[46]

In keeping with the times, error was viewed as resulting from the actions of an individual. Of course, many errors did result from the behavior or decisions of individuals. However, hospitals were already complex organizations, and there was great potential for error from systemwide problems, such as too few nurses, hospital overcrowding, inaccurate or delayed transcriptions, or absence on the floor of important drugs needed for medical emergencies.[47] But somehow the relation of such problems to bad outcomes was rarely made at this time. The tendency was to blame the individual. House officers and staff physicians tended to believe that any bad outcome was the result of their ineptitude, even when larger, systemwide problems were involved. The focus of teaching programs at this time on safety was healthy and good for patients, but it was to await another era for safety considerations to encompass the system as well as the individual.

In summary, graduate medical education involved a moral as well as a cognitive dimension, and training programs took this responsibility seriously. Their aim was to produce complete physicians and surgeons who understood and internalized the full professional responsibilities of being a doctor. As house officers absorbed the message of thoroughness, attention to detail, safety, and absolute commitment to the welfare of the individuals entrusted to them for care, they discovered what made the practice of medicine so special.

THE LEARNING ENVIRONMENT

In theory, medical education could be conducted anywhere patients were treated. Potential sites included doctors' offices, ambulatory clinics, convalescent facilities, and patients' homes. However, for medical education to be most effective, it needed to follow the patients, and by World War I the inpatient hospital setting had become the most important site for the delivery of acute care in America. The old dread of hospitals, widespread in the nineteenth century, had been overcome, and each year more and more patients flocked to hospitals for admission for the treatment of serious illness.[48] The modern hospital is now "the place where anyone, afflicted with any disease or injury that can be relieved by modern medical science, will have a better chance than he could have at home or anywhere else," the trustees of the Massachusetts General Hospital observed in 1928.[49] Small wonder that the acute care hospital became the home of graduate medical education.

Hospitals that sponsored internship and residency programs represented a heterogeneous group, and not all were equally prepared for the task. Many community hospitals, particularly the smaller ones, lacked a clear commitment to education, and they did not have the requisite staff, facilities, and traditions to allow inquiry and learning to proceed at a university level.[50] However, leadership in graduate medical education was provided by the country's "teaching hospitals"—the 100 to 150 of the roughly 6,800 acute care hospitals in existence that provided clinical facilities for medical schools. Teaching hospitals were a motley group, with significant differences among them in size (though all were relatively large), patient composition, ownership, facilities, quality of teaching faculty, and institutional culture. However, among these elite institutions, there were great similarities in their educational qualities. As a group, they provided a highly nurturing environment for graduate medical education, and the stronger the hospital, the closer the learning environment was to the ideal.[51]

One characteristic of teaching hospitals was their diverse and abundant patient population. This was particularly true of larger teaching hospitals in urban areas. One institution with unusual clinical riches was the Johns Hopkins Hospital. A resident in internal medicine described his experience there regarding encountering unusual and interesting diseases. At one point he cared for patients with staphylococcal septicemia, sprue, myasthenia gravis, anorexia nervosa, tetanus, thrombocytopenic purpura, two types of leukemia, constrictive pericarditis, typhoid fever, and one acute and one chronic case of nephritis. “This was almost more than one man deserved,” he exclaimed.[52]

Medical educators noted that the distribution of diseases at a teaching hospital tended not to reflect their prevalence in the general population. However, this was thought to enhance rather than diminish the learning environment of the institution. Consider the case of the Massachusetts General Hospital. The hospital played a major role as a referral center for patients with unusual or especially troubling conditions, thereby giving it a skewed population when compared with community hospitals. In addition, patients tended to flock to the hospital after important new discoveries were made. Thus, the number of diabetic patients admitted there after the introduction of insulin into clinical therapy increased more than three times from pre-insulin days, and the hospital’s leadership in the study of hyperparathyroidism led to more patients being admitted with that condition than anywhere else in the world. New operations were also performed at the Massachusetts General Hospital much more commonly than in the general community. For instance, in 1906 the hospital performed a large portion of the appendectomies and hernia repairs in the Boston area because facilities and trained surgeons in community hospitals were few. Thirty years later, these operations were performed widely throughout Boston, and their incidence at the Massachusetts General Hospital correspondingly decreased (though they continued to be regularly performed). “What was new then is standard now,” the hospital’s executive committee wrote. Instead, hospital surgeons were turning increasingly to chest surgery, endocrine surgery, and neurosurgery. The hospital was justifiably proud of its success in establishing standards, developing new fields of medicine and surgery, and training the next generation of doctors, thereby fulfilling a critically important social mission. In the process, house officers at the Massachusetts General Hospital were not heard to complain of a lack of clinical opportunities.[53]

House officers worked with patients primarily on the inpatient services. Typically, they had outpatient duties as well, but these were relatively few and thought to be of only minor educational value. At this time, outpatient clinics tended to suffer from severe overcrowding, a frenetic pace, and marked understaffing. They ranked low in the hierarchy system of both medical schools and hospitals. Given the ease of admitting someone to the hospital, patients in ambulatory clinics mainly had minor problems. Serious illness at this time required hospitalization, not outpatient management. The chief value of ambulatory departments to many medical educators was in serving as a source of patients to help keep the inpatient wards filled.

A second characteristic of the learning environment was that most patients were charity patients. At voluntary (nonprofit) hospitals like Barnes Hospital, Lakeside Hospital, Presbyterian Hospital (New York), and the Johns Hopkins Hospital, typically 60 to 80 percent of patients were treated on the indigent wards (also known as the "ward" or "pavilion" services). At state-supported teaching hospitals such as the University of Arkansas and University of Michigan Hospitals, the percentage of ward patients was similarly high. At municipal and county hospitals used in teaching, such as Boston City Hospital, Bellevue Hospital, Cook County Hospital, Charity Hospital (New Orleans), and Los Angeles County Hospital, the percentage of ward patients often approached 100 percent. For house officers, the presence of "ward" or "charity" patients was of inestimable value, for these patients provided the "clinical material" from which residents learned to diagnose, treat, operate, and assume real responsibility for patient care. Private patients afforded them few such opportunities. The interchangeability at this time of the terms "charity beds" and "teaching beds" underscored the importance of these patients to the educational and research missions of teaching hospitals.

A third component of the learning environment of teaching hospitals was the deep commitment of the faculty to teaching. Tinsley Harrison, who after World War II became an iconic cardiologist and chair of internal medicine at the University of Alabama, in 1941 described his experience as a house officer at the Peter Bent Brigham Hospital: "The primary emphasis was placed on the training of the house staff," and the residents were inspired by "the deep interest shown by the senior staff in the house staff."[54] Few hospitals could compare with the Peter Bent Brigham Hospital, but the Brigham's commitment to teaching was representative. Indeed, the period between the world wars has been described as the "educational era" of American medical education, in recognition of the importance medical school faculties assigned to the teaching mission at this time.[55]

Teaching in this era had a highly personal quality, and the department chairs were the cornerstones of the process. One did not go to Johns Hopkins to train but to "work under" Warfield T. Longcope in internal medicine, Dean DeWitt Lewis in surgery, or J. Whitridge Williams in obstetrics. Department chairs customarily knew the names of all their house officers—and of their spouses and children as well. Clinical chiefs traveled infrequently so they could keep a close eye on the service. At times they dropped by the wards unexpectedly to check on particular patients, review charts, or round. Even when not physically present, their presence was felt. A surgical resident at Johns Hopkins said of his experience: the chairman "was much in contact with the resident staff and I felt his presence on a daily, if not an hourly, basis."[56] Department chairs typically conducted the morning "residents' report" themselves throughout the year; they considered this responsibility too important to delegate. They were regularly present at other departmental teaching conferences as well, a fact that usually guaranteed high attendance. The bonds they developed with their residents could be exceedingly strong. Evarts Graham, who chaired the department of surgery at Washington University and performed the first successful pneumonectomy for lung cancer, turned down other attractive job offers in large part because he felt too attached to his residents to leave.[57] Clinical chiefs everywhere derived deep personal satisfaction at observing their house officers grow in power and ability as they progressed through the various stages of the residency and assumed greater and greater responsibility.[58]

The commitment to teaching generally pervaded the rest of the department as well. Clinical departments at teaching hospitals typically consisted of a core of full-time clinical scientists, who looked upon education and research as a vocation, assisted by a larger group of voluntary faculty. (Community hospitals rarely had full-time medical school faculty members on their staffs at this time.) The voluntary faculty was composed of outstanding private practitioners in the community who donated their services. The commitment of the private group to teaching was real, the amount of time they gave, prodigious, and their contributions, major. For private physicians, obtaining an appointment to the voluntary faculty was not easy, and many physicians were disappointed by their inability to obtain staff privileges at a teaching hospital.[59] Often there were tensions between the full-time and part-time members of a department, usually relating to the fact that it was the full-timers who were in control. However, even when tempers flared, these tensions were generally kept within the faculty. Instructors were united in their commitment to teaching, and house officers (as well as students) benefited from the variety of viewpoints and perspectives brought to bear on clinical problems.

A fourth component of the learning environment was that sufficient time was available for house officers to do their jobs well. Studying patients in depth, developing the ability to solve unknowns, and learning how to manage uncertainty could be accomplished only if house officers were not rushed. Thoroughness and attention to detail also required time. A great strength of the inpatient wards of teaching hospitals was that they provided sufficient time for studying patients carefully.

Medical educators worked hard to ensure that house officers had enough time for learning, study, and attentive patient care. One way they did so was by hiring far more house officers for the same number of patients than nonteaching hospitals. For instance, one study in 1939 found that teaching hospitals had a ratio of nine patients per intern or resident, compared with a ratio of 25 at community hospitals.[60] To medical educators, limiting the size of a house officer's service was indispensable for both learning and good patient care. As Henry Christian put it, the goal was to provide residents "a varied but not too large a group of patients." Otherwise, a house officer "will be so hurried in his work that he will not have time to do it well."[61]

Medical educators were aided in their efforts to allow house officers adequate time by the lengthy hospitalizations of the era. For instance, the average length of stay at the Johns Hopkins Hospital was 19.5 days in 1925 and 15.4 days in 1940.[62] Accordingly, house officers had the opportunity to study their patients thoroughly, observing the full course of their patients' illnesses. In addition, the lengthy hospitalizations allowed quality control to be present in medical education. Patients were not discharged before the results of diagnostic tests or the responses to therapy were observed. This way, house officers learned if their initial clinical impressions had been correct, and if not, they gained from the experience and sharpened their skills. As one medical teacher observed, there was no substitute for observing the results of clinical decisions "to erase false confidence in diagnosis and treatment."[63] Having a check on a house officer's work provided an indispensable aid to learning.

Of course, taking the time to study patients carefully placed a limit on the number of patients that could be satisfactorily handled. Teaching hospitals were inefficient in terms of seeing the most patients with the fewest doctors in the shortest time. Henry Christian noted, "The more time given to each patient, the less the total number of patients that we can handle per day or per year."[64] This did not trouble medical school or hospital leaders because they defined success by the quality of work, not by the number of patients seen, and quality educational work could not be accomplished on a medical assembly line. Harvey Cushing stated, "Quantity production is well enough in its way, but there are other things far more important for the reputation of a hospital than the numerical turnover of its patients."[65]

The emphasis of teaching hospitals on the quality, not the quantity, of work illustrated a final and critically important component of the learning environment: its suffusion with professional values. Commercialism was antithetical to teaching institutions at this time; professional ideals dominated the culture. Teaching hospitals regularly acknowledged that they served the public, and they competed with each other to be the best, not the biggest or most profitable. "The object for which this institution exists," the Massachusetts General Hospital stated, "is to accomplish the greatest good for the community."[66]

The commitment of teaching institutions of this era to the larger good was illustrated in part by their disdain for commercialism. A midcentury report called academic medical centers one of the country's greatest group of philanthropic institutions, both in regard to the prodigious amounts of free care provided by the hospitals and the professional fees waived by the physicians.[67] For paying patients, teaching hospitals typically sought to keep prices as low as possible. Thus, declared the medical board of Presbyterian Hospital (New York), "A hospital of our size owes it to the community to furnish hospital care at reasonable rates."[68] Competition with community physicians for private patients was unusual. Paying patients, other than those of the voluntary faculty, were seen at the teaching center only on a referral basis, and the patients were returned afterward to their personal physicians. The University of Arkansas explained, "The University Hospital is a charity hospital and should admit pay patients only under conditions that are not in competition with private hospitals."[69] Similarly, the Peter Bent Brigham Hospital had "more patients than it can satisfactorily handle," and accordingly "the last thing it [the hospital] desires is to augment this by patients who otherwise will secure adequate professional service."[70] In Nashville, the chair of medicine at Vanderbilt routinely sent patients to former residents starting their practices, as did clinical chairs at teaching centers around the country.[71] The refusal of medical faculty members to patent their discoveries or accept gifts from pharmaceutical companies, the high standards of intellectual honesty they adhered to, and their open contempt for unusually high-earning physicians stood as other illustrations of the lack of commercialism at teaching institutions at this time.

The commitment of teaching institutions to the larger good was also illustrated by the idealism embodied in their internal culture. The Johns Hopkins Hospital, for example, was widely known for "its sense of service to the patient."[72] Patients trusted the system, believing that the doctors and hospital would do right by them—making every effort to solve their problems, not discharging them before they were medically ready, and placing their interests above the financial interests of the institution. The culture of teaching hospitals was also characterized by creativity and curiosity. Thus, the Johns Hopkins Hospital was known for "always asking the question 'why?'" and for its commitment to the "ever present search for new knowledge."[73] House officers at good teaching hospitals worked in an environment where there was a keen sense of the primacy of the patient, a discontent with the present state of knowledge, and collective pride at being part of an institution that was truly first-rate.

Thus, from an organizational perspective, graduate medical education at good institutions prospered because the learning environment validated the principles medical educators were trying to impart. The institutional cultures were centered on the learners and patients. House officers knew that they were important to their professors and that good patient care mattered. The predominance of charity patients allowed interns and residents to assume responsibility for care, and the presence of time permitted them to be thorough, to reflect, and to wonder. A hospital culture that maximized service, not profits, reinforced the point that there was a moral as well as an intellectual dimension to medical practice.

The above discussion should not be construed as suggesting that teaching hospitals were perfect places. In fact they could be rigid, hierarchical, and authoritarian. Efforts to improve care focused mainly on the work of individuals, not the systems of care, even though hospitals had already become complex organizations. The idea of treating patients as customers had yet to be born. The creature comforts of patients received scant attention, even those of private patients in some instances. The medical board of one prominent hospital found it surprising that so much emphasis "is placed on food served in the hospital . . . when the medical and surgical treatment is the very best."[74] Reflecting the cultural biases of the time, prejudices were often apparent toward African-Americans, Jews, Catholics, and women—both as patients and as physicians.[75]

Nevertheless, teaching hospitals, despite their imperfections, advocated timeless ideals and stood for what was best about medicine. Medical educators recognized that good learning could occur only in an environment in which good patient care was provided. Accordingly, at many teaching hospitals, perfection in clinical care was the goal, and the stronger the hospital, the more explicit was the focus on striving for that goal. At the Massachusetts General Hospital, by World War II America's most admired hospital, it was said that "nothing short of perfection would do."[76] Teaching faculties desired to demonstrate medical care at its finest, giving all house officers a model of excellence to take with them for a lifetime. One former Brigham house officer wrote, "Though now only a memory, it [the Brigham] continues—and will ever continue—to be an inspiration."[77] At its best, the learning environment of teaching hospitals helped inspire residents to want to do their best—both while in training and afterward.

CULTURAL INFLUENCES

Given the highly scientific and technical nature of medical practice, residency training understandably developed in response to intellectual forces within medicine. After all, the need to learn scientific concepts and principles, to develop skills of critical reasoning, to acquire the capacity to manage uncertainty, to master technical procedures, and to learn how to assume responsibility for patient care all reflected powerful professional demands. However, residency training in America developed within a specific cultural context, and these cultural forces indelibly shaped the system as well. Their influence was more subtle than those of the internal forces, but it was just as powerful and important.

Most obviously, graduate medical education in the United States developed within a system of charity care, and it was this fact that allowed the residency system to provide interns and residents the opportunity to assume responsibility in patient care. The United States, like the rest of the industrialized world, used indigent patients as "clinical material." These patients, in keeping with a long-standing Western tradition, received free care in exchange for their participation in clinical education and research. Paying patients (both "semiprivate" and "private"), who were treated in hospitals in growing numbers after 1900, were used only in limited ways in medical education—for histories and physical examinations or for introduction at teaching conferences, and only then when they granted permission. Professional responsibility for their care belonged to their personal physicians, and this responsibility was rarely delegated. Only the indigent patients on the "teaching service" afforded house officers the opportunity to develop management plans, make important therapeutic decisions, and perform surgery and other procedures.

Every indication suggests that ward patients received excellent medical care. Given the difficulty of obtaining a residency position at this time, residents tended to be outstanding individuals—the best of the graduating medical classes. On surgical, gynecological, and obstetrical services, the complication rates on the resident service were generally indistinguishable from those on the staff service. On all services, patients benefited from the close monitoring by the house staff, the extensive discussions about their care, and the fact that house officers (and sometimes students) made important observations that the attending staff had missed. House officers were often fierce advocates for their patients amid a large, sometimes frightening, impersonal system. All this contributed to the ethos of the era that medical education enhanced the quality of patient care.

However, the same high level of quality did not apply to the amenities that ward patients received. In outpatient clinics, there were interminable delays for appointments, overcrowding, hard benches, long waiting times, unappetizing housekeeping, inadequate staffing, and a lack of space and privacy. The inpatient service for charity patients typically consisted of large, open wards of 16, 24, or more beds. Privacy was nonexistent; curtains or screens were used only when the genitalia were being examined. Patients endured noise, commotion, odors, poor food, frequent disturbances, and restrictions on visitors. In addition, ward patients were the ones used as subjects in clinical investigations, sometimes with an absence of informed consent that later generations found shocking.[78] If they died, charity patients were much more likely to die alone, without the comfort of being surrounded by family and close friends.[79]

Paying patients, in contrast, enjoyed far more comfortable amenities. They received their own room ("private" patients) or a room with two beds ("semiprivate" patients), a personal bathroom, soundproofing, sitz baths, showers, better food, much more liberal visiting privileges, and sometimes a sitting room for relaxing or entertaining guests. Typically, they were not asked to participate as research subjects. At the private pavilion of one important Midwest hospital there was a "paid social secretary of the right character" to "look after the relationship between the various men on the staff and the patient" and to "see that the patient is immediately cared for and . . . that consultations are promptly attended to."[80] A prominent New York City hospital hired an individual to improve "the ways and means of making the stay of private patients in this Hospital more enjoyable in respect to non-professional details."[81]

Ward patients also sometimes experienced condescending or demeaning treatment. In 1917, for instance, the entire senior class at the Woman's Medical College of Pennsylvania signed a petition to the faculty deploring the "almost incessant scolding" of the ward patients by the nurses in charge. "We resent the harsh and unsympathetic treatment, the coarse language and lack of consideration of ward patients on the part of Mrs. Murphy, Supervisor of Nurses, and we note that her tyranny is often reflected in the behavior of certain subordinate nurses."[82] How this environment affected the attitudes of house officers and medical students is unknown, though anecdotal evidence suggests that charity patients were most likely to be treated callously at municipal hospitals and that house officers and medical students who trained there became susceptible to developing an insensitivity toward the poor. According to the surgeon Charles W. Mayo:

> At the Mayo Clinic, we used to find that doctors who had been trained in charity hospitals rarely showed the kind of warmth and thoughtfulness toward patients that we value as a doctor. They would tend rather to be brusque and inconsiderate. I used to speculate wickedly on the advisability of arranging, if it were possible, for a few weeks of pain to be part of their curriculum. I can guarantee that it makes a person more compassionate.[83]

Reflecting American society of the period, the most callously treated ward patients were African-Americans. Many teaching hospitals, particularly in the South and in border states, segregated African-Americans into separate "colored wards." In the North, where wards were generally integrated, African-Americans needing hospitalization were often refused admission to a private or semiprivate pavilion, even if they could afford to pay.[84] Grady Hospital in Atlanta was noted for having two patients per bed on its black wards, placed "head to foot," each one hoping to have a small fellow for a bedmate.[85] When interns at Georgetown University Hospital felt they needed more clinical opportunities in obstetrics, the solution was obvious to them: to demand of the hospital "a colored obstetrical ward service to give us better obstetrical experience."[86] African-American professionals suffered as well. Medical school positions for blacks were scarce, residency positions even scarcer, and often black house officers were prohibited from caring for, or even touching, Caucasian patients.[87]

Much of the demeaning treatment of patients on the ward services represented a cultural legacy of nineteenth-century hospitals, in which nurses and administrators strictly controlled the internal environment, dictating precisely what patients could do or say, or not do or say, and when they could do it. Such paternalism resulted from the desire of hospital personnel to improve the "character" as well as the health of their patients, and it was encouraged by the social distance between themselves and their impoverished patients.[88] However, the callous treatment of ward patients, many of whom had recently immigrated to America, also reflected the widespread nativism and xenophobia of post–World War I America, which, among other things, led to the Immigration Restriction Act of 1924. At many teaching hospitals, paying patients insisted on being separated from ward patients, demanding separate waiting rooms and hospital accommodations. Some private patients refused to use the same bathroom or shower facilities as charity patients or to sit on benches or lie on examining tables that had been "contaminated" by the wrong individuals. As always, the culture of teaching institutions reflected the broader sentiments of society.[89]

Yet it would be a mistake not to place American treatment of immigrant and poor patients in a larger context. It should not be forgotten that teaching hospitals were also full of professional and nonprofessional staff members who were genuinely kind and caring with all patients, including charity patients. From the earliest days of scientific medical education in America, leading medical educators regularly emphasized the importance of treating even the poorest patients with dignity. Thus, the famed clinical teacher Austin Flint, for whom the murmur of aortic regurgitation is named, declared, "Manifestations of indifference or harshness toward patients in charitable institutions deserve to be stigmatized as brutal."[90] Of note, numerous first- and second-generation medical educators who had studied in Vienna, Berlin, and other German cities repudiated the inhuman treatment of patients they had witnessed abroad, even as they admired German scientific ideals. John M. T. Finney, a prominent surgeon at Johns Hopkins, was so disgusted and outraged with the cruel treatment of patients he observed in some German clinics that he vowed never to return. He described an operation on one 20-year-old woman:

> She was wheeled into the operating room on a stretcher, then stripped of all of her clothing, lifted to the operating table and tied there by the orderlies with bandages binding her legs together and her arms to her sides, with her head pulled back over the end of the table and tied fast there in a most uncomfortable position. Thus she could not move her head, arms or legs, but could only cry. The whole procedure was brutal. There was no nurse present, only a maid, and the surgical amphitheater was full of doctors and medical students. When she cried from fright and from the rough handling, one of the orderlies would smack her on the side of the face and roughly tell her to shut up. When the surgeon himself came in, she was crying loudly and begging for mercy. He walked over and gave her a resounding smack on the cheek and in turn told her to be quiet. He then proceeded to do the operation, a most painful one, without a drop of anesthetic of any kind, believe it or not. The poor girl screamed and cried until she stopped from sheer exhaustion. The details of the operation are too horrible to relate. I waited until it was over, just long enough to go up and ask the operator—I won't call him a surgeon—why he hadn't given the poor girl an anesthetic. With a shrug of the shoulder he replied, "It wasn't necessary. We could hold her."[91]

It is difficult to justify the harsh and insulting treatment of charity patients that sometimes occurred in American hospitals, but it is safe to say that American hospitals were far from the worst in the world.

If the existence of a two-tiered health care system represented one cultural influence shaping graduate medical education in America, cultural attitudes toward work and family life represented another. Learning and practicing medicine were devouring activities, often presenting what seemed like 36 hours of work to do in a 24-hour day. In arguably his most famous aphorism, William Osler called work "the master-word in medicine."[92] To succeed, doctors needed to focus nearly totally on medicine, to the exclusion of family, friends, hobbies, and a balanced life.

Cultural attitudes of the time supported physicians in their efforts to learn and practice medicine. The United States as a society always had had a high regard for those who could work themselves up to financial and professional success. It was the country's strong work ethic and entrepreneurial spirit that attracted many ambitious immigrants hoping to leave poverty behind. Moreover, during the creation and early development of the residency system, a strong union movement had yet to arrive, and there were no restrictions on the length of the work day or work week or even on child labor. Accordingly, Americans were accustomed to hard work. Few eyebrows were raised when medical students and house officers threw everything into their training and gave up their twenties for their future. As one physician, who took over seven years of training beyond medical school, explained, "I was going through a long training because I wanted to go somewhere in medicine some day."[93]

Attitudes toward marriage and family life reinforced the strong work ethic. Medicine, like virtually all professional fields at the time, was overwhelmingly a male career. Marriage was viewed as women's work; the physician's spouse was expected to support her husband, raise the family, manage the household, and take charge of social affairs.[94] No one expressed this sentiment more clearly than William Osler, who himself did not marry until he was 42. "What about the wife and babies, if you have them? Leave them! Heavy as are your responsibilities to those nearest and dearest, they are outweighed by the responsibilities to yourself, to the profession, and to the public.... Your wife will be glad to bear her share in the sacrifice you make."[95] Of course, not all women found a life of subordinated needs attractive, to which Osler also had an answer: "Marry the right woman!"[96]

Deciding how to balance the intrinsic tension between the professional demands of medicine and responsibilities to one's spouse and family ultimately, of course, was a personal decision. However, cultural attitudes of the period validated the importance of professional work and undoubtedly influenced the choices of almost every physician. Did anyone suffer? Systematic studies of physicians' families were not done, but statements of numerous doctors provide a window into the question. These statements are remarkably consistent, describing neglected spouses and children who often felt alone, even as they might have outwardly professed happiness and contentedness. Consider the observations of the Johns Hopkins surgeon John Finney, who wrote, "So it is that the doctor's family, especially his wife, often has a pretty hard time. She has to bear the brunt of the irregularities and vagaries of his professional life."[97] Or more striking, consider the case of the surgeon Charles W. Mayo. He said, "I rarely saw my children while they were young," and he had to wait until his retirement to spend some time with them, who by then were like "friendly strangers." ("This is the price a father who puts his heart into his career must pay," he added.) Spouses in the Mayo family were also vulnerable to loneliness. Mayo's mother, the wife of Charles H. Mayo, was known for her bubbly personality, happy nature, social charm, and unequivocal support of her husband. Yet she left letters to Charles and his wife, Alice, to be read 15 years after her death. Many of them "expressed Mother's loneliness and longing to be closer to her busy and important husband." Alice "cried like a child over some of them," undoubtedly seeing in them a bit of her own situation. Mayo declared, "I'd never advise a girl to marry a doctor if he is a good one. She will be in for a lot of loneliness."[98]

Lastly, the medical profession did its work largely independent of external forces that became much more conspicuous after World War II. The federal presence in medicine was nonexistent, indeed, not yet even envisioned. Medical education and research were beholden to private donors and state and municipal governments; payment for medical care was the responsibility of the individual. Accordingly, there was little formal accountability. William Welch once told a Senate committee that all medicine asked of Congress was "not to interfere with its progress."[99] In addition, the voice of the consumer in medicine was still muted, even though, as Lisabeth Cohen and Nancy Tomes have shown, the idea of the consumer citizen was clearly arising during the New Deal.[100] The "cultural authority" of medicine was high, doctors had not yet become "providers," patients had not yet morphed into "consumers" or "customers," and conviction remained strong (though not unchallenged) that medicine was a profession and not a business.

Indeed, doctors and the medical profession during this era often acted as if they were above lay criticism, and an attitude that "patients should be seen but not heard" predominated. In many cities, office hours of fashionable doctors began at 2:00 p.m., but patients often waited in the office until 4:00 or 5:00 in the afternoon before they were seen.[101] The poor were not the only ones who endured long waits. Paternalistic attitudes pervaded patient care, particularly in the commonly held belief among doctors that it was often unwise for patients to know the exact nature of their diseases. House officers at the Massachusetts General Hospital were instructed to make sure "that patients are given the information they desire [only] in so far as it is wise."[102] For approval, doctors typically looked to each other, not to their patients. Thus, one young Detroit physician told his mentor, "I care more for the good will of my medical friends than for that of the laiety."[103]

In short, the development of graduate medical education was influenced by cultural conditions as well as by professional forces. A two-tiered system of health care with an abundance of charity patients provided the "clinical material" with which house officers could learn to assume responsibility for patient care. The strong work ethic of the era, a culture in which delayed gratification was the norm for those aspiring to professional success, and the view that marriage was "women's work" made it easier for young physicians to submerge themselves in their training and careers. The muted voices of the federal government and the consumer gave credence to the notion that medicine was above lay accountability and that only doctors could judge themselves. Few medical educators considered these social circumstances in relation to residency training at the time, so much a part of the natural order did they seem. Even fewer contemplated what the implications for residency training might be should social conditions change.

CHAPTER 5
The Life of a Pre–World War II House Officer

Enormous diversity existed among internship and residency programs. There were great variations among the many hospitals that sponsored graduate training: hospitals large and small, privately and publicly owned, with and without medical school affiliations, of varying academic quality, in urban and rural areas, and in different parts of the country. Some hospitals were wealthy and blessed with abundant resources and large staffs; others barely stayed financially afloat. Each had its own traditions and local culture. In addition, the nature of the residency varied from specialty to specialty. Every field had its own temperament, routines, and traditions, and these differences manifested themselves in training programs. Thus, a residency in general surgery was a much different experience from one in pathology or psychiatry. Within an individual program, the culture often changed from year to year—the arrival or departure of a new department chair or group of house officers, giving the program a different personality from the year before. Even within the same cohort of residents, the house officers worked with different instructors, medical students, nurses, and patients. Accordingly, no two house officers ever had the same experience.

Nevertheless, there were many commonalities shared by house officers. All experienced the challenge of choosing a career—a general practice or a specialty, and, if a specialty, which one. All house officers also experienced the anxieties that came with applying for an internship. Once in a program, house officers experienced self-doubt, stress, and fatigue, coupled with exhilaration in the work and considerable pride over their professional growth. The range in the quality of programs was immense, but the best programs provided an environment in which the ideals of medicine were consciously pursued, where standards and expectations were high, where the excitement over studying medicine was palpable, and where house officers experienced joy in the work. Particularly at the prestigious programs, many house officers seemed almost oblivious to the long hours, and those who worked the hardest seemed to be the happiest.

Though most house officers, particularly at university programs, tended to be fulfilled in their work, others benefited from their labors as well. The amount of routine chores grew rapidly in the 1920s and 1930s. Hospitals, as they had since the nineteenth century, continued to profit from the availability of house officers as an inexpensive source of labor. The full-time and voluntary faculty also benefited from the presence of interns and residents, for having house officers staff the clinical service allowed them more time for other activities, such as research or private practice. By World War II, the tension between education and institutional service had become the system's most perplexing and persistent underlying issue.

OBTAINING A RESIDENCY

The life of a medical student was fraught with many uncertainties, not the least of which was the challenge of selecting a career within medicine. Typically, medical students were undifferentiated "stem cells," with the potential to grow into doctors of different types. The best students often had the most difficult time choosing a field since they tended to like everything. One applicant for internship at the Massachusetts General Hospital acknowledged that he "becomes especially interested in every new service," while another described himself as "a child in a toy shop, trying to take everything in at once, but as yet being unable to settle down to one thing."[1] Some students also deeply vacillated between careers in practice and research.[2] It was common for medical students to change their minds many times regarding their ultimate career interests, and frequently they ended up choosing a field much different from what they had thought they might do at the time they started medical school.

Nevertheless, by the fourth year of medical school, medical students generally had achieved some clarity regarding their ultimate career ambitions. As they did, it was clear that some fields were more attractive to them than others. General practice had lost much of its appeal, particularly to the best students. One Harvard medical student applying to the Massachusetts General Hospital for an internship described how his interest had shifted from general practice to internal medicine:

> Then the field of general practice seemed brightest, as I did not like the idea of dropping any part of medicine. I then visited several good hospitals giving rotating services and talked with the internes. I was astounded with the horribly superficial and dabbling training which they received. I decided that I could not be satisfied with covering a field so large that my work in it could almost of necessity be only of mediocre grade.[3]

Among the specialties, some had an easier time attracting students than others. Internal medicine, general surgery, and pediatrics were particularly competitive fields; psychiatry, dermatology, radiology, and pathology were not.

What led medical students to choose the specialty fields they did? This question was never systematically studied, but a fascinating collection of autobiographical statements by intern applicants to the Massachusetts General Hospital in the 1920s and 1930s provides a valuable window. Occasionally students began thinking of a field because of the influence of charismatic teachers they had encountered during medical school. Sometimes pragmatic considerations played a role. For instance, one student was leaning toward psychiatry because he felt the field was less crowded, and hence his prospects for success greater than in other fields he was considering.[4] There was no mention of financial considerations as a factor, and some applicants actually pointed out the unimportance of this to them in choosing a specialty.[5] There was also no mention of workload or lifestyle considerations. What did stand out were intellectual considerations—that is, the intrinsic interest of a field to a student. Thus, one applicant declared: "My hopes for future professional work are easily expressed. I shall eventually settle in that branch of the profession which holds the greatest interest for me."[6] In short, judging from this sample, medical students sought to enter the specialty field they liked the most.

Fourth-year medical students also had to select a specific program, not just a field of study. All students began with an internship—a "straight" internship in a specific field, a "rotating" internship, or a "mixed" internship. After the successful completion of an internship, a young doctor could enter practice as a general practitioner. Those who wished to continue in a specialty residency followed one of two routes. Most began with a "straight" internship, which also typically served as the first year of residency. Some aspiring specialists began with a "rotating" or "mixed" internship. These individuals usually applied to residency programs during their internship, hoping to obtain a position that began immediately at its conclusion.[7] "Straight" internships were found mainly at teaching hospitals, while the more numerous "rotating" and "mixed" internships were sponsored primarily by community hospitals.

What did students look for in a program? Henry A. Christian, the chief of medicine at the Peter Bent Brigham Hospital, in 1924 provided medical students advice about how to select an internship. He suggested that students concentrate their search on hospitals closely associated with a medical school. Here, the educational opportunities were generally the highest, the instructors the best educated and most current, and interest in teaching the keenest. He also urged students to be cautious of hospitals that offered a salary. Hospitals that pay interns do so "because they are unable to get them without salary which is another way of saying that they do not offer internes any adequate educational quid pro quo."[8] Christian also encouraged students to look for hospitals with large numbers of ward beds, high autopsy rates, good esprit de corps among the staff, and a high level of prestige.[9] The aforementioned collection of personal statements by students applying for positions at the Massachusetts General Hospital reveals that these were the characteristics the students themselves considered most important in choosing a program.

Students were also encouraged to visit as many programs as they could. This way, they met staff, administrators, and current house officers and saw the program firsthand. Personal visits often helped students rank their choices. Thus, one surgeon who did his residency at the Cleveland Clinic under George Crile described how meeting Crile while interviewing made his decision for him. "He [Crile] was a sturdily built man of bounding energy who 'filled the room' wherever he appeared. I was captured immediately; I would have waited tables or emptied trash barrels for a chance to work there."[10]

By the 1930s, finding an internship position was not hard. The number of available positions exceeded the number of medical graduates by 25 percent, and new positions were continuing to become available to meet the growing service needs of hospitals.[11] However, obtaining an internship at a high-quality teaching hospital was difficult, particularly a "straight" internship that led to a residency position. In general, students needed to be in the top quarter or top third of their class to be competitive for an appointment at the average teaching hospital. The more prestigious the hospital, the greater the competition, and the stronger the students' credentials needed to be. For top-tier hospitals, students needed to be in the top 10 percent of their class; for iconic programs such as those at Johns Hopkins or the Massachusetts General Hospital, students had to be at the very top. It was said that obtaining an internship at the Massachusetts General Hospital, which in the 1920s succeeded the Johns Hopkins Hospital as the country's most prestigious hospital, "is about as easy as getting into heaven without a harp."[12]

What did hospitals look for in the students they selected? As the director of surgery at the Mayo Clinic put it, they were interested in an applicant's "ability, personality, and character."[13] How best to evaluate these qualities, however, engendered considerable debate among hospital authorities, just as it did among medical school admissions committees trying to identify the most outstanding applicants to medical school. Hospitals used a variety of instruments in assessing applicants, such as medical school grades and class standing, letters of recommendation, personal statements, interviews, research experience, and perceived aptitude for an academic career. Many hospitals also administered written or oral examinations, or both, to intern candidates. The precise emphasis placed on these various factors varied from program to program. As a rule, a teaching hospital tended to favor applicants from its own affiliated medical school, whose work had been seen firsthand and to whom the hospital felt a sense of loyalty. For instance, the medical service at the Peter Bent Brigham Hospital had always sought house officers from the better medical schools, but roughly half each year came from Harvard Medical School.[14] Many teaching hospitals reserved an even higher percentage of places for their own students.

For medical students, the most stressful aspect of obtaining an internship resulted from the fact that every hospital had its own appointment date. Some hospitals made their internship selections as early as November of the students' fourth year of medical school; others waited as long as the following April. In general, community hospitals had earlier appointment dates, and teaching hospitals, later dates. Hospitals expected prompt responses, typically within a week, and a student's acceptance was considered binding. This posed a huge dilemma for students. Should they accept an offer in hand from a less prestigious program or wait to hear from a more desirable program, at the risk that they would end up with no satisfactory appointment at all? This was the fate of 35 excellent students from Harvard Medical School in 1937. They turned down offers from lesser institutions, hoping to land positions at one of the four major Harvard teaching hospitals (the Massachusetts General Hospital, the Peter Bent Brigham Hospital, Beth Israel Hospital, and Boston City Hospital). When they were not offered positions by any of the Harvard hospitals, they found themselves without a suitable internship.[15]

Medical educators frequently criticized the intern appointment system. Evarts A. Graham, the eminent chair of surgery at Washington University, called it "disastrous."[16] Educators were unhappy both with the stresses it created among students and the havoc that it made of the senior year of medical school. Valuable time for study and growth was lost; instead, students were "running around in circles over a period of many months and wrecking their fourth year."[17] In the 1920s and 1930s there was considerable discussion among hospital staffs and within professional organizations about establishing a shared appointment date. In Boston, New York, Baltimore, and other cities certain teaching hospitals agreed to a common intra-city appointment date. However, these informal agreements failed to solve the problem because competing teaching hospitals in other cities, and community hospitals everywhere, had earlier appointment dates, and even within the consortia, hospitals sometimes moved their dates forward. Thus, in Cleveland a group of hospitals twice agreed to a common appointment date, "but someone always cheated and we . . . returned to the old competitive method."[18]

Not surprisingly, students occasionally broke their commitments to hospitals if better positions became available. For instance, Hurley Hospital, a community hospital in Flint, Michigan, reserved four of its 11 intern positions for graduates of the University of Michigan in the upper half of the class. In 1938, each of the four accepted individuals withdrew after obtaining more prestigious appointments elsewhere, leaving the hospital short-handed and irate.[19] Major teaching hospitals were also vulnerable to being jilted. Officials at Strong Memorial Hospital, the teaching hospital of the University of Rochester, were deeply upset when a Johns Hopkins medical student withdrew after later obtaining an appointment at the Johns Hopkins Hospital. Strong, which had refused positions to a number of promising candidates in the expectation that this individual would serve, was left short-staffed for the year.[20] In these situations, angry hospital officials sometimes threatened disciplinary or even legal proceedings, though it does not appear that they followed through on these threats. Interestingly, their understandable wrath was focused on the students, whom they considered blackguards, and not on the appointment system that had led the students to such behavior.

The internship application process was stressful for all students, but for no one more than African-Americans, women, and religious minorities, particularly Jews. This was because good internships, especially those that led to residency positions, were not available to them commensurate with their numbers as medical students. Hospitals that allowed African-Americans and women to work as clinical clerks often did not accept them as interns, no matter how well they had performed as clerks. Residency positions were especially scarce. Before World War II, only a half-dozen hospitals, most notably Freedmen's Hospital (Howard Medical College) and Hubbard Hospital (Meharry Medical College), accepted African-Americans as residents. At that time women were virtually excluded from residencies in certain fields, particularly surgery and the surgical subspecialties. Jews also encountered intense anti-Semitism in seeking internships and residencies, though the presence of excellent Jewish hospitals, most famously Mount Sinai Hospital (New York), gave Jews an advantage that African-Americans and women did not have. Even so, many capable Jewish medical graduates had to be content with less desirable appointments than they merited, and the virulence of the anti-Semitism they encountered in some parts of the medical profession is difficult to exaggerate. Consider the following comment by a medical resident from the Peter Bent Brigham Hospital, writing from a military camp in 1918: "Some of these dam Jews kick but they have their numbers and they get short shrift. Two of them in my crowd were thrown from their horses today, but unfortunately neither was killed. One broke his arm and two ribs. I really think this Country and her Allies could get along without a few of them."[21]

The process of internship selection was stressful for hospitals, not just medical students. All hospitals that offered training programs competed with each other for the best house officers. A strong house staff was indispensable not only for providing good care to patients but also for creating a pool of potential recruits to the faculty or medical staff. Community hospitals, particularly the smaller ones, had the greatest difficulty recruiting interns. With their large patient loads for each intern, scarcity of ward patients, formidable amount of chores, and dearth of teaching activities, many of these programs regularly failed to fill their quota of interns, and some often received no applications at all. To compensate for their lack of educational attractiveness, many of them tried alternative strategies to recruit interns: setting up residencies as "bait" (these residency programs typically were of short duration and bereft of educational value), agreeing to accept individuals as interns without requiring a qualifying examination, advertising in medical journals, or, most commonly, offering a stipend (typically $25 to $75 per month, compared with teaching hospitals, which usually offered no stipends to interns at the time). These strategies generally did not work, as the American Medical Association pointed out, since students made their decisions on the basis of perceived educational quality, not on the basis of the size of a stipend.[22]

Teaching hospitals were not threatened by community hospitals, but they competed vigorously with each other for the best students. They knew they could not rest on their laurels. Many medical schools sought feedback from their recent graduates to ascertain whether they should advise current students to apply to that program or pass it over.[23] If a teaching hospital slipped in its educational work, word got out quickly. In addition, some prominent teaching hospitals bent the rules to overcome their disadvantage of a later appointment date. These institutions secretly pledged internships to unusually capable students in advance of the official notification date, so the students would not feel the need to accept an earlier offer from another hospital. At the Johns Hopkins Hospital, for instance, department chairs had the prerogative to enter into such arrangements with select students "when it is necessary to prevent very desirable men who desire to remain here from going elsewhere."[24] Curiously, medical educators considered this practice "the natural course when competition is not controlled by a plan,"[25] though they did not think circumstances so "natural" when the stated rules were violated by students rather than by hospitals.

Thus, despite the anxieties attendant to applying for an internship, students wielded considerable power. They followed their consciences in making their personal decisions. In an educational free market, they chose specialty fields on the basis of what interested them the most, and they applied to hospitals that they thought provided the best educational experiences. This lesson is worth remembering by those of any era who wish to influence the specialty choices that medical students make.

EXPERIENCING THE RESIDENCY

No two residency programs were alike. Some kept their house officers much busier, some offered their residents much more autonomy, and some demanded much more independent thinking. In an unstandardized system, the work of an intern at one program was often done by a resident at another. The quality of lectures and conferences varied from one program to another, or even within the same program from day to day. Some programs provided a much stronger scientific foundation than others, and these programs experienced greater success at producing clinical scientists and academic leaders. Life as a pediatrician was much different from that of a radiologist or neurosurgeon, and these differences, too, were manifest in the residency experience.

All house officers, however, experienced one thing in common: a total immersion in the institutional culture. They worked, ate, and lived in the hospital. For their efforts they received room, board, uniforms, and a small stipend—$0 to $10 per month for interns, $10 to $50 per month for residents. Interns experienced the thrill of giving rather than receiving orders; residents, of assuming greater responsibility in decision making and the performance of procedures. They experienced the joy of teaching as well. House officers at teaching hospitals spent considerable time with medical students, and they exerted a more powerful influence on the students during their clinical clerkships than anyone, including the faculty. Practicing with a temporary educational license as interns, and eligible to apply for a standard state medical license as residents, they were doctors at last.

Given the important professional responsibilities of house officers, it is ironic that they typically worked under patronizing and demeaning conditions. This represented a legacy of the nineteenth-century hospital's insistence on strictly controlling its internal environment. Interns and residents lived in the hospital in cramped, frugal cubicles, with rooms sometimes smaller and less private than those of a college dormitory. Conditions were especially difficult for women. At the Los Angeles County Hospital, for instance, the women's quarters were shabby and infested with cockroaches, and there were only two toilets and two baths for 20 to 30 women to share.[26] Hospital authorities insisted on strict accountability for the whereabouts of house officers. Thus, particularly during the first quarter of the century, house officers at many hospitals could not leave the premises without first obtaining the permission of the supervisor of nurses. Complaints about poor food, inadequate living quarters, and the lack of opportunity for fresh air and exercise were frequent.[27] In these circumstances, illness among house officers was common, with pulmonary tuberculosis (deemed "the eternal problem" by one leading medical educator)[28] being a particularly notorious scourge.

Marriage was actively discouraged among house officers, owing to the widespread belief that "the work of unmarried men is more effective than that of married men."[29] Specific rules varied from one hospital to another, though some hospitals that did permit marriage still required its married house officers to reside in the hospital along with the rest of the house staff. A particularly curious rule, in place at many important hospitals, held that married individuals were eligible for appointment as interns but that unmarried interns were prohibited from changing their status during their period of service.[30] In 1915, the Henry Ford Hospital in Detroit, Michigan, became the first to appoint married interns.[31] Thereafter, many other hospitals rescinded their prohibitions against marriage, in response to more liberal cultural attitudes and to house staff voices that clamored to be heard. One intern applicant, who planned to marry before beginning his internship, told the Massachusetts General Hospital, "I am aware of the prejudice that is often felt—perhaps justly—against married internes, but in a matter such as this, I do not think that prudence is a primary concern."[32] Nevertheless, through World War II, there was still a strong unwritten rule against the appointment of married individuals. Though some house officers married, the majority did not.

The academic year for house officers tended to have a characteristic seasonality. Summers were exciting but tense, as interns were new and residents less experienced. Data on patient outcomes during various parts of the year do not exist, but it is clear that medical faculties were especially concerned about the beginning of the academic year. Thus, Samuel A. Levine, a cardiologist at the Peter Bent Brigham Hospital famous for his work on thyrotoxic heart disease and myocardial infarction, spoke of just finishing his "arduous month of July" with the new house staff.[33] The Johns Hopkins Hospital started half of its new interns on July 1, the other half on September 1, to lessen the problem of having all interns being new at the same time.[34] By fall, the fruits of determination and hard work appeared, and house officers started to demonstrate a greater sense of self-assurance and a more critical approach to their work. Winters could be challenging because the wards filled with sick patients, particularly with pneumonia and other infectious diseases, and the house officers themselves became vulnerable to fatigue, irritability, and various respiratory illnesses of their own. By spring, the weather had improved, the hospital census had usually fallen, and the house officers had acquired extensive experience, creating a sense of achievement and sometimes a dollop of complacency and overconfidence.[35]

Whatever the season, house officers worked very long hours. Typically, they were "on call" (that is, admitting new patients and handling unforeseen problems with patients already on the service) every other night. Once or twice a month, they had weekends off, which customarily started Saturdays at noon and continued through the following Monday at 8 a.m. Typically, an intern was allowed two weeks of vacation a year, a junior resident received three weeks, and a senior resident got four weeks. Most programs offered sick leave, but some did not. At the University of Colorado, for instance, interns who lost time from work because of illness had to make up that time before they could receive their certificates.[36] Everywhere sleep was a chance commodity, and episodes of sleep deprivation regularly occurred—the resident at the Cleveland Clinic who did not remember being paged the night before, the intern at Johns Hopkins who responded too slowly to a call from the emergency room, or the house officer at the Peter Bent Brigham Hospital who did not respond to a nurse's late-night call, all because of fatigue.[37]

Nevertheless, the pace of work was not consistently hectic. Being on call meant being in the hospital, immediately available for duty. It did not necessarily mean working, or even staying up. Thus, on a slow night with no new admissions and few problems with patients already on the service, house officers slept much of the night. In life-threatening situations, patients typically lived or died on their own, and quickly. House officers did not make use of cardiopulmonary resuscitation, ventilators, dialysis machines, pressers (blood pressure–elevating drugs), antibiotics, or intensive care units, and they did not deal with complex ethical issues attendant to the end of life. Compared with later standards, the pace of care tended to be more leisurely. House officers admitted fewer patients per day, the length of hospital stay was longer, and many patients spent most of their hospitalization in stable condition, convalescing after a major illness or an operation. In the 1920s, two-thirds of teaching hospitals began their scheduled surgeries at 8:30 or 9:00 a.m., and the other one-third scheduled elective surgeries for the afternoons.[38] At some hospitals, interns awoke as late as 8:00 a.m. and ate breakfast as late as 9:00 a.m.[39] Moreover, all house officers were in it together, and the camaraderie provided everyone additional strength. Accordingly, few blinked an eye at the on-call schedule.

What did cause anxiety for the house staff was the unpredictability of the work. Chance always played a role. When on call, house officers never knew whether the night would be peaceful, allowing for sleep, or whether it would be interrupted with one medical problem after another, or even worse, a particularly difficult problem that tested the limits of their knowledge and capabilities. House officers were vulnerable to the vicissitudes of weather. Snowstorms, for example, usually kept volume in the emergency room low. Chance events played a role. Major fires or accidents typically resulted in busy, high-pressure moments in the emergency room and operating suites. If staffing was good, house officers received considerable help with their work, but if nurses, clerks, orderlies, and technicians were in short supply, the house officers on duty found themselves with much more to do in the way of blood drawing, labeling specimens, filling requisitions, transporting patients and laboratory samples, performing laboratory work, bandaging, making telephone calls, and other minor tasks. Even the location of patients made a difference. A house officer's work was always more efficient when his patients were congregated in one area. If the patients were scattered everywhere in the hospital, considerable time and energy were wasted by running all over the premises.

Chance also played a role in determining which individuals house officers worked with. Were the nurses that month knowledgeable and helpful or dictatorial and imperious? Were the medical students for that rotation enthusiastic and involved or detached and disinterested? Were the other house officers hard-working, industrious, and fun, or did they skirt their duties, leaving more work for the rest? Was that month's attending physician kindly and helpful or a tyrant? Such factors influenced the quality of the experience of every intern and resident.

For residents, a particularly keen source of anxiety was the fear of being cut from the program, given the "pyramidal" system in vogue at most residency programs at this time. A typical pyramid was illustrated by the obstetrics and gynecology service of the New York Hospital. In the late 1930s the service consisted of eight first-year residents, eight second-year residents, three third-year residents, two fourth-year residents, and two fifth-year residents.[40] Residents dropped from a program could sometimes find opportunities at another institution to continue their work. This was particularly true for residents not retained at a leading institution. Residents dropped from less prestigious programs had a more difficult time finding another position. Physicians who did not progress far enough in a residency program usually became general practitioners.

Always, there were minor frustrations for house officers: locating missing hospital records (residents often hoarded patient charts, making it difficult for others who wished to use them, including fellow house officers), interpreting illegible handwriting, keeping up with progress notes and discharge summaries, or remembering to sign for verbal orders. On the wards a house officer could understandably be frustrated if a patient admitted to him actually did not require admission; in the emergency room another house officer could be equally frustrated to discover there were no empty beds for a very sick patient he wished to admit. House officers on all services could be annoyed by receiving "inappropriate" requests for consultations from other services or "unnecessary" pages from nurses, especially at night. House officers also faced the challenge of interpreting the whims of their attending physicians. This was particularly true in surgery, for surgeons had the reputation of being highly temperamental. Thus, one successful surgical resident at the Massachusetts General Hospital was praised by the faculty because he "is always at your elbow when you want him and is never under foot when you don't want him."[41]

Residents soon learned that, to succeed, they needed to have "the right stuff." Included in this was the ability to work long and hard without complaining and following all tasks through to completion, expecting no reward other than internal satisfaction. "The greatest squawkers are the poorest doctors," Henry A. Christian declared.[42] This ability to work hard achieved mythic proportion, especially in surgery, where residents sometimes boasted of how well they could perform without sleep. One surgical resident at the Mayo Clinic claimed to have developed a "kind of analgesia" to fatigue and hunger, losing his freshness and alertness only when the work was done.[43] Too many instances occurred of surgical house officers falling asleep while administering anesthesia or holding retractors during surgery to allow credence to be given to surgeons' claims. However, the existence of the myth that doctors, unlike ordinary mortals, did not require rest was an important symbol of what was believed to constitute "the right stuff."

House officers were also expected to embrace the virtues of humility, modesty, and not speaking beyond the limits of their knowledge. One who succeeded in this regard was Paul Beeson, later chair of internal medicine at Emory and Yale. While at the Peter Bent Brigham Hospital, Beeson earned enormous respect from the faculty for being "a very fine fellow with a very extensive knowledge of medicine, and the modesty characteristic of your best men."[44] House officers also needed to learn to work in teams to a degree that is often underappreciated today. For instance, the successful undertaking of the pathbreaking "blue baby" operation to correct the tetralogy of Fallot (a previously fatal congenital heart condition) involved "a team, each member of which must be competently trained and must cooperate and coordinate well," and not just a talented surgeon. "The surgeon, though he plays an important part, depends tremendously upon the pediatrician to make the diagnosis, the physiologist to carry out special tests, the anaesthetist to give a smooth anesthesia, and the assistants to make this difficult and delicate operation an apparently easy one."[45] The most accomplished team players were the radiologists and pathologists, who, though not caring for patients themselves, interacted with every clinical service that did.

Though the hours were long and the work demanding, most house officers quickly became absorbed in the experience. They were finally doing what they wanted to do. Virtually every waking thought was devoted to work. In surgery, for instance, residents thought through operations countless times in their heads, plotting every move in detail, before finally performing the operations themselves. In their quarters, they tied knots by the thousands on the backs of chairs and applied hemostats to loose threads on towels to perfect their basic techniques, much as a pianist practices scales. Despite the many anxious moments along the way, house officers were continually learning and growing, and they enjoyed the satisfaction of knowing that all the years of preparation and hard work were bearing fruit.

Particularly at teaching hospitals, house officers went about their work with a keen sense of intellectual adventure. In these programs, house officers worked side by side with clinical scientists who were studying diseases. House officers quickly learned that their teachers were themselves students, that knowledge must be sought but is never attained, and that there is joy in the search. At Boston City Hospital, Nobel Laureate George Minot often reminded his residents that they were working on the outer boundaries of knowledge and that, to develop as physicians, they must rely on their own critical thinking and not passively accept the teachings of others.[46] The close distance at the time between clinical observations and important questions in clinical research facilitated this sense of incandescent excitement. For instance, myocardial infarction was once a difficult diagnosis, but work at the Peter Bent Brigham Hospital was instrumental in allowing that condition to become an easily recognized clinical entity. This was accomplished by carefully correlating the history and physical findings of patients with changes on their electrocardiograms and pathological findings observed at autopsy—or, as Henry Christian put it, by "careful, simple clinical methods checked by pathological-anatomical studies."[47] House officers were there, witnessing and participating in this important development.

Adding to the sense of excitement, the earlier foreboding about disease greatly diminished, as the fruits of clinical science became more and more abundant. In surgery, surgeons spoke of the thrill of doing operations that "a few years before we should not have thought of attempting."[48] By the 1930s, particularly noteworthy advances had occurred in thoracic surgery, neurosurgery, surgery of the ductless glands, and surgery for impaired circulation in the extremities. These results were made possible not simply by advances in operative technique but by clinical research leading to improved anesthesia, fluid and electrolyte replacement, blood transfusion, oxygen administration, and, beginning in the late 1930s, the preoperative and postoperative use of antibiotics.[49] In medicine, the therapeutic nihilism of the previous generation, so clearly seen in Osler's textbook, gave way to a more hopeful outlook as one major advance after another was introduced into clinical practice. Among these were liver treatment for pernicious anemia, the recognition and treatment of other vitamin deficiency diseases, and hormone replacement therapy for a number of conditions. The discovery of insulin in 1922 was particularly transformational. A year later, one notable clinical chairman observed, "The patient in early coma now recovers and does so within a few hours, in contrast to the previous almost certain death. The hopelessness of feeling when these patients are admitted has entirely disappeared."[50] The introduction of sulfonamides in the late 1930s had a similar effect, allowing mortality in bacterial pneumonia to fall from as high as 40 percent to less than 2 percent. To the noted cancer investigator Lewis Thomas, who was an intern at Boston City Hospital at the time, "The phenomenon was almost beyond belief."[51] Such developments allowed house officers and medical students after World War I a much more optimistic attitude than that of their predecessors, as they saw firsthand that the study of disease at the chemical and physiological level was delivering on its promise of better diagnosis and treatment.[52]

House officers were engaged in a journey of learning and self-discovery. The stronger the program and the better the resident, the truer this statement was. In the best situations, house officers were engaged in intellectual inquiry, not just job training. They were always asking questions, wondering "why?," not just "what should we do?" They regularly experienced the joy of discovering something new—if not to others, at least to themselves. They were treated as professionals, not schoolchildren, and they had the freedom to excel, with no ceiling on what they might learn or accomplish. They were inspired to think beyond the immediate needs of good medical practice to ponder what might be done in the future or how the profession might best fulfill its role in society. The passion some house officers demonstrated was extraordinary. One pediatrics resident at Johns Hopkins wanted to go Christmas shopping but could not find his hat. He then remembered that all he had was a straw hat since he had not been outside of the hospital since early October.[53] A neurology resident at Presbyterian Hospital worked 15 months without a vacation when he finally received 24 days off. He elected to use the time to take a summer course in neuroanatomy.[54]

In short, house officers, particularly at teaching hospitals, found meaning and joy in their work. They absorbed the spirit, not just the content, of medicine. Of course, there were trying and difficult moments along the way, and house officers everywhere were no strangers to stress, anxiety, and fatigue. However, on balance, their spirits usually remained buoyant. Complaints of abuse and expressions of frustration were few. Most felt they were receiving an educational return for their investment of time and energy. The phenomenon of "burnout"—defined as a state of emotional exhaustion, depersonalization, and decreased feeling of personal accomplishment—appears to have been rare.[55] In the language of the psychologist Howard Gardner, they were engaged in "good work"—work that ennobles the human spirit—as residents had been at the early Johns Hopkins Hospital.[56]

Indeed, in some cases, it was not entirely certain that house officers were working. Many felt they were playing. One intern at the Massachusetts General Hospital declared: "Medicine, to me . . . is forever interesting and stimulating. Much of the so-called work in it is really play and interesting recreation."[57] An intern at the University of Pennsylvania described his nights on call as "pure romance," even when repeatedly interrupted from sleep, while a Johns Hopkins house officer described himself as "fulfilled and happy."[58] To Lewis Thomas, who interned in internal medicine at Boston City Hospital in 1937, "No job I've ever held since graduating from medical school was as rewarding as my internship." Thomas insisted that this description of internship represented reality, not nostalgia. "I am remembering the internship through a haze of time cluttered by all sorts of memories of other jobs, but I haven't got it wrong nor am I romanticizing the experience. It was, simply, the best of times."[59] Admittedly, it tended to be outstanding house officers who described their experience in this fashion, sometimes after a lapse of time. However, there is a remarkable consistency in their accounts, and expressions of contrary sentiments do not begin to appear until after World War II.

House officers were aided in this journey by an environment that encouraged them to give everything to their training. Expectations of the resident staff were high; tolerance for shirking duty was low. This attitude was often conveyed by the department chair. At the Peter Bent Brigham Hospital, Henry Christian declared his "disgust for the medical man, who tells you how hard he works instead of telling you how much satisfaction and joy he finds in his professional work and study."[60] For the minority of house officers who married, spouses, as noted earlier, tended to support the high level of commitment to medicine of their physician-husbands. One surgical resident at Stanford wrote to a mentor: "Since I last wrote to you I have been married. This does not interfere with my work."[61] After the Johns Hopkins Hospital decided to allow house officers to marry, one faculty member noted approvingly that this was a good thing because the wives "frequently secure positions to bring in enough money to support their homes, and occasionally assist in the preparation of scientific papers."[62]

House officers also encouraged each other in their journey, as strong friendships grew and camaraderie typically ran high. They worked, ate, and lived together. The "midnight meal" and other occasions provided regular opportunities to discuss everything with each other—the condition of patients, a recent journal article, the large philosophical questions of medical practice, or the latest hospital gossip.[63] They often came to each other's aid—one intern helping an unusually busy fellow intern, knowing the friend would do the same if circumstances were reversed. Esprit de corps was heightened by parties and pranks: being caught and disciplined for staying out late or for some other breach of hospital decorum, getting away with the previous night's raucous party, or, famously at Johns Hopkins, surreptitiously placing a man's hat on the imposing statue of Christ in the hospital's front entrance.[64] A figurative family emerged, as house officers helped each other get through the process, and their friendships proved mutually sustaining in even the most challenging moments.

No one was more important to the metaphorical family than the department chair, who set the tone for the entire program. Chairs had many reasons to be concerned about the quality and well-being of the house staff because it was the house officers who provided the direct care to patients and served as an important pool for potential recruits to the department or hospital staff. But above all, most chairs were interested in their house staff because they enjoyed teaching and derived great personal satisfaction helping their residents mature into excellent physicians. A committed chief set a high intellectual and moral tone and left an imprint on his house officers that lasted for life. Most chiefs made certain that their house officers received credit for their work, as at the Peter Bent Brigham Hospital, where chiefs did not put their names on others' papers when they had not contributed to the work, and where house officers "almost without exception have felt that they would have complete credit for what they did."[65] Chiefs regularly assisted their residents in securing their next position, whether it be further training, an academic appointment, or private practice. And many residents, long after they had secured a permanent position, stayed in touch with their chief—seeking counsel and advice, a word of encouragement, or a photograph to display prominently at home or at the office.

Perhaps no one more fully epitomized the "personal chairman" than Henry A. Christian. To house officers at the Brigham, he was "Uncle Henry," his wife, "Aunt Bessie," and the house staff, "his boys." With his keen intellect, exacting standards, high ideals, and warm personality, it was said that he "created a spiritual atmosphere of the highest character" at the hospital—one in which he was "beloved by his pupils and associations."[66] He was deeply interested in his house officers, not just while they were in training but after they left, regardless of whether they pursued careers in academic medicine or private practice. In turn, his house officers were profoundly loyal to him. "I hope you realize how many men in this great country think of you with the love and reverence that only a father usually receives," one of them told him.[67] "My respect and love for you grow every day, Dr. Christian," said another.[68] His former house officers felt moved to keep him abreast with the details of their lives—the birth of a child, the death of a loved one, a fire in the home, or a professional success or disappointment. As one exuberant former resident wrote to him, "I can't get over the habit of telling you everything that happens to me. The latest is that I've fallen in love."[69] His high standards were imprinted on many of his house officers as a model of excellence for life. One wrote, "My personal admiration for you ever since 'Brigham days' has always led me to evaluate my own ability and accomplishments in terms of what you would think of them."[70] So, too, did Christian inspire his house officers to do their best throughout life. As Eugene Stead told him, "Every Brigham man feels that he must make good because he can't let 'the Professor' down."[71]

Thus, the residency was fraught with hard work, long hours, and innumerable anxieties and pressures. It also contained important mechanisms to help support the residents, including the camaraderie among the house staff and the caring and interest of the faculty. The better the program, the more satisfaction the house staff derived, for they saw that their hard work was bringing results in terms of their growth and maturation as physicians. The ingredients of outstanding programs were readily apparent: superior individuals serving as house officers, equally superior individuals on the faculty, the personal presence of the department chair and other faculty members, the dedication of the faculty to teaching and the welfare of the house staff, an intellectually rich learning environment concerned with the medicine of the future as well as that of the present, and the opportunity to work with intellectual freedom and responsibility. In short, the quality of the residency was ultimately determined by the conditions of work, not by the hours of work.

EDUCATION AND SERVICE

House officers had many important roles. They were learners, but they were also teachers, particularly of medical students and more junior house officers. Some were involved with research. All delivered patient care. Medical educators liked to view graduate medical education as a part of the medical education continuum. From this perspective, house officers were advanced students engaged in patient care as an essential part of their learning. The various educational roles of house officers provided the justification for not paying them salaries. House officers, in this view, were students, not employees. However, house officers had another role that was much less discussed: They were workers. In this role, they provided a variety of mundane services to the hospital for very little cost, and their attentive care of patients provided enormous benefit to the full-time and voluntary faculties.

The multiplicity of roles of house officers resulted from the dual roots of graduate medical education in the United States. The university influence was paramount in shaping graduate medical education, particularly at the residency level, much as it had previously shaped undergraduate medical education. However, graduate medical education also grew from the apprenticeship system, whose imprint was especially notable on the internship. As the internship and residency matured, the remnants of the apprenticeship remained clearly apparent. One leading surgical chief observed, the "germs of the apprenticeship relationship have infected the hospital. The concept of 'you help us and we'll show you how to earn a living,' the implicit *quid pro quo*, still lingers on."[72] Accordingly, virtually every hospital imposed many duties on its interns and residents that had little educational value, and elements of a labor-management relationship were everywhere present.

The worker role of house officers helped account for the remarkable growth of graduate medical education in the 1920s and 1930s. As noted earlier, after World War I the number of internship positions soared, and the number of residency positions grew as well. Though medical and hospital leaders liked to speak of the primary educational function of internships and residencies, in fact it was the work that house officers could do that propelled this rising demand for house officers. As one medical educator observed, "If the purpose of internships and residencies were purely or entirely educational, it is obvious that hospitals would not have increased their house staff members to the present high levels."[73]

All house officers—interns and residents alike—had routine chores. Administrative duties, such as arranging admissions and discharges, tended to be the responsibility of residents, while hands-on work, such as blood drawing or performing laboratory tests, tended to fall to the interns. Every program, of course, established its own specific rules—here, the resident was responsible for the discharge summary; there, it was the intern. However, in general, as the proverb declared, excrement rolled downhill, or, as an important department chair stated more delicately, "There is a tendency in the hierarchy of our staff for each one to shove off on the man of lower grade the chores from which he would fain escape."[74] This meant that most of the menial duties fell to the interns. The program at Vanderbilt was typical. There, according to one house officer, life was "hard on the internes but fine for the resident."[75] At teaching hospitals, the only medical professionals lower in rank than interns were the medical students. Because medical students truly were students—there was no ambiguity about their status as there was for house officers—interns were repeatedly instructed not to pawn off their duties on the students.[76] However, interns frequently ignored that admonition, and students commonly complained of being exploited—receiving too much "scut" (menial tasks) and too little teaching. Arguments could erupt between interns and medical students over the division of chores at any time.

Of course, hospitals were not alike in their attitudes toward house officers as workers. The greatest exploitation of house officers occurred at community hospitals that were not affiliated with medical schools. The smaller the hospital, the more severe the problem, with the greatest exploitation of house officers occurring at hospitals with fewer than 75 or 100 beds. Here, house officers were consumed by activities of little or no educational merit. An important report on graduate medical education in 1940 deplored these conditions. "No intern should be asked to waste his valuable time serving as a high-class orderly in a hospital."[77] Instead, hospitals should hire "salaried house officers," who were not interns or residents, to perform these duties.[78] In the growing competition among hospitals to recruit interns each year, many small hospitals could not fill their positions, despite offering unusually high salaries or sometimes establishing short residency programs as "bait."

However, the economic exploitation of house officers also occurred at teaching hospitals. Consider the internal medicine service at the Peter Bent Brigham Hospital. At the orientation meeting for the house staff each year, interns and residents were told that they should have "a clear understanding that they don't come here only to learn, but also to give service to the hospital. There will be many routines, such as we all have which have to be done even if it may not appear profitable."[79] Much of this work fell to the interns, but the residents also had plenty to do themselves, particularly as the volume of patients and amount of laboratory work grew year by year. In his reports, Henry Christian regularly argued that the service needed more house officers to allow each one more time for reflection and research.[80]

From World War I to World War II, the work required of house officers grew substantially. In part this resulted from greater volume and acuity of care on the clinical services: more patients, shortening length of stay, greater acuity of illness, more surgery, and the growing complexity of operative and medical care. The size of the house staff grew at virtually every hospital in response to these increasing demands, though the programs always seemed to be playing catch-up in trying to obtain enough house officers to keep up with the work.

The work of house officers also grew as diagnostic and therapeutic procedures became more numerous and complex. During World War I, laboratory work was largely confined to performing blood counts, examining blood smears, and performing urinalyses. By World War II, house officers also typed and crossed blood, performed bacteriological cultures, determined pH and oxygen concentrations in the blood, and measured the concentration of certain chemical constituents of blood, such as glucose. Between the wars, house officers began aspirating joints and performing lumbar punctures, thoracenteses (draining fluid from the chest), and paracenteses (draining fluid from the abdomen). The most time-consuming new medical treatment was immune therapy for pneumococcal pneumonia, introduced in the late 1930s. A house officer processed the patient's sputum with rabbit serum to determine which of the several dozen serological types of pneumococcus was involved, then administered a type-specific therapeutic anti-pneumococcal antiserum.[81] Curiously, if house officers ever showed signs of fatigue, older doctors sometimes called them lazy, illustrating the long-standing tendency of the older generation to think that the younger generation was soft.[82]

The great frustration from the house officers' perspective was that much of their work carried little educational value, could be done by others, or both. Phlebotomists or nurses could draw blood specimens and start intravenous lines, and trained technicians could perform laboratory procedures. Physicians were not needed to label specimens, carry specimens to the laboratory, return X-rays and hospital charts, or transport patients. These tasks could easily be performed by clerks, dispatch personnel, and orderlies. Yet these and other similar duties fell regularly to house officers—an unwelcome addition to the many more purely medical responsibilities they had.

Medical educators and residents alike understood that the taxonomy of house officers as either "students" or "employees" was too simplistic. In fact, house officers were both. There was much overlap between their duties as "students" and "employees." No service-oriented activity, such as drawing blood, was devoid of educational value. Performing such routine tasks provided house officers additional opportunities to be with their patients, perhaps allowing them to detect a change in condition that might otherwise have been missed. In addition, for house officers to be responsible for their patients' management, they had to be willing to perform chores: holding retractors during surgery, wheeling a patient to the X-ray department at midnight because no orderlies were on duty, or running an important specimen to the laboratory because a dispatcher was not immediately available. However, the problem for house officers was the excess of such chores and the expectation that they would provide such services for all patients, not just their own. Thus, they regularly drew blood from patients throughout the hospital because there were too few phlebotomists, made blood smears for patients they did not know because there were insufficient technicians, or held retractors late in the day on patients who were not theirs because the surgeon needed an extra pair of hands.

By the 1930s it was clear that hospitals and faculty alike benefited from the work of house officers. Hospitals benefited financially, much as they did from the work of student nurses. With house officers, hospitals needed to hire fewer clerks, dispatchers, orderlies, laboratory technicians, and phlebotomists. Private practitioners, both at teaching and community hospitals, knew that skilled physicians were watching their hospitalized patients. A good house staff allowed them more efficient days in the office and calmer, more restful nights and weekends at home. Full-time faculty similarly benefited. Relieved by house officers from many details of patient care, they were freed to devote more time to research and scholarship. Robert M. Heyssel, president of the Johns Hopkins Hospital from 1983 to 1992, pointed out that William Osler probably could not have written his textbook if not for the house staff being constantly on call and working up every new patient.[83] Every full-time clinical faculty member subsequent to Osler similarly profited from the efforts of house officers.

From World War I to World War II, graduate medical education grew and spread rapidly. In the process, hospitals and the medical profession were themselves transformed. During World War I, a house staff had been a luxury for hospitals. By World War II, a house staff had become an indispensable factor in the running of all but the smallest of hospitals. This fact was noted by the Massachusetts General Hospital.

> It would be utterly impossible to get the vast amount of detailed work which modern care of hospital patients demands, such as record taking and other paper work, examinations, routine and special, technical, diagnostic, and therapeutic procedures, laboratory work, assisting at operations, manning the emergency ward, and being on call for any bedside necessity, by means of a volunteer visiting staff. Were there no internes a paid permanent staff would be necessary.[84]

The average citizen had little idea of the critical role that house officers played in the daily work of American hospitals.

Before World War II, there were few complaints leveled against the residency system. House officers liked it. At the better programs, they felt they were getting a solid educational return that justified the hard work. In addition, they knew that a privileged position in society awaited them on the completion of training, making it difficult for them to identify with other groups of struggling laborers. Hospitals liked it as well. Having a house staff allowed them to provide better patient care and to save money in the process. Private practitioners and full-time faculty received important services that saved them considerable time and worry. The country became populated with excellent practitioners. However, as the residency system developed, the medical profession became vested in maintaining the educational status quo. That was because any change that might relieve house officers of nonprofessional duties would be costly to hospitals and faculty members in terms of time, money, or both.

CHAPTER 6
Consolidating the System

By the 1930s, the residency had become the most prestigious route to specialty practice in America. However, as seen earlier, it was not without competitors. Study in Europe, formal graduate study at a university, volunteer work in a specialty clinic at a teaching hospital, assisting an established specialist, attendance at postgraduate courses, and self-declaration provided alternative routes. Only with the emergence of the specialty boards in the 1930s did the residency become the sole route to specialty practice in America. This represented the second major reform in American medical education, analogous to the creation of the university medical school a generation before.

The residency system served the profession and country well, allowing great advances in both clinical science and the quality of specialty practice. Ironically, however, though the residency system arose as a manifestation of the university ideal in medical education, the university lost control of the residency system. Graduate medical education ultimately became hospital-based, unlike medical school, which remained under the aegis of the university. And though every patient could now take much greater confidence in the quality of care he or she received from a certified specialist, deeper concerns began to arise about the ability of the residency system to serve the broader societal needs of the American health care system.

THE SECOND REFORM OF MEDICAL EDUCATION

By the 1930s, the residency system was recognized as the soundest form of specialty training. Its success spoke for itself. Large numbers of excellent practitioners had been trained in the system, as had the overwhelming majority of younger academic leaders. The contrast between specialists trained in the residency system and earlier "specialists" was profound. In surgery, for instance, Allen O. Whipple, director of the surgical service at the Columbia-Presbyterian Medical Center, observed, "It is evident that carefully selected graduates from our own and other medical schools, with a year of training in general medicine and three to four years in surgery, are far more experienced and better trained than the former two-year intern finishing with a four to six months' service as House Surgeon."[1] The residency system was widely considered America's most unique contribution to medical education, and many gave it credit for the country's emerging leadership in medicine internationally.[2] As one sign of the growing strength of the residency system, the number of positions in "long residencies" (that is, three or more years of training) increased from 332 in 1934 to 1,791 in 1939.[3]

As the residency system grew in importance, other pathways to specialty practice declined in popularity. One was earning an advanced degree in a medical specialty through formal graduate study. Most medical graduates wanted to continue their studies as doctors, as they could in the residency system. Accordingly, formal graduate study faded away as a pathway of specialty training. In 1937, for instance, the faculty at Columbia ended its degree-granting program and merged it with the residency, and in the late 1930s other important institutions, such as the Massachusetts General Hospital, also concluded that the route to specialty training should exclusively be through the residency system and not a degree-granting program.[4]

Another pathway to specialty practice that lost popularity was study abroad. After World War I, American doctors resumed travel to the clinics of Germany and Austria for training in a clinical specialty, but in much lower numbers than before the war. This approach was taken mainly by medical graduates, especially Jewish physicians, unable to obtain residency positions in the United States. Learning a specialty through volunteer outpatient work in a hospital specialty clinic or as an assistant to an established specialist in practice also greatly declined in popularity, largely because these approaches were considered vastly inferior to the residency.

Nevertheless, through the late 1930s two alternative routes to specialty training remained vibrant, posing stiff competition to the residency system. One was the so-called short residency, offered largely by community hospitals. The standard "long residency" involved study of no fewer than three years of study. The "short residencies," most of which were twelve months in duration (Table 6.1),[5] provided far less time in study than the standard residency. In addition, they provided little teaching, meager exposure to research or the basic sciences, and much less responsibility for patient care. Some did not even have a program director.[6]

Table 6.1 SHORT RESIDENCIES IN THE UNITED STATES, 1934–39

Year	12 Mo.	18 Mo.	21 Mo.	24 Mo.	30 Mo.
1933–34	1,209	78	34	383	12
1934–35	1,819	53	35	237	7
1935–36	2,153	27	45	222	—
1936–37	1,163	65	50	766	8
1937–38	1,730	97	38	525	10
1938–39	1,695	60	24	980	6

The other route that remained popular, especially among established general practitioners who wished to become specialists, was taking short courses in a medical specialty. These courses, which typically were each two to six weeks in length, were offered by one of the country's thirty or so postgraduate medical schools, the majority of which were for-profit proprietary institutions. After completing "study" at a postgraduate school, physicians "graduated" and declared themselves specialists in that field. Self-declaration as a specialist was permissible and legal because possession of a state medical license granted the privilege to practice any area of medicine or surgery the physician wished. Some general practitioners took self-declaration a step further, limiting their practice to surgery or obstetrics or ophthalmology even without taking a course.

The problem with shortcuts to specialty practice was that patient interests were not served. This was true in every specialty. However, nowhere was it more evident than in the surgical fields, largely because poor results from surgery were immediately observable and could easily lead to maiming or death. Prominent university teachers of surgery generally maintained that a minimum of 1,000 hours of operating time over a six- or seven-year period was required to produce a highly qualified surgeon.[7] Yet many self-declared "surgeons" acquired their skills though a one- or two-week surgical course at a proprietary postgraduate school, where operations were conducted on cadavers or dogs but not human patients.[8] Moreover, university instructors of surgery regularly taught that surgical judgment was more important than operative technique. In a good residency, surgeons developed excellent diagnostic skills, shrewd clinical judgment, the knowledge of when not to operate, and the unwillingness to go beyond their ability or to tackle problems they were not qualified to address. The short specialty courses at proprietary schools did not teach these attitudes and skills.

An example of the horrors that could be wrought on patients by self-designated specialists involved a young woman in Chicago who had gone to a self-declared "plastic surgeon" to have an operation for what she thought were bowlegs. In fact, she did not have any curvature in the bones of her legs; she merely had more fat on the outer sides of her legs than on the inner sides, giving the false appearance of bowlegs. The normal anatomy of her bones would have been recognized by any legitimate orthopedist or plastic surgeon. However, the normal anatomy did not stop this "surgeon" from operating. He used a special orthopedic saw to cut the bones straight across at the midpoint of the shins. This instrument was never intended to be used for cutting bones crosswise; rather, it was meant for cutting bones lengthwise, as in taking out bone grafts. Misusing the instrument, the surgeon cut through the tibia and fibula of both legs, severing the blood vessels and nerves below each knee. Shortly thereafter, the woman developed gangrene of both legs, requiring bilateral amputations above the knees to save her life. All this for an operation that any well-trained orthopedic surgeon would have recognized should not have been done in the first place.[9]

Accordingly, to medical educators in the 1930s, specialty education in America stood desperately in need of reform. They believed that the public needed to be protected from superficial training and commercialism in graduate medical education, just as medical educators a generation before had argued that the public required such protection in undergraduate medical education. Medical educators deemed it morally unacceptable for physicians to practice beyond the limits of their training; they believed that doing so represented a profound violation of the public trust. Thus, they embarked on a campaign to make the "long residency" the sole method of entry into specialty practice, and they took dead aim at eliminating the "short residency," the brief postgraduate courses, and self-declaration as acceptable qualifications for specialty practice. The reform of specialty training became just as much a moral crusade to them as the reform of undergraduate medical education had been to their predecessors prior to World War I. This second reform movement was more muted in tone than the first, given the profound improvements in medical education that had already occurred and the absence of a muckraker comparable to Abraham Flexner. Nevertheless, the ideals and values were the same: the necessity of protecting the public and the importance of placing patients' interests first. Just as the reform impulse continued in American politics after the official "closing" of the progressive era during World War I, so it continued in medical education as well.[10]

These attitudes could be found among educational leaders in all medical specialties. However, no group of educators spoke more emphatically about the need to limit specialty training to graduates of the "long residency" than teachers of surgery. Eminent surgeons (and the major surgical organization, the American College of Surgeons, founded in 1913) became the leaders of the campaign to reform specialty training. They spoke repeatedly of the importance of proper training in surgery and all the surgical specialties; they regularly pointed out that completion of medical school and an internship, which typically prepared an individual well for general practice, did not qualify an individual to undertake major surgical operations. Surgical leaders viewed safe surgery as a moral and humanitarian goal, not as a strategy calculated to benefit surgeons. As one surgical teacher explained, the concept that surgeons should be thoroughly trained is based "on the principle that individual or private interests must be subordinated to public welfare," and he argued that specialty training, like undergraduate medical education, must serve "the public good."[11]

To underscore the reform spirit of champions of the residency, it is helpful to note that their efforts on behalf of the residency were intertwined with efforts to reform other aspects of the practice of specialty medicine. Once again, this was seen most clearly in surgery. As surgical leaders and the American College of Surgeons led the campaign to upgrade surgical training, they also lobbied vigorously against the widespread practices in surgery of advertising for patients, charging exorbitant fees, fee splitting (essentially a kickback from the operator to the referring physician), and ghost surgery. In addition, in its work in surgical education, it became clear to the American College of Surgeons that the training of a surgeon could not be separated from the level of excellence of the hospital in which the training occurred. For instance, the College discovered a deplorable condition of patient records at many hospitals. Surgeons at these institutions were not required to document the presumed diagnosis or reason for operating in the patient's chart, nor were they required to write daily progress notes. Thus, the College began its Hospital Standardization Program, with the goal of elevating standards at hospitals and providing accreditation to deserving institutions. In 1951 the Hospital Standardization Program evolved into the Joint Commission on Accreditation, which continued thereafter as the organization responsible for accrediting the nation's hospitals and as an important prod for improving the quality and safety of care.[12]

Thus, specialty education in the 1930s bore more than a few similarities to undergraduate medical education in the years before the Flexner report of 1910. In the early 1900s, the university medical schools were beginning to thrive, but they still faced stiff competition from dozens of proprietary medical schools offering inferior education to poorly prepared students willing to pay the fees. By the 1930s, commercialism had been contained at the level of the medical school but not in graduate medical education, where educationally undesirable pathways continued to compete with the residency system. The great challenge confronting graduate medical education on the eve of World War II was the lack of uniformity of specialty training and the low standards of entry to specialty practice. The residency system was proving a resounding success, but many so-called specialists were self-declared and poorly trained. To medical educators of the period, ensuring the qualifications of specialists assumed the dimensions of a moral crusade, just as ensuring the qualifications of general practitioners had been to medical educators a generation before.

THE RISE OF THE SPECIALTY BOARDS AND THE TRIUMPH OF RESIDENCY

In the 1930s, with the major problems of undergraduate medical education solved, medical educators focused increasingly on graduate medical education. Here, they found many similarities with the challenges they faced a generation before. The reform of undergraduate medical education required not just the creation of strong medical schools and teaching hospitals. It also required the elimination of the educationally inadequate proprietary schools. The problem of graduate medical education was similar. Comprehensive reform in specialty education demanded not only the development of a sound educational pathway—the residency—but also the elimination of unsound shortcuts into specialty practice.

The movement to reform specialty training in the United States was led by the specialty boards. These were professional organizations composed of representatives of the Council on Medical Education and Hospitals of the American Medical Association and the various specialty societies (for instance, the American College of Physicians for the American Board of Internal Medicine and the American College of Surgery for the American Board of Surgery). The first specialty board, the American Board of Ophthalmology, was organized in 1917; in the 1930s specialty boards in the other major fields appeared (Table 6.2).[13] Their work was aided by the Advisory Board for Medical Specialties, an umbrella group established in 1933 whose membership consisted of all the specialty boards.

The task of the specialty boards was two-fold. Most conspicuously, they evaluated candidates who wished to be certified as specialists in a particular field. This they did through administering a rigorous examination testing the candidates' knowledge and abilities. Each board determined the rules

Table 6.2 APPROVED EXAMINING BOARDS IN MEDICAL SPECIALTIES—1940

Name of Board	Year of Activation
American Board of Ophthalmology	1917
American Board of Otolaryngology	1924
American Board of Obstetrics and Gynecology	1930
American Board of Dermatology	1932
American Board of Pediatrics	1933
American Board of Orthopedic Surgery	1934
American Board of Psychiatry and Neurology	1934
American Board of Radiology	1935
American Board of Internal Medicine	1936
American Board of Pathology	1936
American Board of Anesthesiology	1937
American Board of Plastic Surgery	1937
American Board of Surgery	1937

and details of its own examination, and procedures frequently changed over time, but at the start the boards conducted their examinations in two parts: a written examination customarily taken at the time a candidate completed training, and an oral examination taken after several years of practice. In addition, the boards also specified what prior experience was necessary to qualify an individual to take the certifying examination. In the late 1930s, the Advisory Board for Medical Specialties adopted the requirement that, after 1942, all candidates for certification must have completed a satisfactory residency of at least three years in duration. By this decree, the "long residency" in an approved hospital became the sole acceptable route to specialty certification. In the late 1930s and early 1940s, the various alternative routes to specialty practice simply faded away.

What constituted an approved residency? Much more was involved than merely the length of time in study. It was necessary for the program to provide the residents graded responsibility in patient care, under the careful supervision of highly qualified instructors. It was also necessary for programs to meet specified standards in terms of the hospital staff organization, the educational program, the inpatient and outpatient clinical facilities, and the quality of the library, hospital laboratories, and pathology department. It was particularly important that the residency programs made provisions for instruction in the basic medical sciences related to the particular field, consisting of both didactic teaching and opportunities for independent study. The 1942 standards of the Advisory Board for Medical Specialties required a period of up to 18 months to be devoted to "graduate training in anatomy, physiology, pathology and the other basic medical sciences which are necessary to a proper understanding of the specialty in question."[14] An approved residency was expected to foster "the development of well-rounded clinicians able to appreciate and to assist in the advancement of medical science."[15]

The standards established for residency programs represented process measures, not outcome evaluations. No studies were performed comparing the results of residency training with any of the other approaches to specialty study, any more than randomized, double-blinded clinical studies were conducted to test the usefulness of insulin or penicillin. To observers at the time, the results were just too immediate and obvious to warrant further thought. As one report said of the value of the residency system, "The number of leaders in practice today who have been so trained is an adequate answer to it."[16] Accordingly, the goal in approving residency programs was to ensure that the identifiable components of a strong teaching program were all in place. The idea was that future specialists would receive the same opportunities that the leading current specialists had received.

The process measures put in place were considered inviolable. This was especially true of the specified length of training, which was required to be no less than three years in any specialty and as many as five years or more in the various surgical fields. At a time that a high school diploma was considered excellent preparation for most careers in the workplace, a few began to worry about the prolonged length of medical training. They argued that residency programs should focus on a person's actual attainments and not simply on the amount of time spent in training.[17] However, these pleas went unheeded. Medical educators almost universally felt that a graduate physician could not acquire proficiency in a specialty in a shorter period. Any effort to shorten the length of medical training, in their view, should focus on the medical school or premedical years.[18]

Who approved residency programs? At the start this issue caused considerable confusion. The boards offered one definition, the Council on Medical Education and Hospitals another, and the various specialty societies yet another. In general, the specialty societies placed greater emphasis on the training in the basic medical sciences than did the Council or the individual boards. This confusion was brought to an end by the creation of the Residency Review Committees (RRCs) in the various specialties. RRCs evolved from predecessor organizations, but in 1953 RRCs were officially organized in several fields, and soon thereafter every field had its own RRC. RRCs were tripartite committees; each RRC consisted of representatives from the Council on Medical Education and Hospitals, the specialty society in that particular field, and the corresponding specialty board. With the creation of the RRCs, a clear separation of responsibilities occurred in the governance of residency training: RRCs became responsible for the review and accreditation of programs; the specialty boards, for the examination of candidates.[19]

Major transitions are rarely easy, and such was the case with the establishment of the board certification system. In addition to the confusion surrounding the definition of an "approved" residency, considerable controversy ensued regarding the status of highly proficient specialists in practice whose education had preceded the establishment of the board system. In some cases, their formal study was not long enough to satisfy the new rules. A 45-year-old pediatrician or neurologist, for example, might have taken a university residency in the 1920s that at the time involved two years of study rather than three. Or that same 45-year-old individual might have taken a three-year residency that met the new requirements but had felt gunshy about taking an examination after so many years away from formal schooling. "One does not easily go back to that sort of thing [taking an examination] after being out of school for 24 years,"[20] one such individual remarked. Ultimately, many of these individuals were "grandfathered" as board certified, though fierce debates erupted over precisely which individuals merited "grandfathering," and many disappointed physicians had their requests for "grandfather" status rejected.[21] In addition, for many years the boards experienced intense pressure from doctors in practice to reduce standards or even to abandon their work.[22] However, the boards stood fast. In the late 1940s and early 1950s resistance to the boards from within the profession finally abated.

With the triumph of the residency system, the landscape of American medical education permanently changed. Proprietary postgraduate medical schools closed, as proprietary undergraduate medical schools had the generation before. Legitimate postgraduate schools, such as the New York Post-Graduate Medical School and Hospital, either discontinued operations or evolved into the continuing medical education department of an affiliated medical school. These institutions had labored hard and honestly during a simpler era in medicine, and their passage marked a sad, poignant moment. Short residencies, assisting established specialists, and other alternative routes to specialization disappeared. The language of graduate medical education became standardized. Everywhere the terms "intern" and "resident" came to connote the same specific level of experience and responsibilities, while the hodgepodge of alternative terminology ("extern," "resident intern," etc.) vanished. By the end of World War II, the new system was fully rationalized.

With the implementation of the new system, the home of graduate medical education became the hospital, not the medical school or university. This was a natural consequence of the need to study medicine where medical care was being provided and of the rise in importance of the hospital as the most important locus of patient care. However, the movement of graduate medical education into hospitals did not invalidate the notion that graduate medical education was a university activity. The emphasis of residency programs on the study of the basic sciences and on clinical research led to the view that residents were essentially indistinguishable from graduate students. Francis G. Blake, chair of the department of internal medicine at Yale, observed, "Graduate teaching of an excellent character, of course, already exists in the interne, resident, and fellowship programs as they have been developed in our better teaching hospitals throughout the country, even though it is not formalized under university auspices and does not lead to a doctorate in the medical sciences." Blake considered the residency system to represent "informal graduate teaching." He felt that formal study toward a graduate degree would "add little except another series of letters after a man's name."[23] His views were widely shared.

The triumph of the residency system did not occur without costs. Many older specialists, trained under earlier systems of instruction, found their stature in the profession to be diminished, for the public and profession now deemed them to be practicing beyond their level of competence. As one report carefully pointed out, the indictment of earlier methods of specialty training did not represent a criticism of the physicians themselves. Rather the indictment was of a casual system of specialty training that would not be acceptable in the future.[24] Nevertheless, the professional standing of these older specialists fell.

In addition, general practitioners fared poorly in the new system. The boards were created not to impose legal limitations on anyone's medical practice but to provide transparency, so that the public could recognize those specialists who were truly well trained. However, at the local level, board certification began to confer many advantages. In the post–World War II Veterans Administration medical system, certified specialists received higher pay. At many hospitals, particularly in larger communities, general practitioners were either denied admitting privileges or prohibited from operating on their patients or attending deliveries. Thus, George Heuer, one of Halsted's surgical chief residents and later chair of surgery at the University of Cincinnati and then Cornell, played a heroic role in the history of surgery for his numerous contributions to upgrading surgical education and practice.[25] However, he was detested by many general practitioners for his successful efforts to exclude them from performing much of the surgery that they formerly had done.[26]

Residency programs also learned there were costs associated with having a new regulatory system overseeing their work. Once the boards and RRCs were in place, residency programs, even the finest programs at the Massachusetts General Hospital, the Johns Hopkins Hospital, the Peter Bent Brigham Hospital, and other notable institutions, were bound to obey the new rules and dictates. Almost immediately medical educators began to complain about the rules the regulatory agencies sometimes passed. Evarts A. Graham, a great chest surgeon at Washington University who spearheaded the creation of the American Board of Surgery (he held certificate number one from the board), said later of the board he had helped establish, "I think we should encourage variations and departures from the more or less rigid schedule of training set down in the Board's requirements.... Let's not make every young surgeon do the goose step."[27] An important report in 1940 declared, "The emphasis should be on standards, not on standardization."[28] Yet the overarching direction was toward standardization. The same rules now applied to every program; there would be no exceptions. Medical educators were pleased to see that the new system, in effect, created a floor for specialty training—that is, minimum standards existed for all programs and all individuals. However, they began to worry that a ceiling might be imposed on outstanding programs that wanted to innovate or try something unconventional. Their concerns about the stultifying effects of regulatory bureaucracy did not diminish with time.

Medical schools, too, learned that there were costs to the establishment of new regulatory agencies. With this step, control of graduate medical education moved from the medical schools to the profession at large, unlike undergraduate medical education, which remained under the jurisdiction of the medical schools and their professional organization, the Association of American Medical Colleges. Medical school faculty members, of course, remained exceedingly influential in the new regulatory organizations. However, theirs was not the only voice, and many decisions were made that the academic representatives thought unwise. Curiously, this transfer of control of residency training from the university to the profession at large occurred by default, not by intent. Since World War I, major specialty organizations, including the American College of Physicians and the American College of Surgeons, had urged medical schools to assume corporate responsibility for all of residency training.[29] Medical faculties were warned, "If the schools do not take this responsibility [of regulating residency training], then the special certifying boards or other professional bodies will."[30] However, medical schools demurred, believing the task was too large. Accordingly, regulatory control, as predicted, fell to the profession as a whole—a circumstance many academic physicians later regretted.

The triumph of the residency system represented a major contribution to the nation's health. Patients were assured of high-quality specialists, just as a generation before they were assured of high-quality general practitioners. Of note, the initiative for the second reform of medical education came almost entirely from within the medical profession, unlike the first reform of medical education, where foundations, philanthropists, state governments, and the public at large clamored in support of the educational policies shaped by academic leaders. Also of note, the second reform of medical education demanded much greater courage on the part of medical leaders. Unlike the Flexnerian reforms, in which all doctors benefited from the imposition of higher standards, the triumph of residency pitted some doctors against others, and many physicians saw their practices suffer in this cause for the greater good. Doctors, in this case, regulated themselves, thereby demonstrating the capacity of the profession to work proactively for the public interest.

GRADUATE MEDICAL EDUCATION AND THE PUBLIC GOOD

By the end of World War II, the residency system had proven a spectacular success. During World War I, the US military found that the overwhelming majority of physicians calling themselves "specialists" were scandalously unqualified, and most were not permitted to serve.[31] In contrast, during World War II the high quality of American specialists allowed for unprecedentedly low death rates among sick or injured US troops.[32] Residents themselves benefited enormously. They received an excellent education and, once they completed a program, particularly at a notable teaching hospital, their futures were secure.[33] Patients also benefited. The quality of specialty care in the communities improved enormously as graduates of residency programs entered practice. For instance, Detroit was once considered to be "in the mire medically," but medical conditions in the city rapidly got better as an influx of young graduates of residency programs began "pushing things."[34] Clinical investigation prospered as well, as many products of the residency system began choosing careers in academic medicine. Early in his career, Henry A. Christian helped establish the American Society of Clinical Investigation (ASCI). However, as a result of the residency system, the number of clinical investigators grew so large that the ASCI could no longer accommodate young investigators. Accordingly, in the early 1940s Christian established the much larger and more democratic American Federation for Clinical Research so that all clinical investigators might belong to a professional society.[35] For all these reasons, one medical school dean in 1944 called graduate medical education "the outstanding feature of American medical education today."[36]

The residency system developed in response to the growth of specialization. Of note, in every case there were specialists before there were specialties. That is, the earliest specialists created a field themselves through their own investigations and practice. These imaginative pioneers were not formally trained in a specialty; rather, they were self-educated. Only later, as a field gained recognition, did leaders of that field establish residency programs and a specialty board. This process of informal beginnings followed by the creation of training programs and specialty boards occurred in every area of medicine and surgery before World War II and in all the specialties, subspecialties, and sub-subspecialties that proliferated with ever-increasing rapidity after the war.[37]

Specialization represented a logical response to the growth of medical knowledge, the development of new instruments and technologies, and the increasing complexity of medical practice. As Harvey Cushing put it, the various medical and surgical fields consistently "grow so large that they tend, through a process of mitosis, to separate off as independent units."[38] Medical specialization resonated with university scholars, so familiar themselves with the idea of discovering new knowledge and the resultant need to focus their investigations. The idea also resonated with the general public, for specialization and the division of labor were still part of the cultural and political mantra. Specialization also was fostered by changing social and economic conditions, such as the rapidly expanding populations of cities, which allowed doctors more opportunities to see cases that were statistically unusual.

However, more than the accumulation of knowledge accounted for the development of specialization. In particular, the boundaries of specialties typically represented contested terrain. Was child psychiatry a subspecialty of pediatrics or of psychiatry? Was dermatology a subspecialty of surgery or of internal medicine or a field of its own? As Rosemary Stevens has pointed out, these issues were hotly contested, and customarily the outcome was determined politically.[39] A particularly illustrative example of the negotiation of a field (or "social construction," using language popular among sociologists and historians of science) was the case of gynecology. From its beginning, the development of gynecology was closely associated with that of surgery and obstetrics—as evidenced by the title of the important journal *Surgery, Gynecology & Obstetrics* (or the "blue journal," as aficionados often called it, in reference to the color of its cover).[40] However, the identity of gynecology was fiercely debated. Variously, at different institutions at different times, it was its own department, a division of a surgery department, a division of an obstetrical department, or a co-equal with obstetrics in a combined department of obstetrics and gynecology. Only in the late 1950s did the debate end and the convention of a combined department of obstetrics and gynecology become established.[41]

The growth of specialization threw into sharp relief the long-standing tension in medicine between the holistic and the focused approach to patient care. From the time specialization began in the mid-nineteenth century, professional leaders warned against adopting too narrow a view of the patient, and they encouraged physicians to enter a specialty only after acquiring a sufficient knowledge of general medical principles. For instance, a report on graduate medical education in 1940 argued that "the specialist should be a broadly trained and well-educated physician first and a specialist second."[42] Along the way, however, the definition of "generalist" narrowed. Consider the case of gastroenterology. Before World War I, leaders of internal medicine regularly argued that a doctor must be a good general physician first, and only then a general internist. After World War I, professional leaders argued that one could not become a good gastroenterologist without first being a sound general internist. After World War II, the argument changed again: A physician must be a good general gastroenterologist first, and only then should that individual concentrate on hepatology (diseases of the liver). Later still, the view emerged that one must first be a good general hepatologist before subspecializing further in viral hepatitis, autoimmune hepatitis, cirrhosis, or some other specific disease of the liver. This inexorable march toward increasing specialization proceeded in every field of medicine, with generalism continually on the defensive and specialization always on the offensive.[43]

How many specialists did the country need, and what was the appropriate mix of specialists? This thorny question became increasingly problematic as the many forces promoting specialization grew stronger and stronger. General practice was declining in prestige, the public demand to see specialists was growing, and more and more medical students were hoping for careers as specialists. (Indeed, with its greater prestige, higher income, shorter hours, and fewer house calls, specialty practice carried a strong appeal to medical students.) No one knew how many specialists the country needed, or even how best to make that calculation. However, the consensus among medical educators and policy makers was that general practitioners would and should continue to provide the bulk of medical care in America. Estimates varied, but authorities typically maintained that

10 to 20 percent of the country's doctors should be full-time or part-time specialists.[44]

A great triumph of the residency system during the first half of the century was that it succeeded in meeting the perceived needs of the country in terms of the number of specialists produced. In 1938, of the country's 169,628 physicians, 33,618, or 19.8 percent, limited their practice to a specialty—a figure that included many older, self-named specialists.[45] In 1947, of the nation's 165,000 physicians, roughly 20,000, or about 12 percent, had been certified by a specialty board.[46] This congruence between the number of residents trained and the perceived national needs for specialists occurred because residency training programs practiced birth control. Specialty training programs intentionally limited the number of residents they accepted to allow close tutelage and to ensure that those residents seeking academic positions would have a reasonable chance at obtaining one. Hospitals and training program leaders believed it was in the best interests of society and of the profession as a whole not to attempt to make residencies available to all who desired them. As one report put it, "A man entering his internship has no assurance that he may later be able to obtain a satisfactory residency."[47] In this way, the aspirations of individual medical students for residency positions were subjugated to the larger goals of society—an unusual occurrence in a highly individualistic culture that much more often strove to expand rather than limit opportunities for the individual.

On the other hand, graduate medical education did much more poorly when it came to the geographic distribution of doctors. Since the beginning of the twentieth century, there had been a growing maldistribution of doctors between urban and rural areas, with cities attracting the lion's share of the physician workforce. This was true of general practitioners, not just specialists, despite the popular image of general practitioners as rural doctors. In 1947, nearly half of the country's general practitioners practiced in large cities with populations greater than 100,000.[48] To the Commission on Medical Education, a major study group sponsored by the Association of American Medical Colleges in 1932, "The greatest health problem of the country is that of making modern medical services available to the entire population."[49]

All century long, medical educators had found this situation deplorable, and many exhorted students and house officers to consider establishing rural practices. However, these efforts were to no avail. As another major study demonstrated, physicians' choice of a practice site reflected their response to professional, social, and financial incentives, and in these regards cities offered many more advantages than rural areas.[50] Physicians, in other words, had the same wants and needs as everyone else. Americans as a people were rapidly migrating to the cities, and the country as a whole was losing much of its rural character. These circumstances were beyond medicine's ability to control. Of course, with regard to where they practiced, doctors had a choice, unlike entry into a specialty, for which they had no guarantees. As physicians chose a location to practice, free-market forces reigned. There were no central controls, individual choices trumped perceived social needs, and rural areas suffered.

It would be a mistake to be too harsh on graduate medical education for the maldistribution of doctors, given the individual's freedom to choose a location of practice and the powerful market forces favoring cities. However, in another aspect of its work, graduate medical education was much more vulnerable to criticism. House officers practiced medicine in an extravagant fashion, regularly obtaining tests, X-rays, and procedures because they were there rather than because they were needed. The result was a conspicuous and unnecessary elevation of the costs of care—both at the teaching hospitals in which house officers trained, and subsequently in practice as doctors followed practice patterns they had learned as house officers.

Some escalation in testing was inevitable and appropriate. Scientific medicine had advanced tremendously, and with this the laboratory had become much more important in clinical care than before. Clinical research had provided one important contribution after another toward the diagnosis and treatment of disease, and these various tests and procedures were quickly transferred from the research lab to the clinical laboratory. House officers by 1940 needed to understand abnormal metabolism, blood changes, the results of bacteriological cultures, and chemical abnormalities within the body, along with an expanding menu of radiological procedures—all new developments of the preceding 25 years. In addition, some extra testing was necessary for learning purposes. House officers might debate on rounds whether a patient was borderline jaundiced and then order a serum bilirubin level to find out, in the process sharpening their clinical acumen whatever the result. And, of course, since they practiced at teaching hospitals, house officers frequently cared for unusually sick or complex patients, who required much more in the way of studies and procedures.

However, archival records of teaching hospitals consistently demonstrated a flagrant excessiveness in the test-ordering habits of house officers. If a patient was transferred from internal medicine to surgery, or from surgery to internal medicine, it was common for the resident staff to repeat all tests and examinations, even those just done.[51] At New York's

Babies Hospital, the pediatrics unit of the Columbia-Presbyterian Medical Center, authorities estimated that 70 percent of the laboratory studies ordered by house officers were of questionable value. They urged that routine examinations be reduced by at least one-third and that laboratory work be ordered much more discriminately, mainly in those specific situations where there was "some definite diagnostic or therapeutic need."[52] At the Hospital of Woman's Medical College of Pennsylvania, it was noted that "the calls for laboratory work are greatly in excess of those actually needed" and that "most of these superfluous tests are ordered [by house staff] on ward patients."[53] At Johns Hopkins, one authority complained that countless X-rays and laboratory tests "are ordered without any particular indication."[54] The most severe critics of house staff ordering practices, not surprisingly, were hospital administrators, charged with the task of paying for the care the residents provided to ward patients from the institution's habitually precarious charity budget. At Johns Hopkins, the hospital director pointed out that the "great extravagance" of house officers in ordering tests was the chief cause of the hospital's deficit.[55] Hospital costs before World War II were low enough that most hospitals managed to scrape through. However, interns and residents were learning extravagant practice styles.

Excessive testing by house officers usually reflected the way they were taught by the attending faculty. Faculty often labored under the erroneous view, described by one neurologist at the Columbia-Presbyterian Medical Center, that they owed patients "all the necessary tests and even some which were considered unnecessary," all for "the sake of completeness."[56] The stereotypical attending physician of the era was much more likely to scold a house officer for failing to obtain a test, even an obscure one, than to discuss with the house officer why certain tests might not be needed. At Johns Hopkins, Winford H. Smith, the hospital director, discussed this situation in detail. According to Smith, an inordinate amount of unnecessary studies was ordered "simply because the young house officer is afraid the chief or someone of his superiors will ask for it and will call him down if he hasn't it already." The solution, according to Smith, was for faculty to adopt a different, more careful approach with interns and residents. "If the younger staff members [house officers] were made to feel that they would be called down by their superiors just as hard for ordering X-rays, electrocardiograms, laboratory examinations, etc., which were not definitely indicated, this would save a lot of time and considerable money."[57] Ironically, Smith advocated exactly what the original Johns Hopkins faculty had stood for: teaching a parsimonious, problem-solving approach to patient care in which tests would be obtained only if they influenced management. Few faculty members in subsequent generations, at Johns Hopkins or elsewhere, upheld that ideal.

Medical educators before World War II took deserved pride in the work they were doing. They repeatedly pointed out that setting high standards in teaching, research, and patient care represented major contributions to the public good, and they were right. However, medical educators tended to look at medicine narrowly, with little concern for the costs or availability of care. So dedicated were they to their immediate work with patients, so high the cultural authority of medicine, so quiet the consumer voice, that at times it seemed as if all they wanted was for the public to support their important work and then leave them alone. A few warned of the danger of ignoring public sentiments or concerns. The internist Lewellys F. Barker of Johns Hopkins argued in 1942 that failure of the profession to assume leadership in addressing the broader issues of medical care "might lead to sudden and unwise legislation that would be harmful both to the profession and to the public."[58] For now, however, such pleas fell on deaf ears within the medical profession. It was for later generations of physicians to learn that the public could indeed express its wrath if it felt that the profession was heedless to its interests.

CHAPTER 7

The Expansion of the Residency in an Era of Abundance

After World War II the United States enjoyed unprecedented prosperity. The nation had become the world's preeminent economic, military, and political power. The citizenry now accepted a much larger, more active role of the federal government, and the country had evolved into a highly urban, technological, and industrial nation. Hopes and aspirations were high, as America rebuilt Europe, developed an interstate highway system, and sent a man to the moon.[1]

Fueling much of the postwar optimism was America's faith in science and medicine. Scientific research had been central to the country's military success. The physical sciences had produced radar and the atomic bomb, while medical research and care had paid off spectacularly in terms of saving lives, alleviating suffering, and helping the wounded recover. After the war the country's faith in scientific research, and in higher education more broadly, was tangibly demonstrated by the creation of the National Science Foundation, the expansion of the National Institutes of Health (NIH), and the enormous growth in the size, functions, responsibilities, and complexity of the research university, which Clark Kerr, the president of the University of California, famously named the "multiversity."[2]

For a generation following the war medicine basked in glory. The public image of physicians rose to unprecedented heights, and hopes for the future seemed limitless. In the 1950s and 1960s such faith seemed justified by the success of penicillin and other antibiotics, the development of the polio vaccine, and the invention of remarkable new technologies such as renal hemodialysis and cardiac catheterization. The dean of Harvard Medical School, writing in 1966, declared, "The fruits of medical research have outstripped even the most optimistic predictions of a generation ago, and a better-informed, better-educated public is insatiable in its demands for more knowledge and new victories over disease."[3]

In a prosperous nation, this faith in medicine brought renewed attention to health care. The result was a huge private and public investment in medical research, the spread of voluntary private medical insurance plans, and the enactment in 1965 of Medicare and Medicaid. Just as the research university evolved into the multiversity, medical schools and teaching hospitals were transformed into academic medical centers—large, complex institutions with greatly expanded roles in the delivery of medical care, medical research, research training, graduate medical education, and the instruction of allied medical personnel.

In this context new pressures were placed on the residency system. The demand for medical care was rapidly increasing, medical knowledge and technologies were growing with stunning speed, medical practice was becoming increasingly specialized, and hospitals were evolving into complex temples of technology. As a result, hospitals required more and more residents to ensure their effective operation. Faculty, with growing research and clinical responsibilities, also needed help from a larger resident staff, as did private practitioners, whose own practices were becoming busier and more demanding. Medical students aggressively sought out residencies, shunning careers in general practice for those in a specialty. After completing a residency, many pursued subspecialty training as well. Very quickly, a vastly expanded system of graduate medical education was in place.

From the beginning of the postwar expansion, the country's system of graduate medical education operated with distinction. America's acknowledged superiority in medicine was attributed in no small part to the residency system. The country's specialists and subspecialists were considered the best in the world. However, new challenges arose, in large part because of the tendency of doctors to concentrate on immediate professional concerns while giving less consideration to the problems of the health care system or the needs of the broader society. Most notably, as general practice precipitously fell in popularity as a career, many thought leaders and public officials began to worry that the country had too many specialists and too few primary care physicians. No one doubted that changing medical practice required more specialists than before, but the concern arose that graduate medical education had overshot the mark. In addition, residency training continued to occur in an environment of abundance where the resources were seemingly present for physicians to perform whatever tests or treatments they wished. The creation of third-party payers (insurance companies, Medicare, and Medicaid) only enhanced this sense within the profession that America was a society without limits. The result was the perpetuation of a wasteful practice style that created substantial unnecessary costs. Few people yet worried about the expense of care, and there were many reasons for rising medical costs beyond physicians' profligate practice styles. However, the forces leading medical costs to escalate were already in place, and one of the major reasons could be found within medical education.

FROM PRIVILEGE TO RIGHT

During World War II the residency system had been stretched to the limits. Both graduate and undergraduate medical education adopted accelerated programs of instruction to increase the output of physicians. Hospitals operated with skeleton house staffs because most residents had their hospital appointments interrupted to serve in the military. Faculty and nursing ranks were depleted as well, as many volunteered to serve in the theaters of war. Residents were in such sort supply that many hospitals, like the Cleveland Clinic, acknowledged looking for residents "with wooden legs, glass eyes, tuberculosis, and other lesions which incapacitate them for military service."[4] Somehow, academic medical centers continued to do good work. This resulted in no small part from the efforts of the house staff, which, in the view of leaders at the Massachusetts General Hospital, kept "the whole machine from breaking down."[5]

Medical educators knew that graduate medical education would be challenged after the war as well. Physicians who had served in the military would need refresher courses to become familiar with the scientific and clinical developments that had occurred during the interim. Accordingly, one medical center after another made plans to establish refresher programs for returning medical veterans to facilitate their return to practice.[6] In addition, physicians who had had their residencies interrupted would need opportunities to complete their residencies after returning home. Thus, teaching hospitals typically made plans to increase the size of their resident staff to accommodate returning veterans who had started in their programs.[7]

Most medical educators expected the pressure on graduate medical education to last for only a few years. They did not expect it to take long for returning veterans to take the necessary refresher courses or complete their residencies. Medical educators anticipated that most medical veterans would enter or reenter general practice. Accordingly, educators believed that the greatest pressure on faculties would be in providing continuing medical education courses to medical veterans. For instance, the Council on Medical Education and Hospitals of the American Medical Association (AMA) expected that the most important postwar work in graduate medical education would be providing "opportunities for individuals desiring refresher courses as a basis for reentering practice" and that the postwar pressures on graduate medical education would last only "temporarily."[8]

To the surprise of medical educators, this proved not to be the case. Overwhelmingly, medical veterans wanted residencies, not refresher courses. Over two-thirds of military physicians expressed a desire to become certified specialists. This figure included large numbers of older physicians who had been in general practice for many years prior to enlisting in the military.[9] A chastened Council on Medical Education and Hospitals acknowledged that it had greatly underestimated the strong demand for residency positions that followed the war.[10]

World War II irrevocably altered physicians' attitudes toward specialization. In the military, doctors who were certified specialists or well along in their residencies received higher rank, more pay, and greater professional responsibility than general practitioners. Specialists and advanced residents received preferred assignments in military hospitals, while lesser-trained physicians generally became battalion surgeons or were assigned to induction stations. Seniority, age, or extensive experience in general practice did not matter to the military officials; specialty training did. As a result, specialists found their professional status suddenly upgraded, while general practitioners experienced a corresponding diminishment. After the war, thousands of returning medical veterans sought to become specialists, stimulated largely "by the great importance given to it [specialization] in the armed forces during the war."[11] By 1951 the number of certified specialists had tripled from 1940.[12]

The demand for residency positions proved not to be temporary. In 1947, an official at one state medical school noted that its students "decry preparation for general practice,"[13] a phenomenon now observed at most medical schools. By 1963, 83 percent of graduating medical students sought careers as specialists rather than as general practitioners.[14] The reasons for this were not hard to find—the rapid expansion of medical knowledge, the growing procedural complexity of medical practice, the increasing disparity in income and social prestige between specialists and general practitioners, and the replacement of generalists by NIH-trained subspecialists as attending physicians, thereby providing students fewer role models of physicians comfortable managing a broad range of illnesses on their own.[15] Now, through the military, the federal government had given its stamp of approval to specialization.

Although the demand for residency positions became intense after World War II, the desire of physicians to specialize was not new. Rather, what was new was the enormous increase in the opportunities for specialty training. The spread of private medical insurance after the war, coupled with the growing complexity of hospital-based medicine, led to hospitals becoming much busier. Before the war hospitals successfully operated with small house staffs; now they needed many more house officers to tend to the vast amount of moment-to-moment care. Attending medical and surgical staffs supported (and lobbied for) the enlargement of their house staffs, knowing that delegation of clinical responsibility to house officers allowed them more time for research, practice, other professional duties, or leisure. Accordingly, both community and teaching hospitals clamored for more and more interns and residents. By 1970 US hospitals offered 46,250 residency positions, compared with 5,796 in 1940.[16] New York was the state most prominent in graduate medical education, offering one-sixth of the country's internships and one-sixth of the residencies.[17]

Some of the expansion of the residency system occurred at existing teaching hospitals. During the postwar years, the "pyramid" system gave way to the "parallel" system, introduced before the war at the Mayo Clinic, in which every individual admitted into a program had the opportunity to complete the program.[18] In 1927, when the first list of approved internships was published, there were three times as many interns as residents in the country. By the 1960s, there were three times as many residents as interns.[19] At most academic medical centers, the number of house officers soon exceeded the number of medical students in the hospital. For instance, by 1952, the Columbia-Presbyterian Medical Center had 229 residents; by 1955, the New York Hospital had 178.[20] There seemed to be no end to this expansion. Thus, in 1979 the Massachusetts General Hospital had 390 residents, 203 clinical fellows, and 137 research fellows.[21]

With the number of residents growing so rapidly, many academic medical centers began to worry about being able to provide their house officers enough clinical experience. This was a particular concern in general surgery, the surgical subspecialties, and obstetrics and gynecology, where the limiting factor in the number of residents that could be trained was the amount of surgical "material" available for actual operating experience. Accordingly, academic medical centers began to develop affiliations with carefully selected hospitals in order to obtain enough patients to serve the educational needs of their residents. Typically, residents at the teaching hospital took rotations at the affiliate, while the affiliate, if it had its own residency program, sometimes sent its residents to the teaching hospital for instruction. A prominent example was the affiliation between the

New York Hospital-Cornell Medical Center and the North Shore General Hospital in Long Island. During this period the Veterans Administration hospitals became important educational partners with academic medical centers, ultimately accommodating roughly 10 percent of the country's residents. Municipal hospitals continued their important role in residency training. Some, such as Boston City Hospital, were major academic centers in their own right with their own house staffs; others, such as St. Louis City Hospital, were affiliated with nearby medical schools, which sent them residents.

Academic medical centers, of course, had no monopoly on graduate medical education. Most of the expansion of the residency system occurred at community hospitals unaffiliated with medical schools. Indeed, in 1955, 80 percent of approved residencies were found at such institutions.[22] Some of these provided excellent educational opportunities. The Newark Beth Israel Hospital, whose history has been skillfully recounted by Alan and Deborah Kraut, was one such institution.[23] However, large numbers of community hospitals sought residents mainly for prestige, the work they could provide, and the conveniences they could offer the private medical staff. Such programs met stated requirements regarding the adequacy of the physical facilities, the number of beds, the quality of the clinical laboratories, and the size of the professional staff, but they exhibited a marked indifference to education. House officers there received little autonomy, teaching, or inspiration, and the educational reputation of these institutions suffered. Positions at many of them often went unfilled.

At all hospitals, the expansion of the residency programs was driven by the need to provide clinical services. In every specialty at every hospital, growing clinical demands led to calls for more interns, residents, and specialty fellows. If good educational opportunities could be provided, so much the better, and the leading hospitals did an excellent job of keeping their teaching responsibilities in focus as they grew larger and busier. However, even at the most prominent teaching institutions, the driving force for growth was a larger and busier clinical service. Time and time again, the chief of pediatrics here, neurology there, and radiology somewhere else sought additional house officers—all because of a larger number of patients, the increased severity of illness, and the growing complexity of care.

Fueling the expansion of the residency system were the financial resources and political support that only a wealthy country that valued medical care could provide. Graduate medical education was becoming expensive to support—not only because of the need to pay faculty, keep malpractice premiums current, and provide educational resources, but also because house officers had begun to demand and receive salaries. These expenses were paid for by revenues hospitals received for patient care—initially, from Blue Cross and other private insurers; after 1965, from the Medicare program as well. In addition, many new opportunities for specialists to practice were becoming available. The Hill-Burton Act of 1946 provided matching federal funds to communities wishing to build a hospital. The result was a building boom in hospital construction, particularly in smaller communities. This provided physicians a strong inducement to pursue a residency, now that the facilities they needed to do quality work in a specialty were more widely available.[24]

Particularly important in the financing of residency training was Medicare, which quickly became graduate medical education's largest funder. Medicare provided hospitals payments for both the salaries of house officers and teaching faculty ("direct" graduate medical education payments) and the additional expenses hospitals incurred by virtue of being teaching institutions, such as a sicker patient mix with longer lengths of stay ("indirect" graduate medical education payments).[25] By the 1970s, graduate medical education had become a major financial item for hospitals, accounting for 3 to 4 percent of the operating budget. In the late 1970s, for example, the residency program was a $5,000,000 item at Presbyterian Hospital (New York) and a nearly $7,000,000 item at the Massachusetts General Hospital.[26]

The residency, of course, was related to the internship. Gone was the potpourri of internships of different lengths of time; now internships were universally one-year experiences typically taken immediately following medical school. In the postwar era, medical students wishing to specialize usually chose "straight" internships in a particular specialty. "Straight" internships, though called "internships," in fact represented the first year of a multiyear specialty residency. (A small number of aspiring specialists still took "rotating" internships followed by a residency.) Competition for positions was fierce, putting both hospitals and medical students on edge. Hospitals wanted to fill their quotas with outstanding students. That way they could provide patients excellent care and also have a strong pool for future recruitment to the faculty and clinical staff. Students, in turn, wanted the top programs, both for their immediate educational value as well as for a head start for the future. Having a distinguished educational pedigree and prominent faculty supporters helped open professional doors.

Although the recruitment of interns caused considerable nervousness everywhere, the process became organized and much fairer with the creation of the National Intern Matching Program, colloquially known as "the Match." The Match arose from the pronounced dissatisfaction students and some hospitals had with the traditional rat race where students scrambled to find an internship and were often pressured by hospitals to make early commitments. In the new system, which was developed with considerable student input, the Match served as a clearinghouse for the preferences of both students and hospitals. Students provided the Match a list of hospitals where they wished to be considered, ranked in order of preference, and hospitals supplied the Match a ranked list of the students who had applied to them for positions. Students were "matched" to the highest internship on their list that had an opening for them. Whether there was an opening for a student was determined by whether positions had been filled by applicants that the program had ranked higher. The new system, deemed "a democratic plan in the American tradition,"[27] assured students that they would receive their best choice available, and it was also fair to hospitals. After a trial run in 1951, the Match was implemented for the 1951–52 academic year. Satisfaction among all participants with the new system was high.[28]

Hospitals competed vigorously with each other to attract the best students. Students took many factors into consideration when compiling their rank lists, such as geographical location, the vibrancy of the city, housing, the neighborhood surrounding the medical center (in this regard, some important academic centers like Johns Hopkins and Columbia-Presbyterian began finding themselves at a disadvantage because of the deteriorating neighborhoods in which they were located),[29] proximity (or distance) from family, the institutional culture, the degree of camaraderie within the program, and opportunities for spouses. As house officers began receiving salaries, the fierce competition for interns allowed students to consider salary levels as another ingredient of their decision making. Thus, the University of Arkansas, which at the time was paying the lowest intern salaries in the South, found it had to increase compensation to become more competitive in recruitment.[30] Word of mouth also mattered. For instance, one graduate of the Boston University School of Medicine had a wonderful experience as an intern at Beverly Hospital, an excellent community hospital in Beverly, Massachusetts. The following year one-third of the graduating class of Boston University applied for an internship at that hospital.[31] As always, students and house officers voted with their feet, and collectively they had considerable power to influence training programs.

What mattered most to students seeking internships, however, was the quality of a hospital's educational program. As the Council on Medical Education and Hospitals noted, in the selection of a training hospital for internship, "Apartments, tennis courts, and television do not replace graded clinical responsibility under first-class teaching clinicians and scientists."[32] In this regard teaching hospitals enjoyed significant advantages over community hospitals. The lure of teaching hospitals had always been present, but the Match demonstrated that point convincingly. Each year, most teaching hospitals filled their positions, having to turn away many applicants in the process. Competition for places at the elite teaching hospitals was particularly formidable. In 1959, the department of medicine of the Massachusetts General Hospital received 178 applications, all from students at the very top of their respective classes, for 12 internal medicine internships.[33] In contrast, many community hospitals could not attract a single intern, and some did not receive a single application. In 1954, of roughly 800 hospitals participating in the Match, 146 completely filled their positions, while 284 hospitals did not get a single intern. The Council on Medical Education and Hospitals spoke of these two groups as "the 'alls' and the 'nones'"—the "alls" being mainly teaching hospitals, the "nones" consisting entirely of community hospitals.[34]

As the demand for house officers increased, a shortage developed, particularly for interns. In 1952, for instance, approximately 10,500 internship positions were available, but there were only 5,800 medical graduates to fill them.[35] As a result, many hospitals, particularly community hospitals, began to recruit foreign medical graduates to their house staffs. This practice intensified after 1965, when the Immigration and Naturalization Act Amendment terminated the national quota system previously in effect. This bill also assigned preferential immigration status to professionals in areas presumed to be in short supply nationwide, one of which was medicine. The result was an even greater influx of graduates of foreign medical schools, especially from underdeveloped countries, into the United States for internship and residency training. By the late 1960s, roughly one-third of interns and residents in the United States were graduates of foreign medical schools. Even so, the demand of hospitals for house officers could not be fully met, and 20 percent of approved internship and residency positions still went unfilled.[36]

With the expansion of graduate medical education, the residency system became much different from what it had been at the beginning. The residency of Osler and Halsted was intended for a small number of carefully selected individuals with exceptional scientific ability. The residency at that time proved a fertile training ground for those wishing to pursue careers in clinical science and academic medicine. The post–World War II residency became open to any US medical graduate who desired to enter specialty practice. Thus, the residency system became "democratized."[37] Not surprisingly, relatively few physicians progressed from residency into clinical investigation, a fact lamented by some academicians. On the other hand, virtually everyone who entered medicine was capable and dedicated, even those without the attributes necessary to be successful at clinical research. The transformation of residency from a privilege into a right allowed all doctors the opportunity to pursue their interests and to work to the maximum of their capability.

As the residency system became democratized, traditional barriers based on religion, gender, and race dramatically lessened. For instance, in the 1950s religious quotas ended. Talented Jewish physicians, who formerly had flocked to Mount Sinai Hospital (New York), making it one of the leading teaching hospitals in the world, began passing over Mount Sinai to pursue residency opportunities at prestigious teaching hospitals affiliated with strong medical schools. Accordingly, Mount Sinai had to build its own medical school so that it could remain competitive as a teaching institution.[38] Similarly, women physicians, though still few in number, found that virtually all hospitals were now willing to accommodate them as house officers, although some fields, such as pediatrics, were more hospitable to female residents than others, such as surgery.[39] African-American physicians, even fewer in number than women physicians, also found doors opening at most teaching hospitals, a process that was cemented in the late 1960s after the civil rights movement had gained momentum. Howard University Hospital, once the crown jewel of graduate medical education for blacks, began losing desirable candidates to other academic medical centers, and other traditionally important black teaching hospitals, such as Homer G. Phillips Hospital in St. Louis and Kansas City General Hospital Number 2, were forced to close.[40] For both women and African-Americans, full equality required a supportive environment and equal treatment with white males—all of which were much slower to arrive. With residency positions becoming more widely available, however, a start had been made.

As always, there were inevitable tradeoffs in the expansion of the residency system. As the system grew, its regulation became increasingly rigid and bureaucratic. Control of the internship and residency remained fragmented among a large and confusing array of agencies: the specialty boards, Residency Review Committees, Association of American Medical Colleges, and AMA, among others. As before the war, regulating bodies remained focused on time requirements and educational processes. The result was considerable inflexibility. For instance, there was no acknowledgment that some trainees might be able to advance more quickly than others; all residents were bound to the same lock-step rules dictated by the boards. Many young physicians were refused the opportunity to take board examinations because they lacked two or three weeks of the prescribed training time. Programs that wished to try new designs and educational approaches found it difficult to do so.[41]

In the regulation of graduate medical education, the university had little say, compared with its pronounced impact on undergraduate medical education. Medical schools and universities, of course, greatly influenced the content and methods of graduate medical education. However, they did not evaluate, monitor, or regulate it since before the war they had ceded that responsibility to the profession at large. In 1966 two widely publicized reports—the Millis report of the AMA and the Coggeshall report of the Association of American Medical Colleges—urged universities to assume greater responsibility for the conduct and control of the entire continuum of medical education.[42] However, the die had already been cast, and the regulatory landscape of graduate medical education remained unchanged. In 1973 a close observer of graduate medical education spoke of its "dysmorphic accreditation system."[43]

As the enterprise of graduate medical education grew, it also became dependent on the third-party payers that funded it. After its enactment, Medicare became the most important payer. Ironically, Medicare funding allowed programs to do excellent professional work, but in the process it caused them to become hidebound. Medicare's direct and indirect graduate medical education payments were tied to the care that house officers provided to hospitalized patients. These payments did not cover the work that house officers did in any ambulatory sites outside of the hospital's teaching clinics and emergency rooms, such as in health maintenance organizations, doctors' offices, or community clinics. Medicare regulations thus made experimentation in ambulatory settings extremely difficult financially for teaching institutions, even as the need to provide residents ambulatory experiences grew over time. Beginning in the 1970s, many calls were made to reform this aspect of the payment system, but these calls have been ineffectual.

The transformation of residency from a privilege to a right reshaped the contour of medical education. Originally, the MD degree stood as an indicator of a physician's readiness for assuming full professional responsibility. For the majority of doctors who now pursued specialty training, the professional degree in medicine was being awarded halfway through the required course of study or, in many specialties, less than halfway. Medical educators observed that most of the knowledge, skills, attitudes, and behaviors of doctors in their day-to-day practice of a specialty were determined by their residency and fellowship rather than their experiences in medical school.[44] Whereas the purpose of medical school was once to prepare medical students for practice, its function now was to prepare medical students for residency.

THE MATURATION OF CLINICAL SCIENCE AND THE CREATION OF SUBSPECIALTY FELLOWSHIPS

The multiversity of Clark Kerr fostered the rapid expansion of knowledge in all areas of scholarship. Research, of course, had long been a growth industry at US universities, but the NIH, National Science Foundation, and other public and private funding agencies allowed the pace of discovery to accelerate rapidly. Specialization became a necessity in all fields, fostered by the explosion of knowledge and the increasing sophistication of research methods and techniques in every area of human inquiry.

Medicine, of course, participated in the proliferation of knowledge. During the postwar period, clinical research became much more scientifically sophisticated. Observational studies of patients yielded less and less in the way of new fundamental knowledge. Instead, biochemistry, physiology, immunology, and, increasingly, molecular biology and cellular physiology provided the dominant routes to medical discovery. Clinical science became more and more "reductionist," with its gaze shifting to ever-smaller particles, such as genes, molecules, proteins, antibodies, receptors, and chemical agonists and antagonists, and with investigators studying mice, bacteria, viruses, and tissue cultures. As one manifestation of this change, increasing numbers of researchers with PhD degrees began receiving appointments in the clinical departments of medical schools. As early as 1953, the Massachusetts General Hospital already had more than a score of research scientists with doctorates in its clinical departments who devoted their entire time to laboratory investigation—a number that continued to grow larger over time.[45]

The increasing sophistication of clinical science greatly affected the residency system. It became clear that physicians could no longer acquire the scientific expertise during residency to emerge as mature, independent clinical investigators. "The day when a few animal operations provided the basis for a surgical contribution is forever past,"[46] surgical residents at the Peter Bent Brigham Hospital were told in 1953. Indeed, the legendary chief of surgery at the hospital, Francis D. Moore, criticized those departments that required every resident to go to the laboratory or publish a certain number of papers: "This has produced laboratory drones rather than scholars and trash rather than literature."[47] In short, the residency system, originally created to prepare scientific leaders, now found that much of its value as preparation for an academic career had diminished. Residency still provided invaluable clinical training but not the concomitant preparation for a career in clinical science.

This is not to say that research disappeared from residency programs. Many faculty leaders continued to emphasize the importance of research for residents. Particularly at the better teaching hospitals, residents in every specialty could be found conducting clinical studies, engaging in laboratory projects, and sometimes publishing. Unlike before, however, such experiences were not intended to prepare a person for a career in clinical research. Rather, they were meant to enhance the educational value of residency and provide a way whereby residents could decide if they wished to pursue further training in clinical research. Thus, surgical house officers at the Peter Bent Brigham Hospital were told that every surgical resident "should spend a part of his time asking questions about surgery. . . . It makes little difference whether or not he plans investigative surgery as a career."[48]

The proliferation of knowledge also reshaped the traditional clinical goals of the residency system. For many decades, residency training had brought medical graduates to the cutting edge of specialty care. After the war, that objective could no longer be met. Increasingly, it became clear that no one could master a broad specialty like pediatrics, surgery, obstetrics and gynecology, or internal medicine. Instead, specialties began to divide into smaller units. Internists began to subspecialize in rheumatology or cardiology; obstetricians and gynecologists, in high-risk pregnancy or infertility; ophthalmologists, in diseases of the retina or cornea. Even the most talented clinicians had to subspecialize if mastery of a particular area was their objective.

The creation of subspecialties, like that of specialties, began informally. There were subspecialists and, soon, sub-subspecialists before there were subspecialties and sub-subspecialties. As described by W. Bruce Fye, the research interests of investigators in a specialty led them to focus on smaller and smaller areas within that specialty. Eventually, a critical mass of clinical knowledge, special techniques, and professional leaders was achieved, allowing subspecialty training programs to be organized, accreditation of programs to be granted, and board certification to be offered.[49]

The case of thoracic surgery is illustrative. Originally, the American Association for Thoracic Surgery was open to investigators in any area who had advanced knowledge relevant to chest surgery. This included internists, radiologists, physiologists, and others. The founders of thoracic surgery, such as Evarts Graham of Washington University and Edward Churchill of Massachusetts General Hospital, were self-trained in the field. These early leaders opposed the formation of a subspecialty board in the field, an idea that one called "an abomination."[50] However, many others quickly entered thoracic surgery, the field advanced, and soon formal training programs and a subspecialty board were organized. Membership in the American Association for Thoracic Surgery became limited to board-certified thoracic surgeons. To Churchill, the new membership requirement marked "the death knell of the Association as I have known it."[51]

To meet the scientific and clinical challenges imposed by the prolifera tion of knowledge, an additional training step after residency—the clinical fellowship—appeared. After the war clinical fellowships became the standard vehicle for entry into a medical subspecialty. They provided both an educational experience for those who wished to practice a clinical subspecialty and an opportunity to acquire advanced research training for those considering a career in clinical research. Thus, they represented what residency had once been: an advanced clinical experience for mature physicians to become expert in a defined clinical field and an opportunity to acquire laboratory skills for those hoping to pursue an academic career. Subspecialty fellowships in a few fields had been offered before World War II, but after the war they proliferated and became formally integrated into the structure of graduate medical education.

The route to subspecialty practice depended very much on the field. In internal medicine, pediatrics, neurology, and other nonsurgical fields, physicians took a clinical fellowship after the completion of their residency. Upon finishing the fellowship, individuals became eligible to take the subspecialty board examination in their field for certification. In the surgical fields, subspecialty fellowships also appeared. However, the greater length of time of residencies in general surgery and some surgical subspecialties offered more opportunity for research than residencies in nonsurgical specialties. In the surgical fields, particularly at prominent teaching hospitals, residents continued to engage in research for one or two years as part of the residency experience. Accordingly, many surgeons became better prepared during residency to engage in independent research than their counterparts in other disciplines. Thus the imperative for a fellowship after residency was less, at least from the perspective of learning how to do clinical research. It was not until a generation later that the practice of taking additional fellowship training following residency became a more common occurrence in surgery.

Clinical fellowships shared certain features in common. At the beginning, they were short—often one year in length, sometimes two. By the 1970s some subspecialty fellowships were two years in length, and many by then were three years. Subspecialty fellowships typically offered both advanced clinical training and a sophisticated experience in clinical research. These components were usually demarcated. In a typical three-year fellowship, the first year was heavily clinical, while the last two years were devoted mainly to research. Those aspiring to academic careers often found the research experience of even a clinical fellowship to be insufficient. Accordingly, many undertook additional scientific study, obtaining a PhD in a basic science or spending another two or three years in a laboratory at the NIH.

Subspecialty fellowships also represented the most variable part of medical education. Fellows during their research years worked with a particular mentor on a particular problem, much as doctoral students worked closely with a particular PhD adviser. Fellows enjoyed a close day-to-day relationship with their adviser, and no two fellows had the same experience. Unlike graduate study leading to a PhD degree, there were few formal requirements, little that resembled a schedule, and nothing in the nature of a formal examination. By and large, the success of the fellowship was judged by the future productivity of the fellow.

Subspecialty fellowships grew in number with amazing rapidity in the two decades following the war. Within a generation there were more fellows than residents at many teaching hospitals. For instance, in 1964–65, there were 246 subspecialty fellows at the Massachusetts General Hospital, compared with 180 residents.[52] Fueling the growth of subspecialists was the NIH, which provided medical faculties with training grants to support subspecialty fellows, particularly during the research years. (Fellows doing clinical work were usually supported by patient-care revenues.) Many private foundations also helped fund fellowships. For instance, in the early 1960s, the Josiah Macy Jr. Foundation, whose important role in medical education is often underappreciated, provided certain departments of obstetrics and gynecology with training grants to prepare young specialists in the field for careers in academic medicine.[53] Also fueling the growth of the subspecialty fellowship system was the intense desire of residents themselves to pursue subspecialty training. In the 1950s and 1960s, subspecialty fellowships, like residency positions, became a right, not a privilege, of trainees. Fellowship positions became available to virtually everyone who wanted one—if not in one's desired field or hospital, then at a second or third choice.

Like residency positions, subspecialty fellowships were initially intended for exceptional individuals with academic aspirations. The fact that much of the funding for fellowship programs came from the NIH and that fellows typically were paid by the university (in contrast to residents, whose paychecks customarily came from the hospital) underscored that point. However, the fellowship system proved inefficient at producing clinical investigators. As the number of fellowship openings soared, and as opportunities became available for the rank and file, the great majority of physicians saw subspecialty training as a route to private practice rather than to an academic career. In the 1970s, for instance, the Johns Hopkins faculty discussed how few cardiology fellows nationwide were entering academic medicine and how many gastroenterologists were devoting their time mainly to performing endoscopies.[54] It was estimated that only 6 percent of subspecialty fellows in internal medicine departments were serious about academic career.[55] Subspecialty fellowship programs produced many fine investigators and teachers, but they represented only a small fraction of those who took fellowships.

Both specialization and subspecialization in medicine occurred by a process that some called "specialization by addition." In other words, training in a subspecialty was added on to training as a specialist, just as the internship and residency were added on to the four years of medical school. Although this lengthy period of education maximized the likelihood that a subspecialist would enter practice thoroughly prepared, it also exacerbated a long-standing problem in medical education: the growing length of training. This was not a new concern, but in the 1950s many professional leaders began to worry more than ever that the process of medical education was taking too long. Some were concerned that the length and expense of medical education were discouraging able young individuals from less affluent backgrounds from entering the profession.[56] However, no one had any solutions, and the problem continued.

The emergence of subspecialty training changed the culture of both medical education and medical practice. Within the academic medical center, subspecialty fellows now competed with residents for patients and responsibilities. In theory, subspecialty fellows were consultants to residents. In practice, however, fierce jurisdictional battles often erupted as both groups competed with each other to make decisions about patients. Within medical practice, turf battles among different specialties and subspecialties became more spirited than ever as the scope of so many fields became smaller and smaller and as overlapping responsibility inevitably occurred. Should women with ovarian hormonal disturbances be treated by a gynecologist or an endocrinologist? Should carotid angiography be performed by neurosurgeons, radiologists, or neurologists? Did pediatric psychiatry "belong" to pediatrics or psychiatry? Was the emerging area of adolescent medicine part of pediatrics or internal medicine? Would thoracic surgeons or pulmonologists receive responsibility for bronchoscopies, and would abdominal surgeons or gastroenterologists perform colonoscopies? Such battles, fueled by ego, professional aspirations, and growing financial considerations, did not reflect the best side of doctors. Turf warfare clearly illustrated that the development of specialty and subspecialty practice was shaped by more than the proliferation of medical knowledge alone.

The growth of subspecialty fellowships also inflamed long-standing tensions between generalism and specialization in medicine. There was no doubt that subspecialists were well trained and that having a sufficient supply of qualified subspecialists was a public good. However, the gaze of the profession narrowed. Some critics worried that doctors would soon forget general principles or fail to take the whole patient into account. "We are becoming so subspecialized that I am afraid that we are losing sight of the fact that we are practicing medicine and must deal with the patient and not just the right index finger," one faculty member at the Cleveland Clinic maintained.[57] Others worried that physicians were spending so much time in scientific training that they were not acquiring an adequate understanding of the cultural and historical forces that have shaped modern civilization, an understanding deemed essential for the most productive service to society.[58]

Always, there were those trying to defend generalism against the onslaught of specialization. In 1961, for instance, the chief of internal medicine at the Peter Bent Brigham Hospital decided to maintain the medical service at the hospital as a general medical service—that is, patients with all conditions continued to be mixed together on the wards, in contrast to segregating patients into different areas by virtue of their medical problems, such as one area for cardiac patients and another for patients with cancer.[59] In 1972, George Zuidema, the chief of surgery at Johns Hopkins, shocked the 15 third-year clinical clerks meeting with him when he told them that he was not a surgeon. The stunned students sat there in silence until Zuidema proceeded to explain that he was an internist who just happened to use his hands for therapy. The point that sound specialty and subspecialty practice depended on a firm foundation in general medicine was indelibly imprinted on those students.[60]

However, even as Zuidema and others defended generalism, the increasing subspecialization and fragmentation of medicine was proceeding unabated. In Zuidema's own specialty of surgery, for instance, the field was already becoming increasingly partitioned into many competing subspecialties, and the fragmentation did not end there. The surgical subspecialty of orthopedics, for example, was beginning to divide into sub-subspecialties like hands and feet, shoulder, neck, spine, joint replacement, orthopedic oncology, sports medicine, pediatric orthopedics, and trauma. Soon, some orthopedic surgeons would concentrate on particular operations or conditions within the sub-subspecialty. As always, specialization won every victory, and generalism sustained every defeat. The result was a medical profession that sometimes appeared more like an array of competing fiefdoms than it did a cohesive profession.

THE ASCENDANCE OF SPECIALTY PRACTICE

As the residency and subspecialty fellowship programs expanded in the 1950s and 1960s, the composition of the physician workforce changed.

The percentage of specialists and subspecialists soared, while the percentage of general practitioners precipitously fell. The numbers bore witness to the harsh reality. According to one study, in 1931, 84 percent of practicing physicians classified themselves as general practitioners; in 1960, 45 percent; and in 1965, 37 percent. More ominously for the future of general practice, half of that 37 percent was over 65 years of age. In 1967, only 15 percent of medical students planned to enter general practice, and that number was rapidly dwindling every year.[61]

Curiously, in the 1950s most students entered medical school with the intention of *not* specializing. The majority thought they would become general practitioners. However, as the classic sociological study of medical education led by Robert Merton demonstrated, the career intentions of medical students frequently changed during the course of their training. By their senior year, when it was time to select a field within medicine and enter the Match, their career preferences overwhelmingly had switched to specialty practice.[62]

Why did medical students decide to pass over general practice for specialty careers? Both the Merton study and a second important study, conducted by the Association of Teachers of Preventive Medicine,[63] identified the same overriding reason: Medical students found specialty practice much more intellectually exciting and professionally fulfilling. In medical school, students developed a growing appreciation of the complexity of modern medicine and an increased awareness of their inability to master all of medicine. Most medical students wanted to feel that they were in command of their area of practice, and they also wanted to experience the excitement of being at the cutting edge of a field. Specialty practice appealed much more to medical students in these regards than general practice. In their minds, specialty practice held more opportunity to satisfy their professional ambitions and fulfill their desire to do "good work." As the Association of Teachers of Preventive Medicine put it, general practice permits "only a superficial and unsatisfactory approach to the problems of diagnosis and therapy.... This type of environment is not attractive to physicians of professional or personal ambition."[64]

Students' views on the relative merits of general and specialty practice were reinforced by the attitudes of those around them. Many medical faculty members regarded specialty practice as a much higher calling than general practice, and this perspective was not lost on students. Most major teaching hospitals did not even offer rotating internships, and many leading residency programs refused to award positions to applicants who had taken such internships.[65] In the world of private practice, the scope of general practice began to contract, as services once performed by general practitioners became the province of specialists. Thus, at many hospitals general practitioners lost the privilege of doing surgery, delivering babies, administering anesthesia, or treating more complicated problems in internal medicine, pediatrics, or neurology. To the general public, general practitioners were increasingly viewed as the doctors to see for a cold or constipation, but specialists were perceived as the physicians of choice for serious problems.[66] A prominent general practitioner lamented, "If such exclusion is insisted upon he [the general practitioner] will in effect become the 'scut boy' of the profession—as such, how can we attract competent men in this field?"[67]

Of note, financial considerations did not appear to be a factor in the decision to specialize. That was the conclusion of the teachers of preventive medicine. In 1949, the mean income of a general practitioner in private practice was $8,835, compared with $15,014 for a specialist. To the study group, it was not clear that the added earning power of specialty practice offset the personal and financial sacrifices of undertaking several years of residency training at a nominal salary. The teachers of preventive medicine concluded that the choice between general practice and specialty medicine was much more influenced by an individual's professional interests, qualifications, and aspirations than by economic factors.[68]

In the era of abundance, medical students received the right not only to specialize but also to choose their area of specialization. Here again, students made decisions based on their sense of how much intellectual excitement and professional satisfaction a field offered. For instance, in the 1960s ophthalmology was much more popular than otolaryngology, despite great similarities in income, lifestyle, and social status. The difference reflected the much greater sophistication and technological capacity of ophthalmology at that time. One surgical chair commented, "It is difficult to get good house staff in otolaryngology as the field is not sufficiently challenging."[69] Throughout the 1950s, 1960s, and 1970s, internal medicine was the most popular and competitive field, attracting up to 80 percent of students elected to Alpha Omega Alpha (the medical honorary society) at many schools.[70] Radiology, psychiatry, anesthesiology, pathology, and certain surgical subspecialties like orthopedics and urology encountered the most difficulty attracting applicants. The competitive position of radiology improved dramatically in the 1970s—not because of any change in the lifestyle or income of radiologists, but because the advent of noninvasive imaging (for instance, ultrasonography and CAT scanning) transformed the field into a hotbed of intellectual excitement. Many factors influenced specialty choice, but high among them was a student's desire to find a field that provided enjoyment and satisfaction in work.

The decline of general practice might not have occurred had graduate medical education continued to practice birth control as it had before World War II. However, in allowing residency training to become the right of all medical students, it ceased to do so. The transformation of residency from a privilege to a right embodied the virtues of a democratic free enterprise system, where individuals were free to choose their own careers. In medicine, there were now no restrictions on professional opportunities. Individual hospitals and residency programs sought house officers on the basis of their particular service needs and educational interests, while students sought the field that interested them the most. The result was that specialty and subspecialty medicine emerged triumphant, while general practice languished.

Some in medicine, most notably the AMA, attempted to halt the decline of general practice. The AMA's idea was that graduate medical education should continue to practice birth control. The AMA proposed that a quota system be established for internships—one that would allow teaching hospitals far fewer interns than they presently had and that would grant smaller community hospitals many more. The AMA's membership, which consisted mainly of general practitioners, stood to benefit greatly from this plan because it would provide more intern coverage at the smaller hospitals, which was where most general practitioners admitted patients. General practice as a field also stood to benefit because community hospitals offered mainly rotating internships, which usually led to careers in general practice. However, the academic community ridiculed this idea as serving only the interests of the AMA, and the proposal never gained traction. In the 1950s, the AMA's proposal to establish intern quotas at teaching hospitals, together with its lackluster support of federal appropriations for medical education, earned it considerable disfavor within academic medicine. As a consequence, the organization lost much of the credibility and influence in medical education that it once had deservedly enjoyed. Yet, for all the criticism, the AMA was the only major medical organization at the time to question whether the proliferation of specialty and subspecialty practice was an unqualified public good.[71]

The ultimate triumph of specialty practice came with the decision in 1970 to eliminate the freestanding rotating internship. Effective July 1, 1975, the internship officially became the first year of an integrated residency program; the rotating internship ceased to exist as an independent, culminating educational experience. This step was prompted in part by the Millis report of 1966, which argued for the greater involvement of medical school faculty in graduate medical education.[72] Ironically, this report was sponsored by the AMA. This event sounded the death knell of general practice, which was converted into the new specialty of family medicine, complete with its own three-year residency program and certifying board.[73]

In a free society, physicians had the right to choose not only a specialty but also where to practice on the completion of training. Here, too, physicians had clear preferences, choosing urban locations over rural communities by a wide margin, as they had all century long. Even general practitioners, commonly perceived as country doctors, chose urban settings much more frequently than often appreciated. In 1948, nearly one-half (49 percent) of general practitioners practiced in communities with populations of 100,000 or greater.[74] For most physicians, the economic, cultural, and professional advantages of cities proved too alluring. Many medical faculties, particularly at state schools, encouraged their students and house officers to practice in rural locations, but these efforts invariably failed. One such faculty at the University of Arkansas, after decades of trying, acknowledged the problems it encountered in this area: "We realize full well that the College of Medicine has little control over the personal and socio-cultural elements which determine where our graduates will practice medicine, nor are we ethically or legally able to forcibly place our graduates in needy areas."[75] Once again, individualism trumped societal needs.

By the 1970s graduate medical education faced a perplexing predicament. More and more doubts began to surface about whether graduate medical education was producing the types of doctors the country needed, particularly in regard to specialty mix and geographic distribution. No one doubted that having well-trained specialists was critically important to the nation's welfare, but many began to fear that graduate medical education had overshot the mark. Ironically, no one knew for sure what the proper mix of specialists and generalists should be; most spoke with humility on that subject. A popular consensus was a 50–50 mix, but that was purely a guess. No one knew either what the proper distribution among specialties should be or even how many doctors as a whole the country needed. Similarly, concerns were increasingly expressed about the scarcity of doctors in rural and inner-city areas, though, once again, precisely how many doctors ideally should practice in those locations was uncertain. One thing was clear, however: The sum of individual decisions was not meeting perceived public needs.

At the root of the problem facing graduate medical education was that fundamental American values conflicted with each other. On the one hand, the ascendance of specialty practice served as a testimony to the power of American individualism and personal liberty. Hospitals and medical students made decisions on the basis of their own interests, desires, and preferences, not on the basis of national needs. The result was the proliferation of specialty practice to the detriment of primary care (as it became known in the 1970s) and the medical overpopulation of the cities. The rest of the Western world avoided this problem by making centralized decisions to match specialty training and the geographic location of physicians with perceived workforce needs. The United Kingdom, for example, limited (and still limits) the number of physicians who can undertake specialty training, and primary care and specialist physicians alike have restricted choice in where they can practice, if they wish to participate in the National Health Service.[76]

On the other hand, by not producing the types of doctors the country was thought to need, there was increasing concern that graduate medical education was not serving the national interests. This would be a problem for any profession, given the fact that a profession is accountable to the society that supports it and grants it autonomy for the conduct of its work.[77] This posed an especially thorny dilemma for medicine, in view of the large amounts of public money medical education began receiving after World War II. Some leaders of medical education began to worry that if the profession itself could not achieve a specialty and geographic mix more satisfactory to the public, others would do it for them.[78] Various strategies were suggested or tried—for instance, loan forgiveness or higher compensation for those willing to work in primary care or an underserved area. However, none of these strategies succeeded—in no small part because of the professional lure of the specialties and the cities to physicians, and because of the traditional American reluctance to restrict an individual's right to make his own career decisions. Thus, the dilemma continued.

THE PROPAGATION OF WASTEFULNESS

Since the nineteenth century, the technological imperative has affected medical care. Instruments, procedures, and laboratory tests were developed, and doctors felt compelled to use them. In the first part of the twentieth century, as research in clinical science began to expand the menu of available laboratory tests, complaints that physicians were ignoring the patient's history and substituting laboratory studies for a physical examination were common. Such observations were made with even greater frequency after World War II and with still greater intensity and frequency after 1970, as the emergence of noninvasive imaging studies transformed radiology and offered physicians even more studies to choose from. Stanley J. Reiser has described this issue as medicine's "reign of technology."[79]

One manifestation of the technological imperative in graduate medical education was the excessive use of tests and procedures. As seen earlier, the greatest educational deficiency in residency training prior to World War II was the failure of medical educators consistently to live up to their own ideals of producing "scientific practitioners" who obtained tests and procedures when dictated by a patient's particular circumstances. Instead, house officers learned to practice wastefully, obtaining tests simply because the tests were available, not necessarily because they were needed. It was easy for this behavior to be carried with them as they established their own practices.

After World War II this behavior continued unabated. Residency training propagated wasteful behavior as house officers everywhere engaged in an exceedingly profligate practice style without being taught the proper use of resources or being challenged for their excessiveness. Formal studies were not conducted, but the archival records of one teaching hospital after another show that wastefulness was the order of the day. At Johns Hopkins, the New York Hospital, Presbyterian Hospital (New York), and many other places, faculty members observed the continual overordering of tests.[80] At Jefferson, the faculty estimated that house officers had obtained three times the number of tests that were actually needed.[81] At Mount Sinai Hospital (New York), the "excess ordering of routine tests" forced the hospital to spend $100,000 to hire additional laboratory technicians.[82] At University Hospitals of Cleveland, the laboratory director repeatedly complained about the lack of discrimination of house officers in requesting laboratory work. Studies should be obtained "because they are needed," he wrote, not because "they are readily available."[83] Year by year the magnitude of testing grew, as illustrated by the experience at Presbyterian Hospital (New York) in Table 7.1.[84] Particularly notable was the immediate utilization of new technologies, such as brain scans and coagulation studies in 1967, which augured their rapid proliferation in use in the years that followed. Nationwide, the amount of laboratory tests at academic medical centers in the late 1960s increased at a rate of 20 percent per year.[85]

In the 1960s, as medical costs continued their inexorable rise, some faculties became increasingly concerned about the wasteful practices of their house staff. Many solutions were attempted—here, a committee of chief residents to discuss excessive laboratory utilization; there, the dissemination to the house staff of the cost of various tests and procedures; elsewhere, feedback to the individual house officers as to how much they

Table 7.1 ROUTINE DIAGNOSTIC TESTS,
PRESBYTERIAN HOSPITAL, 1963–67

Laboratory	1963	1964	1965	1966	1967
Clinical Chemistry	238,220	297,791	313,532	346,428	385,196
Clinical Pathology	440,972	453,301	495,522	516,056	596,538
Bacteriology	85,898	95,609	108,227	107,418	123,309
Blood Bank	186,047	187,200	190,922	204,804	279,501
Serology	25,760	26,013	25,767	26,886	30,488
Cytology	19,434	23,330	25,735	26,838	29,620
Mycology	2,702	3,228	3,489	3,385	3,628
Cardiology	21,014	23,953	26,775	28,924	30,094
EEG	6,302	6,820	7,097	7,818	7,770
EMG, Nerve Conduction	—	—	1,223	1,245	1,262
Brain Scan	—	—	—	—	3,154
Coagulation	—	—	—	—	533
Acid-Base (Peds.)	—	—	—	—	11,093
Acid-Base (Surg.)	—	—	—	3,543	5,243

were spending. However, such efforts had little effect. This was illustrated at Johns Hopkins in the 1970s when an unusually outstanding intern was told that his practice patterns were among the most costly of his peers. The proud intern interpreted this as another indication of his excellence, and he boasted of this "recognition" to the students he had with him at the time.[86]

The failure of these efforts could have been predicted because they did not address the chief reason for the lack of parsimonious care provided by house officers: flawed medical teaching. As before the war, attending physicians seldom taught discrimination in patient management or the fact that it was often better for patients *not* to do particular tests or procedures. Rather, teaching physicians tended to encourage doing everything available, whether needed or not, and criticize house officers if they failed to do so. In 1964 John H. Knowles, the general director of the Massachusetts General Hospital, made this point in his annual report. "Medical faculties have not taught by rewarding restraint and thoughtfulness in the use of tests but usually have condemned the house officer when he missed one determination." To Knowles, medicine would be better taught "by explaining why certain tests are not needed rather than resigning ourselves to a trial and error method on the part of the house staff."[87]

Always, of course, there were exceptions. A particularly notable example was J. Willis Hurst, the chair of internal medicine at Emory University and Hospital from 1957 to 1986, the cardiologist to President Lyndon B. Johnson, and a gifted and caring clinician and teacher who was sometimes likened to William Osler. For three decades Hurst emphasized the importance of rigorous problem analysis and decision making to his house officers. He regularly differentiated between "could" and "should," telling his house officers, "A physician should have a good reason for ordering a diagnostic test or procedure."[88] He taught the importance of knowing that in some situations "a problem should not be solved."[89] He met regularly with his house officers, not just in conference situations but at patients' bedsides. He was known for appearing on the floor at odd hours—nights, weekends, holidays—not just to check their work but to check their thinking. As Hurst put it, a true teacher should "look into their [residents'] minds and determine how they arrived at their conclusions and what they plan to do about them. This is very different from giving a mini-lecture."[90] Unfortunately, for medical education and the public, there have been few Willis Hursts.

There had been earlier instances in the history of residency training when house officers practiced with greater discretion. Particularly during the height of the Depression and World War II, when money and supplies were limited, house officers tended to be highly judicious in their decision making, consistently foregoing unnecessary items, and earning the praise of hospital administrators for doing so.[91] However, these moments were few and short-lived. In the environment of abundance of postwar America, the concept of limits, constraints, or rationing seemed distant and far-fetched. It was easy for faculty to overlook indiscriminate ordering habits, just as it was easy for them to succumb to the technological imperative, engaging in a medical arms race to obtain any and all new technologies. As the president of one major teaching hospital put it, "The major question concerning new technology acquisitions is *how* to acquire rather than *if* to acquire."[92]

Medical faculties after the war were no more lax in their ability to teach a judicious approach to patient care than they were before the war. What had changed was that the menu and cost of items were rapidly growing, making the economic consequences of wasteful practice styles more consequential. In an environment of abundance, it was easy for house officers to assume that good medical care involved doing everything imaginable, especially when more and more patients had insurance, hospitals always seemed to have money, and few faculty members seemed to care about waste and inappropriateness. Of course, there were exceptions. A noted neurosurgeon warned, "Unless these [excessive] costs are controlled promptly by the profession the control will pass largely from our hands."[93]

However, such views were seldom expressed and, even less frequently, acted on. In the 1950s, 1960s, and 1970s, faculty members, house officers, and practicing physicians continued to engage in a profligate practice style, seemingly oblivious to the ominous upward spiral in the country's medical costs and seemingly equally oblivious to the fact that their own wastefulness had contributed to the problem.

CHAPTER 8
The Evolving Learning Environment

The generation between 1940 and 1970 witnessed extraordinary changes in America's health care system. Physicians entering medicine in 1940 did so with the doctor-patient relationship a dyad; they left medicine in 1970 or the years that followed with a third-party payer standing between them and the majority of their patients. Most physicians entering medicine in 1940 did so with the expectation of providing considerable charity care; by 1970 free care from physicians was rapidly becoming a rarity. In 1940 the traditional two-class health care system of paying patients and charity patients defined health care in America. By 1970 health care had come to be seen as a right, the majority of Americans had medical insurance of some type, and traditional charity patients had declined greatly in number.

The years between 1940 and 1970 were also notable for major changes in medical knowledge and practice. In 1940 infectious diseases still reaped terror, with the recently released sulfa drugs the only available antibiotics. By 1970, earlier fears of infectious diseases had considerably abated, thanks to the development of penicillin and its derivatives, other effective classes of antibiotics, and the polio vaccine. In the place of infectious diseases, the leading causes of mortality in America became cancer, cardiovascular disease, neurological illnesses, and other chronic conditions. During this period clinical science reached the cellular, subcellular, molecular, and genetic levels, allowing the development of a host of new diagnostic and therapeutic modalities. Among them were medications for high blood pressure, anti-arrhythmia drugs, cancer chemotherapy, and prednisone and other anti-inflammatory drugs. The old fear of the surgeon's knife practically disappeared, a result of better intra operative anesthesia, more effective postoperative care, fewer and more easily treatable operative infections, and the safer and more widespread use of blood transfusions. Developments in operative technique, coupled with advances in anticoagulation and immunosuppressive therapy, transformed the focus of surgery from excision to repair and implantation. Ventilators, hemodialysis, cardiopulmonary resuscitation, and intensive care units also arrived—developments applicable to all branches of medicine and responsible for saving countless lives.

Thus, in this period there were profound changes in the health care system, characterized by new payers, new relationships with patients, and new attitudes defining health care as a right. There were also major changes in medical science, diagnosis, and treatment. These new conditions posed marked challenges for residency training. The rise of third-party payers weakened the traditional ward services of teaching hospitals that had been so essential for clinical learning, and the growing scientific complexity of medicine made it increasingly difficult for residency training to incorporate cutting-edge scientific training into a fundamentally clinical experience. Nevertheless, the residency system responded constructively to these challenges. The key to doing so was its ability to adapt its practices to the changed cultural and scientific environment without sacrificing its core academic and ethical values: intellectual rigor and an unswerving commitment to serving patients.

THE DECLINE OF THE WARD SERVICE

The evolution of graduate medical education in the United States, as pointed out earlier, was "culturally contingent"—that is, it was shaped by cultural conditions, not just by scientific developments alone. Nowhere was this more apparent than in the use of the charity wards of teaching hospitals for medical teaching. The charity wards provided a wonderful educational laboratory for house officers and medical students because of the high degree of responsibility they were allowed in treating indigent patients. One surgeon trained in this system recalled that it "was the charity patients' job to let us use their bodies to learn on. The patient expressed no resentment and we felt no guilt."[1] Private patients, in contrast, were used only sparingly in medical education. This two-class system of medical care represented the social contract of poverty. Charity patients received free care in exchange for being used for medical education.[2]

After World War II, teaching hospitals found it increasingly difficult to maintain their charity wards. The chief problem was financial. Reimbursement from municipal and state authorities had always been far less than the costs of care. In earlier times, when medical costs were relatively low, these deficits were typically made up by philanthropic gifts, endowment income, or small profits from caring for paying patients. After the war, however, medical costs began to escalate rapidly. As a result, by 1965 most teaching hospitals were financially hemorrhaging from the burden of providing free care.[3] Gone were the days when a wealthy hospital trustee could pull out his checkbook to cover the hospital's operating loss from the year before; the amounts of money were just too high. For instance, at Moffit Hospital (the teaching hospital of the University of California, San Francisco), the 483-bed teaching patient unit at 80 percent occupancy lost nearly $3 million in 1952, compared with its 250-bed private patient unit, which at the same 80 percent occupancy broke even.[4] The problem of growing deficits from free care was also illustrated by the experience of the Massachusetts General Hospital (Table 8.1).[5]

After World War II, as the country prospered, the number of patients able to pay for medical care began to grow substantially. Initially, this occurred because of the spread of private medical insurance. The search for collective medical security had deep roots; the Blue Cross and Blue Shield organizations were established during the Depression. Following the war, however, private medical insurance became much more widely available, as Blue Cross and Blue Shield gained many more individual subscribers and as employer-based medical insurance became a standard benefit of employment.[6] The direct result was that millions of middle-class

Table 8.1 INCOME, DEFICITS, AND FREE CARE, MGH, 1940–64

Year	Operating Income	Operating Deficit	Endowment Income Community Fund	Loss from Free Care
1940	2,084,000	891,000	720,000	434,000
1945	2,726,000	1,156,000	849,000	360,000
1950	5,884,000	879,000	799,000	1,137,000
1955	8,658,000	1,318,000	1,299,000	1,896,000
1960	15,270,000	1,877,000	1,400,000	2,811,000
1964	23,163,000	1,691,000	1,497,000	4,328,000

individuals who once would have been treated on the ward service of a teaching hospital by the interns, residents, and fellows under the supervision of members of the medical faculty now found themselves able to pay for their hospital care.

For both teaching hospitals and patients, the arrival of private medical insurance proved a great boon. With the costs of care soaring and the provision of charity care taking an ever-increasing toll, hospitals found a much-needed source of income. Patients, too, found the new system of medical economics immensely to their liking. Insured patients received the amenities of private patients and did not have to stay in large, impersonal wards. Accordingly, voluntary (that is, private, nonprofit) hospitals everywhere began converting ward beds to semiprivate beds (two, three, or four beds per room) to accommodate the growing number of insured patients. (Single occupancy private rooms required self-pay or additional payment from an insured individual to cover the difference in cost between a private and semiprivate room.) At the Peter Bent Brigham Hospital, for instance, ward patients occupied only 50 percent of the beds in 1953, compared with 85 percent in 1944.[7] A similar conversion of ward to semiprivate beds occurred at virtually every teaching hospital in the country.[8]

To medical educators, the movement to prepaid medical insurance caused much alarm. Educators appreciated the financial and social advantages of prepaid medical insurance, and they knew that medical students and house officers had much to learn from private patients. However, ward beds were considered teaching beds, while private beds were not. As before World War II, private patients, whether self-paying or insured, usually did not consent to be used in medical teaching, and when they did, it was typically for demonstrative purposes, not to let residents make important decisions or perform surgery. The limited involvement of private patients affected both undergraduate and graduate medical education, but it was a particularly pressing problem for residency training because of the educational necessity that house officers assume responsibility in patient care. Residency training in every specialty was affected, but especially the surgical fields and obstetrics and gynecology because of the need for house officers to perform enough operations and procedures to satisfy the requirements of the boards.[9]

As the number of insured patients rapidly increased, renewed attempts were made to involve private patients more effectively in medical education. For instance, many programs established policies allowing only interns and residents to write orders in the charts of private patients, thereby conferring more responsibility to house officers in managing these patients. However, such efforts typically failed to provide house officers enough responsibility to satisfy the dictates of graduate medical education. At the New York Hospital the faculty observed that "teaching on a semi-private service leaves much to be desired," while at the Massachusetts General Hospital private patients were used for resident training but "not very successfully."[10] At the Columbia-Presbyterian Medical Center, the staff found value in assigning house officers to rotations with private patients, provided those experiences were limited to one or two months a year. Beyond that, "No further intellectual gain is accomplished by increasing resident time spent for private patients."[11] The faculty there summarized the prevailing viewpoint among medical educators: "The present system of ward service teaching is eminently superior to any type of private patient teaching."[12]

Accordingly, medical educators viewed the decline of the ward service as a huge threat to residency training. There was uniform agreement in the educational community that if the ward service were to disappear, the quality of graduate medical education would deteriorate. As the Johns Hopkins faculty put it, "This potential dearth of service patients is an exceedingly serious problem, and if unresolved will spell the doom of The Johns Hopkins residencies."[13]A staff committee at the Massachusetts General Hospital felt similarly: "Ward patients are diminishing—they may well disappear completely. Were this to occur, the teaching of the house staff would be the most difficult because of their need for assuming responsibility with patients."[14] Great teaching hospitals considered their ward service their "soul,"[15] and they feared that attrition of the ward service would mark the descent of medical education to mediocrity.

Concerned about these developments, many faculties, particularly at university teaching hospitals, took a variety of steps to ensure that house officers would continue to have sufficient opportunities with ward patients. Some academic medical centers attempted to raise funds to endow teaching beds.[16] With the cost of care soaring, this approach was at best a stopgap measure, but it did underscore the strong commitment of medical educators to do everything possible to maintain a rich learning environment. A much more common, and much more viable, approach was to establish or strengthen affiliations with veterans and municipal hospitals. At these institutions, house officers were permitted graded responsibility under faculty supervision just like on the charity wards of university teaching hospitals. For many residency programs, the use of veterans and municipal hospitals became an important tool for ensuring that house officers had the opportunity to make medical decisions, perform procedures, and operate, even as the private services at the primary teaching hospitals grew larger.

The most important approach was to negotiate arrangements with Blue Cross and other private insurers whereby certain ward beds would qualify for semiprivate reimbursement rates without a hospital's losing the right to use them as teaching beds. This was accomplished by redefining what was meant by being a "private" patient. Formerly, private patient status had been conferred simply by a patient's ability to pay for the hospitalization, either by self-pay or insurance. Under the new criteria, a "private" patient was one who not only paid for the hospitalization but also had a private physician of his own on the hospital staff. For patients without a private physician, insurance companies agreed to let house officers "represent" their attending physicians, thereby allowing hospitals to collect insurance payments for these patients without changing their educational practices. By the early 1960s, such patients accounted for roughly one-half of the patient days on the ward services of teaching hospitals. This approach provided a viable educational and financial solution to allowing house officers to continue assuming responsibility in patient care.[17]

Even as the ward service reached an accommodation with private insurers, however, it became endangered from another front: the emerging attitude that medical care was a right, not a charitable gift. This new attitude was part of a larger civil rights movement that, among other things, emphasized the dignity of all individuals, regardless of race, class, creed, or gender. As part of this cultural shift, almshouse medicine became increasingly indefensible, as did a two-class system of medical care. The ultimate manifestation of these forces in medicine was the enactment of Medicare (for the elderly) and Medicaid (for the poor) in 1965. This legislation did much more than extend medical insurance coverage to millions of vulnerable Americans. It also represented the culmination of a social revolution that viewed separate systems of medical care as intrinsically unequal and undeserving of public support. The legislation was a product of the same forces that led to the Civil Rights Act of 1964, the Voting Rights Act of 1965, and the war on poverty.

For residency training, and for all of medical education, the passage of Medicare and Medicaid was a momentous event. Medicare and Medicaid provided academic medical centers enormous amounts of clinical income for services they previously had been providing for free or below cost. The result was financial strength, explosive growth, and an exponential rise in the amount of clinical care they provided. Medicare and Medicaid also catalyzed the formation of "faculty practice plans"—multispecialty group practices consisting of the full-time faculty of medical schools. As faculty practice plans grew, so did the financial compensation of faculty, which soon rivaled that of physicians in private practice. House officers, too, benefited, as the tsunami of clinical income allowed hospitals to escalate rapidly the salaries they paid interns and residents.[18]

Patients also benefited immeasurably from Medicare and Medicaid. Millions of people, who otherwise might have gone without, received care. In addition, all hospitalized patients soon came to be treated with much more courtesy and dignity. Within a decade, the large 16- or 24-bed (or larger) hospital wards were gone, in response to Medicare requirements that patients be assigned to semiprivate rooms containing two, three, or four beds as a condition of payment. Medicare and Medicaid also brought about the end of racial segregation in American hospitals. Segregation was already declining in medicine, but now, to receive reimbursement from Medicare and Medicaid, hospitals had to integrate patient care in the institution as a whole as well as in the assignment of individual rooms.[19] Outpatient departments were renovated, appointment systems were introduced, and inpatient facilities were modernized and made more comfortable. Even the terms "ward service" and "teaching service" were abandoned, to be replaced by euphemisms such as the "university clinical service." These linguistic changes were symbolically important, much as the substitution of "black" (and later "African-American") for "Negro" and "health care" for "medical care."

Medicare and Medicaid, however, also created major challenges for graduate medical education. They threatened the viability of the ward service, much as the rise of prepaid medical insurance had done earlier. The reasons were the same: the requirement that Medicare and Medicaid patients be treated as private patients. This meant that there had to be a responsible senior physician, not just a resident, in charge of the case, if professional fees under Part B of Medicare were to be paid. Once again, medical educators worried that the ward service would be destroyed, teaching programs critically damaged, and house officers unable to receive sufficient responsibility to become adequately prepared for independent practice. These worries were identical to those they had experienced when private medical insurance first appeared. However, medical educators feared that the erosion of the ward service would be carried much farther under Medicare than it had been with private insurers. As one physician at the Massachusetts General Hospital predicted, federal medical care programs for the elderly might "wipe out the medical ward teaching service with a stroke of the pen."[20]

Quickly, however, prophesies about the end of the residency system proved unfounded. An accommodation was reached that satisfied federal officials that Medicare and Medicaid beneficiaries were receiving private medical care while leaving the residency training system intact. The key to this rapprochement was the same that had been used with the private insurance companies: redefining a "private patient" as one who had a private physician, not simply as one who had the ability to pay. Thus, for Medicare and Medicaid patients without private physicians of their own, the faculty attending physician became the private physician of legal record, and house officers were allowed major responsibilities in clinical management as representatives of the attending physicians. This arrangement allowed house officers to continue to receive supervised independence. John H. Knowles, the general director of the Massachusetts General Hospital, observed after Medicare and Medicaid had taken effect that "there has been considerable worry, although, still no proof of damage."[21]

The chief consequence of the arrival of Medicare and Medicaid for residency training was the burden of paperwork imposed on faculty attending physicians. With private insurers, the faculty had to document their involvement in the hospital charts, but under Medicare and Medicaid, documentation requirements became more stringent. The precise rules of documentation for billing purposes varied from hospital to hospital—here, countersigning a resident's note; there, a separate note by the attending physician. Medicare regularly sent out clarifications of the conditions that had to be met for teaching physicians to be eligible to bill for professional services. These requirements frequently changed: yesterday, notes by the attending physician three days a week; today, daily notes. Over time, documentation requirements became increasingly onerous, and faculties regularly sought ways to lessen that burden. As hospital costs continued to rise, Medicare officials scrutinized the documentation of faculty services ever more closely.

From an educational perspective, however, the debate over documentation was a sideshow. The chief difference in residency training after Medicare was the more careful documentation by attending physicians of the supervision they had provided house officers. What was important educationally was that the principle of the assumption of responsibility survived relatively unscathed. Ward patients were given new names, hospitalized in more comfortable quarters, provided more amenities, and treated with greater courtesy. However, as before, they were still cared for mainly by the house officers, who continued to act with considerable independence. Once again, the residency system survived intact in the face of the changing pattern of medical practice.

That the residency system—and, specifically, the principle of graded responsibility—continued was clearly in the national interest. As mentioned before, there was no avoiding the moment when a doctor operated or assumed the management of complex patients for the first time without the direct supervision of a more experienced physician. The only question before medical education and the public was the circumstances in which this would happen. Among both medical educators and knowledgeable public leaders there was unanimity on this matter. They believed it far better for this moment to occur as part of the graded responsibility of residency, where help could be immediately summoned, rather than to wait until physicians were in practice, where help might not be immediately available and where mistakes from inexperience on their unsuspecting first patients would pass undetected. Medical education could not avoid its traditional ethical dilemma: balancing the needs of the individual, who benefited from being treated by the most experienced doctor, with those of the community, whose interests resided in having the most junior doctors gain experience so that down the road there would be well-trained doctors for everyone. The graded responsibility of the residency system seemed the best way to achieve a proper balance.

What was not achieved, however, even after the federal government became involved with financing health care, was the creation of a true one-class system of care. In medical care, as in the rest of American society, social justice was not fully achieved. Most medical teaching and learning continued to occur on the vulnerable—those with lower incomes and less social status. In contrast, in a true one-class system of care, all patients would be used equally in teaching. In such a system, the surgical resident might operate on the bank president, while the patient on Medicaid would have the same opportunity as a wealthy individual to have his operation performed by the hospital's most experienced surgeon.

In short, neither medical educators nor the public had figured out a way to involve private patients more fully in medical education, particularly at the level of residency training. Some educational leaders tried, arguing that the quality of care provided by residents at major teaching hospitals was so good that no properly informed individual would wish to be denied "the privileges of being used for teaching."[22] However, private physicians liked maintaining control of their own patients, most well-to-do patients did not wish residents to replace their private doctors, and there was little national will to change the system any more. The modified two-class system of care continued—and has not been modified further. Part of the challenge of achieving greater social justice in America in the future will be to determine procedures for using all classes of patients equally in medical education.

THE PRESERVATION OF EDUCATIONAL QUALITY

After the war residency training faced challenges beyond the declining number of ward patients. There was now much more that medical and surgical care had to offer, and larger numbers of patients had insurance to pay for hospital services. The result was a great expansion in the clinical work of academic medical centers, with rapidly growing demands on the time of both faculty and house officers. Some medical educators worried that there might not be enough faculty available to teach or that the expanding clinical duties of house officers would drown out the intellectual aspects of residency training.

Medical educators met these challenges quickly and effectively. As the demands of clinical care increased, so did the size of full-time faculties at medical schools. Fueled by research as well as by clinical dollars, the number of full-time faculty members at US medical schools grew from approximately 3,500 in 1951 to more than 17,000 by 1966.[23]

Although medical school faculty members in the 1950s and 1960s were torn often by the growing demands of research and clinical responsibilities, large numbers still had the time and commitment to teach. For instance, at one major Midwestern medical school, one-third of overall faculty effort was devoted to clinical teaching at some level, though that figure varied considerably among individual faculty members.[24] Fortunately for graduate medical education, there was no shortage of capable instructors and role models.

Teaching at many residency programs was also immeasurably aided by physicians in private practice who donated their services in exchange for admitting privileges to the hospital. At this time, admitting privileges to university teaching hospitals remained extremely difficult to acquire. This was an honor reserved for only private practitioners of the highest caliber. Some members of the voluntary staff rivaled any full-time faculty member in knowledge, judgment, and analytical abilities, and many outstanding teachers came from their ranks.

A particularly notable example occurred in St. Louis, where I. Jerome Flance and Michael Karl became fixtures in the internal medicine training program at Washington University from the 1950s through the 1980s. Founders of the Maryland Medical Group, a premier group practice in internal medicine located close to the medical center, Flance and Karl were brilliant diagnosticians, gifted teachers, and kindly souls who inspired generations of Washington University residents and students. Flance published many clinical observations and case studies, once identifying a new syndrome, thesaurosis, a toxic lung condition caused by a propellant commonly used in hair spray in the 1950s, that ultimately led the Food and Drug Administration to ban the use of that agent.[25] On another occasion he diagnosed the acute rupture of the myocardial wall in a patient recovering from a heart attack at the patient's bedside. He saved her life by sending her directly to the operating room, where the chest surgeon he had summoned was waiting. Had Flance taken the time to obtain radiological studies, she would have died before getting to surgery. Karl, who published regularly as well, introduced the liver biopsy to St. Louis, remaining for decades the local expert in the procedure. He gave dozens of exemplary discussions at clinical-pathologic conferences, not once missing the diagnosis. He possessed unparalleled wisdom about both medicine and life. Both Flance and Karl ultimately were honored with multiple "teacher of the year" awards from the medical school, masterships from the American College of Physicians, and honorary degrees from Washington University.

The clinical demands on house officers also proved to be less of an educational distraction than some had feared. After the war, as before, medical educators understood the educational importance of house officers being assigned a manageable number of patients. Only in this fashion could there be sufficient time for interns and residents to reflect on their work and to discuss and debate issues among themselves. There was a widespread understanding that assigning house officers too many patients at one time was just as deleterious to learning—and more dangerous for patient care—as too few.[26] Accordingly, many programs took measures to ensure that the growing size of the clinical service remained aligned with educational goals. Virtually all programs increased the size of their house staffs, with many leading teaching programs appointing more house officers than needed for clinical care so that residents would have a better educational experience. For instance, Presbyterian Hospital (New York), which was deeply committed to advancing house staff education, increased its resident staff from 125 in 1941 to 247 in 1959, during which time the combined ward, semiprivate, and private bed capacity increased only from 1,259 to 1,498 and the number of outpatient clinic visits remained unchanged.[27]

A particularly illustrative example of the efforts to keep educational needs in focus was the internal medicine program at Duke under Eugene A. Stead Jr. Stead's residents worked incredibly hard, and the program was notorious in some circles for its "on-call" schedule of five nights out of seven, compared with every other night at most programs. However, Stead made certain that there were more house officers on call each night than were needed for clinical coverage because he believed that having more residents in the hospital increased the opportunities for learning. In Stead's system, routine work was diluted among a larger group, residents could more easily exploit educational opportunities, and house officers usually got more sleep than house officers at other programs. Two former residents recalled:

> Duke hospital [*sic*] could have gotten by with only one or two house officers [in internal medicine] in house, but Stead knew that much of the fun and excitement of medicine occurred during the evening hours. By being in the hospital at night, the house officers could attend their patients who got sick, and could share interesting clinical experiences with their colleagues. Often over a midnight supper, house officers would discuss the findings of patients admitted late at night; afterwards several of them would go to listen to an unusual heart murmur, palpate a vascular thrill, or feel an abdominal mass. *Those learning opportunities would have been lost if only the minimal number of staff were on duty at a given time. Busy with routine tasks, they would never have a chance to explore new phenomena or exchange ideas.*[28] (Italics mine)

The time demands on house officers also grew as changes in medical practice led to shorter hospitalizations and a more hurly-burly pace. From 1946 to 1962, the average length of stay at acute-care hospitals fell from about 16 days to 10 days.[29] Many medical educators began to worry that the turnover of patients would become so great that house officers would no longer have sufficient time for reflection.[30] Work demands with each patient also grew because there were so many new treatments and technologies. Nevertheless, the average 10-day hospitalization of this period still allowed house officers the opportunity to get to know their patients as individuals and to study the patients and their diseases. Hospitalizations were also long enough for educational quality control to be present. Residents were able to observe the results of tests they had ordered, procedures and surgeries they had performed, and therapeutic strategies they had initiated—and to make adjustments in the diagnosis or management of a patient's illness if necessary, and then to observe whether the adjustments had worked and make other changes in care if they had not.

Educational quality control also remained in the work schedules of residents. After a night "on call" (which often allowed for at least a few hours of sleep), house officers went home the next day when the work was done and not according to the dictates of an arbitrary call schedule. Typically this occurred in the late afternoon of a "post-call" day. Thus, work schedules allowed admitting house officers to see the results of the diagnostic tests they had ordered and to make the next set of decisions based on them. This practice was clearly good for residents' education, but it was also good for patient care because no other house officer could know a patient as well as the resident who did the complete admitting workup. As one intern attested, "It's almost impossible to pick up pieces on patients you haven't worked up."[31]

The residency system also faced the challenge of adapting to the growing scientific sophistication of clinical science, which now depended more on quantitative biology than on medical training. The ideal of graduate medical education was reiterated by the medical faculty at Johns Hopkins in 1956: "One of the cardinal principles in higher education is the encouragement of the thorough mastery of knowledge through participation in the process of discovery. It inevitably leads to emphasis upon scholarly teachers, upon free time, upon depth of study, and upon the cultivation of individual initiative."[32] As seen before, however, in the postwar era it became extremely difficult for residency training to prepare a medical graduate for specialty practice and at the same time provide the scientific tools for a career in clinical research. It would have been an easy matter for residencies to concentrate on clinical instruction alone. However, that would have created the danger that the residency system would so devalue scientific instruction and research that it would devolve from a university-level educational experience into apprentice-style practical training.

Fortunately, that did not happen. Medical educators, particularly at the better teaching hospitals, took effective steps to ensure that residency programs would continue to adhere to high intellectual standards. The key to this effort lay in making certain that residency training continued to take place in a rigorous intellectual environment where questions were asked, authority was regularly challenged, and debate was encouraged. Components of this environment included a spirit of inquiry, dissatisfaction with present knowledge, intellectual honesty, and a commitment to service. In such an environment medical educators continued to infuse residency training with the intellectual and philosophical considerations traditionally of concern to the university. Stated another way, in the postwar period the residency system completed its journey from its beginnings as university-based, research-oriented graduate education to its new state as professional education. The system evolved, but it remained a part of the university and avoided assuming the characteristics of a trade school that provided only practical learning.

For some house officers, research did remain a component of the residency. This was particularly true in the surgical disciplines, whose longer training periods made more provision for research experiences, and for house officers in all specialties who wished to acquire exposure to clinical investigation. The difference in the 1950s and 1960s was that laboratory projects became elective opportunities for those who desired them, not formal requirements. This new attitude was expressed by Francis D. Moore, the iconic chair of surgery at the Peter Bent Brigham Hospital from 1946 to 1976, who encouraged but did not require his residents to spend time in the laboratory. "I felt that research was a little like playing the piano," he wrote. "Some people were good at it and some were not. There was no use forcing everybody to practice three hours per day."[33] Moore thought that the best approach was to make research opportunities available for those who desired them, support handsomely those individuals whose work was promising, and allow the others to return to the clinical service without prejudice if the laboratory was not a strong point for them.[34] Like many leaders of academic medicine, he understood that true scientific creativity could not be mass-produced.

All house officers, including the great majority not planning careers in clinical investigation, continued to study the scientific foundations of their fields. Indeed, after the war, as before, the specialty boards continued to emphasize the medical sciences as fundamental to satisfactory preparation for any specialty. It was thought that ongoing scientific exposure would enhance the doctor's ability to figure out problems and adapt to new situations and to reduce the dependence on memorized facts. The goal was to produce "sound clinicians," defined by their problem-solving skills. A "sound clinician," as one important leader of internal medicine put it, was "not measured by his capacity to recognize the exotic in medicine" nor by "authoritarian omniscience" but by the ability to "discern the essence of a problem and recognize how to seek and where to find pertinent information."[35]

Medical educators of this era sharply distinguished between education and training, and they insisted that the residency experience should be the former. In their minds, education meant acquiring the ability to adapt to the future, not merely to learn for the here and now. It meant an emphasis on the higher-order cognitive skills of analysis, synthesis, and problem solving, not the lower-order cognitive skills of recall and recognition. It meant reading to build knowledge, explore problems, and deepen understanding, not just to acquire isolated facts. It meant understanding *why* something should be done, not just knowing what to do. It involved the cultivation of critical skills, a distrust of authority, a recognition of what was not known, and the ability to tolerate and manage uncertainty. Education required inquiry and curiosity to be part of the daily learning environment, in contrast to training, which could occur in isolation from research. Education also required learners to teach, in contrast to training, where learners learned but rarely taught. Education was value-laden, involving reflection on the values of the profession, the type of doctor a trainee wanted to be, the role of the doctor and the profession in the community, and the responsibilities of the profession to create a better health care system and a healthier society, all in contrast to training, which was much more content-driven and value-neutral. In short, professional education involved intellectual inquiry, not merely practical training for the forthcoming job.

The defense of graduate medical education as professional education was led by department chairs at the leading medical schools and teaching hospitals. In internal medicine, no one defended the importance of intellectual rigor in residency training more vigorously than Stead, the chair of internal medicine at Duke from 1947 to 1967 and arguably the most iconic figure in American medicine since World War II. Stead was a multitalented individual who built his house with his own hands, became a savvy stock-market investor, and founded the physician assistant movement. He did part of his residency as well as his early faculty work at the Peter Bent Brigham Hospital, where he came under the influence of Henry A. Christian and Soma Weiss, whose values he later passed on to his own students and house officers, first at Emory (1942–46), later at Duke. He conducted world-class clinical research, particularly in the area of cardiovascular disease. He was also a legendary critic, reviewing every manuscript written by members of his department prior to submission for publication, as well as a generous mentor who often removed his name from the scientific papers of students and residents working with him who were carrying out his ideas. At both Emory and Duke, he taught "Sunday school"—informal teaching conferences on Sunday mornings that were heavily attended not only by residents and students but also by faculty and community physicians. If a medical student "aced" him, he bought that student a cup of coffee and offered him an internship. Stead was famous for his terse aphorisms, known as "Steadisms," such as "What this patient needs is a doctor!" and "What you're telling me is that life is hard. I already know that." Thirty-three of his residents went on to chair important departments of internal medicine.[36]

Stead was also a professional educator concerned with how people learn, retain, and use information. He regularly described the qualities that distinguished the great residency programs from the mediocre, publishing articles with such titles as "Training Is No Substitute for Education" and "The Role of the University in Graduate Training."[37] He believed a good clinical education emphasized thinking, problem solving, and learning from new experiences—and not memorization. He regularly pointed out the value of exposing house officers to controversy because it forced them to think critically and distrust authority. He thought it much more important to develop the resident's "ability to learn from a new situation" than to focus on "the catholic covering of all clinical experiences."[38] He also insisted that house officers should engage in teaching—medical students and each other—because "learning is an active process and each of us learns more when we teach than when we are taught."[39] In selecting faculty, he emphasized the importance of seeking individuals who were much more interested in conveying attitudes than in transmitting facts. "Select those who are more concerned with what is not known about a subject than in the transmission of current knowledge," he advised.[40] What was a "safe doctor" to Stead? It was someone with "the ability to comfortably say *I don't know but if it's important I'll find out*."[41]

In surgery, perhaps the most ardent proponent of residency training as professional education was Francis H. Moore at the Peter Bent Brigham Hospital. Moore was a prominent academic spokesperson and a renowned clinical investigator (he was elected to the National Academy of Sciences in 1981 for his pioneering work using radioactive tracers to determine the composition of fluids and chemicals in the body and for his contributions to kidney transplantation). Most of all, he was a surgical teacher. Moore disdained what he called the "high volume, low knowledge" residency product. In his words, "It is possible for a Resident to have carried out many vagotomies and pyloroplasties and emerge at the end of his five years knowing almost nothing either about the physiology of the stomach, the measurement of gastrin, the evidence for neurological innervation by the vagus of the parietal cells, the actual influence of this on the pylorus, let alone any concept of the simple statistical formulations by which followup studies can be evaluated."[42] To Moore, mastery of surgery involved not just technical skill but also scientific understanding and exquisite clinical judgment. A successful operation on the kidney, for instance, "may hinge equally on a well-tied knot or on a thorough understanding of the biochemistry of the obstructed nephron."[43] He believed that the importance of manual dexterity in surgery had been overemphasized; instead, he urged that much more attention in training be given to judgment, timing, case selection, and the surgeon's mental processes. "The most important thing I do about an operation is what I think about it before I start," he wrote.[44] He relished controversy and debate on his service, demanded that his house officers take seriously the teaching of students and each other, and expected all of his residents to study some clinical problem, if only a review of the literature or preparation of a case report.[45]

Of course, there was great diversity among residency programs, and not all achieved the same level of educational success. The strongest programs were the university programs, while the weakest were at community hospitals. That there were large differences among these programs can be seen by the results on specialty board examinations. In the 1960s, for instance, 72.7 percent of examinees from university teaching hospitals passed the internal medicine examination on the first attempt, compared with 57.8 percent from community hospitals with a university affiliation and 35.6 percent from community hospitals without a university affiliation.[46]

What accounted for these differences among residency programs? Certainly, it was not with anything that could be readily measured. All programs had adequate physical facilities, enough beds and teachers, good laboratories and libraries, and sufficient formal lectures and teaching conferences. Had they not, they would not have been accredited by the relevant Residency Review Committee. The structural characteristics of residency programs did not provide the answer.

Rather, the differences in educational quality among residency programs resulted from differences in their learning environment. Facts and procedures could be taught in school-child fashion from lectures and demonstrations. This was not the case, however, for higher intellectual abilities such as clinical judgment, analytical rigor, creative capacity, or the ability to manage uncertainty. As Moore put it, clinical judgment "cannot be learned from books."[47] Rather, it involved informal learning from conversations, discussions, reflection, role modeling, and absorption of the values and attitudes of the faculty. The better these elements, the stronger the residency program.

The most important informal learning was that acquired from discussions about specific cases. Examples of such exchanges included conversations with attending physicians or consultants about complex patients in whom the treatment of one problem might exacerbate another, discussions with fellow house officers (and sometimes faculty) at dinner or at the "midnight meal," conversations with the attending surgeon while scrubbing or during the course of an operation, informal discussions with a faculty member about the flaws in a recent paper or about his current research, or discussions at residents' report about not just how to make the diagnosis of systemic lupus erythematosus but also about whether there was sufficient evidence to make the diagnosis and begin treatment in the patient admitted last night (and if not, what needed to be done to make the diagnosis or establish the presence of a lookalike condition). One study of 27 hospitals observed that discussions at teaching hospitals regularly explored the underlying science, examined the rationale for current practices, fostered critical thinking, and encouraged exploration of the unknown. In contrast, teaching at community hospitals rarely engaged in those activities, focusing instead on practical topics, particularly patient management of the more common problems.[48]

In short, excellence in residency training was not a matter of formal curricula, lectures, or books, as valuable as these devices might have been as educational supplements. Rather, excellence depended on the intangibles of the learning environment: the skill and dedication of the faculty, the ability and aspirations of the house officers, the opportunity to assume responsibility in care with a manageable number of patients, the freedom to pursue intellectual interests, and the presence of high standards and high expectations of the house staff. With these elements properly in place, excellence was assured, and residency training could continue to occupy a legitimate place in the university.

MAINTAINING THE MORAL MISSION

Graduate medical education, as discussed earlier, had a moral as well as an intellectual dimension. The core of this ethic involved the primacy of the patient: the physician's obligation to do everything possible for the patient, refraining from doing harm, and always placing the interests of the patient before his or her own. This, of course, was the ethic of the profession more generally. These values were acquired during a doctor's medical education, and primarily during residency—just as a physician's intellectual and technical competence. Fortunately, the moral dimension of graduate medical education, like the intellectual dimension, remained intact during the decades that followed World War II, despite major changes in the practice of medicine, the financing and delivery of health care, and the broader cultural fabric.

Typically, actions speak louder than words, and so it was for the moral dimension of residency training and medical practice. The strength, or lack thereof, of a physician's professional values lay in his or her behavior. Above all, two principles guided ideal physician behavior: thoroughness and assuming responsibility for the patient's welfare. In the 1950s, 1960s, and 1970s, medical teachers not only championed these principles in their residency programs but also illustrated them in their personal behavior. The result was that house officers continued to receive the opportunity to absorb the highest values of the profession.

Thoroughness in the care of patients was the first principle taught by medical educators of this period, as it had been by their predecessors. By "thoroughness" they did not mean obtaining every conceivable test and procedure (although, as described already, graduate medical education did remain guilty of promoting overtesting). Rather, by this term medical teachers meant a compulsive attention to detail and a refusal to cut corners. This began with a complete history and physical examination for every newly admitted patient. Such attention to detail was in patients' interests. A careful examination might reveal large lymph nodes or a big spleen in an asymptomatic individual, allowing early diagnosis and more effective treatment of an unsuspected lymphoma, or fresh hemorrhages in the retina on funduscopic examination that indicated the patient's high blood pressure had turned malignant. Thoroughness also involved close attention to detail in the ongoing management of patients. In most specialties, for instance, house staff teams typically made late afternoon chart rounds on every patient to be certain that ordered tests and procedures had in fact been done, to check the results, to act if necessary on any abnormality, and to review the notes of nurses and consultants.

The strongest champions of thoroughness tended to come from internal medicine and pediatrics, undoubtedly because of the comprehensive scope of those fields. Perhaps no one embodied thoroughness more fully than Philip A. Tumulty of Johns Hopkins, a graduate of the Johns Hopkins School of Medicine (1940) and A. McGehee Harvey's first chief resident in internal medicine at Johns Hopkins (1946–48), who was a superb clinician, teacher, and champion of the humanistic approach to patient care. Bursting with charisma, humor, tact, and kindness, for over four decades he personified to Hopkins medical students and house officers the power of the Oslerian approach to patient care—a meticulous history and physical examination, coupled with a thoughtful, reasoned approach to diagnosis and management. Tumulty taught that the greatest sin of a clinician was that of superficiality, for a physician will be judged and trusted solely in terms of "the thoroughness of his approach to the problem."[49] He told students and residents, "Regard yourselves as indomitable gatherers of clinical evidence. Hunt for it anywhere it might be hidden, in the history or physical examination, by some special test, or in conversation with a family member, or tucked away in some previous medical report, for hidden anywhere it may well be."[50] He particularly emphasized the importance of not just talking with patients but of listening and of having repeated conversations over time. Frequently, "One accomplishes more with subsequent conversations than with the initial, as rapport develops and first tears fall away."[51] He also recognized that a physician could be thorough only with sufficient time. He wrote, "Effective conversation with patients . . . can't be accomplished in a hurry. Time is its essential ingredient, and hence the physician must not overschedule himself to the degree that a meaningful dialogue with patients is impossible."[52] Tumulty described his approach to patients most fully in his book, *The Effective Clinician* (1973),[53] a gift not only to learners of his era but also to posterity.

Though innumerable examples from virtually every hospital in the country could be given, the value of thoroughness was illustrated in 1972 on the Osler Service (the traditional ward medical service) of the Johns Hopkins Hospital. Kenneth L. Baughman, then an intern, later to become a renowned cardiologist, had just admitted a woman with respiratory complaints. As part of his admission workup, he performed a pelvic examination, during which he detected a small ovarian mass. The patient was asymptomatic from the mass, but a biopsy revealed it to be malignant. Fortunately, the ovarian cancer was small and still curable, and the woman's life was saved with surgery. Baughman became the buzz of the Osler Service for his thoroughness, and all the medical students on ward medicine at that time vowed that they wanted "to be like Baughman" when they "grew up."[54]

Medical teachers of the 1950s, 1960s, and 1970s, like their predecessors, also continued to stress that physicians should feel absolute responsibility for the care of their patients. The term "responsibility," like that of "thoroughness," requires clarification. It did not mean attempting to care for a patient alone. Doctors had long known that medical practice is a team sport, with physicians from different specialties, nurses, therapists, social workers, dieticians, and many others all having something important to contribute to the care of an individual patient. Rather, the term meant that a patient should be able to identify one person as in charge, as coordinating, and as always available in the event of an emergency or major complication. Trust was a major component of this relationship, for patients needed to be confident that their physicians were working on their behalf and doing everything possible to solve the problem of the moment.

Surgeons most commonly articulated the importance of assuming full responsibility for their patients' care from admission to discharge. For example, Francis A. Moore of the Peter Bent Brigham Hospital considered this idea to be a "basic concept in the organization of Brigham surgery."[55] To Moore, the essence of high-quality clinical care consisted of "the assumption by a physician (be he attending man or intern) of complete, undivided personal responsibility for one patient despite the divided and complex problems, knowledges [*sic*] and skills which go into that patient's care."[56] In a hypothetical dialogue Moore described to his residents the absurdities that could easily result when no one was clearly responsible for a patient:

> "Who's in charge of this patient?"
> "Well, he was admitted to the ward service when Dr. Jones was on visit but since then Dr. Smith has come on. The Residents have changed this week, Dr. Doe is studying his peripheral oxygen tension, and I am new here myself. Of course, Dr. Coe is Chief of Service and Dr. Blotz is the Resident."

> "Yes, but who is making the final decisions about his care?"
> "No one knows."[57]

Moore insisted that for every patient in the hospital "there must be one individual in close daily touch with the patient who is in full possession of all the developing data, who makes the decision[s] and to whom all others are responsible."[58] Moore taught that an operation was an important tactical feature of a broad plan to get a patient well. Thus, he explained, in this light the terms "pre and postoperative care" lose their significance, and the ethical surgeon becomes as responsible for the nonoperative aspects of care as for the operation itself.[59]

During this era the moral message of graduate medical education made a powerful and lasting impact on most house officers. This was because the message was reinforced by the institutional culture in which they worked. Throughout this period, academic medical centers continued to emphasize the importance of service to patients. Hospital authorities regularly spoke of the relief of suffering, the welfare and well-being of individual patients, and the role of the teaching hospital in making medicine better in the future—and not of such goals of a later era as the capture of market share or the maximization of financial profitability. As John H. Knowles put it, "The hospital should exist for the patient and not the patient for the hospital."[60] The implicit atmosphere of the "hidden curriculum" reinforced the values that medical educators were trying to impart.

Part of this culture consisted of a disdain toward commercialism. Academic medical centers retained an arms-length relationship with industry, medical researchers generally did not patent their discoveries, and medical faculty members accepted salaries significantly lower than those of their counterparts in private practice for the privilege of being able to engage in teaching and research.[61] Leading teaching hospitals derided the practice of selling medicine, such as by offering annual comprehensive examinations for business executives, as money-making devices beneath the dignity of the profession.[62] Indeed, the trustees of the Massachusetts General Hospital went to great lengths to differentiate hospitals from commercial businesses. In 1954 the trustees wrote:

> Like a business, a hospital... operates much better financially with high volume than with low volume. Unlike a business, it does not view an increase in volume with certain satisfaction. If the increase is due to more illness in the community, though the hospital is needed and benefits financially, the cause is a public calamity.[63]

As another sign of their disdain toward commercialism, academic medical centers, as before the war, did not compete with community hospitals for patients. Teaching hospitals regularly addressed the issue of how large they should become, and they concluded that they needed only to be large enough to have sufficient numbers and varieties of patients to meet the necessities of medical education and research. As Georgetown University Hospital put it, "The basic objective of the Hospital is to develop and sustain a program of patient care which will meet the requirements of the faculty for teaching and research."[64] This behavior of academic medical centers was part of the broader postwar pattern of "hierarchical regionalism," in which federal health policy encouraged one or more teaching hospitals to serve each region of the country, providing consultations to smaller hospitals and specialized care to any patient who needed it.[65] In accordance with this idea, teaching hospitals of this period sought to support and maintain the health care delivery system, not to be the delivery system.

Teaching hospitals of this period also remained important philanthropic institutions. The amount of free care they provided continued to be prodigious. In the 1950s, teaching hospitals frequently lost six-figure amounts each year from charity care, and in the 1960s, annual losses often reached the low seven figures. The New York Hospital in 1955 was one of many teaching hospitals that prided itself "on never turning away a patient . . . who needed care."[66] A well-publicized report on medical education in 1953 highlighted the charitable work of academic medical centers. "No other profession or group of educational schools matches this achievement," declared the report.[67] This characterization remained true throughout the 1950s and 1960s.

Teaching hospitals of this period, as always, competed vigorously with each other. In 1967, when a national magazine listed the Massachusetts General Hospital as the nation's best hospital and the Johns Hopkins Hospital as second, signs appeared throughout the Johns Hopkins Hospital saying, "We try harder," invoking a popular advertising slogan from Avis Car Rental.[68] This competition was on the basis of the quality of patient care and the level of education and research. Teaching hospitals strove to be the best, not the biggest. They measured themselves by the quality of their work, not by their physical size, number of patients, balance sheets, or profitability. At top-flight institutions such as the Massachusetts General Hospital and the Johns Hopkins Hospital, the stated goal of clinical care was perfection. Medical educators knew that the conditions of practice at a teaching hospital could rarely be reproduced elsewhere, but their goal was to provide learners with a model of excellence that would continue to inspire them throughout their lifetimes in practice.

Academic medical centers of this period were hardly perfect places. The main problem was that the high quality of care they provided pertained to the professional aspects of care, not the comforts of being cared for. Teaching hospitals were widely perceived as cold and impersonal, despite their technical excellence. Ward patients suffered the most, with crowded conditions, substandard food, loud noise, a lack of privacy, occasionally unkempt or decrepit facilities, and sometimes demeaning treatment by medical and hospital staffs. Even private patients sometimes had to endure difficulties. For instance, at the New York Hospital, telephones and television sets were routinely provided to private patients only in 1969.[69] At all hospitals, for private and ward patients alike, informed consent had not yet been defined or implemented, either in clinical care or clinical research.[70] Occasionally, minor transgressions of the truth were permitted, such as the common practice of the era of introducing medical students to patients as "Doctor."[71]

Nevertheless, the atmosphere of most teaching hospitals reinforced the notion that the welfare of the patient came before all other considerations, even though hospitals adhered to a professional rather than a consumer definition of quality. There were always lapses, of course, as human beings and institutions are both imperfect. However, the fact that the primacy of the patient continued to flourish as the ideal spoke volumes as to the values of residency programs and teaching institutions. Medical educators, hospitals, and the profession at large did not often forget that they existed to serve, and most patients continued to believe that doctors and the medical system were on their side.

CHAPTER 9
The Life of a Post–World War II House Officer

As noted already, medical knowledge and practice changed considerably during the generation following World War II. So did the health care system and the values and attitudes of the broader society. Not surprisingly, the residency experience also changed in response to these developments. House officers after the war had a more frenetic life, greater clinical and educational responsibilities, and new groups of patients to care for. Residency programs grew enormously in size, many house officers married and started families, and virtually all began living outside the hospital. As a result, much of the earlier sense of personal intimacy within residency programs began to disappear.

However, there were many aspects of the residency experience that changed little, even as medical and surgical practice continued to evolve. House officers of the 1950s and 1960s continued to enjoy great camaraderie and the exhilaration of knowing that their clinical competence was growing perceptibly on a virtually daily basis. House officers of this era also experienced many of the traditional stresses of residency, such as long hours, hard work, sleepless nights, and the sense of vulnerability to unpredictable forces like the weather or nursing shortages. Though complaints among house officers were common, most residents believed they were receiving a tangible educational return for their sacrifices.[1] The key to a successful residency experience lay, as always, in the overall quality of the educational environment and not in such preoccupations of a later era as the number of hours worked per week or the length of a call shift.

Two traditional concerns of graduate medical education continued to loom large, however: the challenge of providing house officers adequate clinical supervision and the tendency of many hospitals to exploit their house officers as a source of cheap labor for nonprofessional chores. These ongoing concerns represented the underside of an exceptionally fine educational system. Their solution represented no simple matter. In supervising house officers, it was not easy to achieve the appropriate balance between protecting patients and not stultifying clinical maturation. Nor was it easy to resist the temptation to pile more chores on the best workers in the hospital, especially when faced with rising costs and limited revenues. To most medical educators and hospital officials, it was easier to ignore these problems than to address them. Some educational leaders appeared oblivious to the fact that these were issues at all. These repetitive concerns of graduate medical education could not be ignored, however, and how medical educators addressed them would ultimately shape the course of residency training in America.

CHANGES AND CONTINUITIES

Medical students had always tried to obtain the best internship and residency appointments they could. This was just as true during the post–World War II generation as it had been all century long. Changes occurred in the reputations of many teaching hospitals, however. Some academic medical centers once considered no more than ordinary matured into prominent teaching institutions. Examples included Southwestern, Stanford, and the University of California, San Francisco. Other academic medical centers created after the war, such as those at the University of Washington and the University of California, Los Angeles, soon became important educational centers. Excellence in residency training was migrating westward, in response to population shifts, improvements in communications, and the rise of air transportation. Some programs that later blossomed continued to languish in mediocrity. For instance, surgical training at the University of Pittsburgh, which a generation later became internationally renowned, at the time remained poorly respected among surgical leaders because it had few "teaching beds" and had never attracted a surgeon of stature.[2] In the 1950s and 1960s some of the finest residency programs were still found at municipal hospitals closely affiliated with medical schools. Beginning in the late 1960s, however, municipal hospitals lost much of their earlier educational luster. Many of them closed (for instance, Philadelphia General Hospital), while others contracted their educational programs (for example, Boston City Hospital)—the victims of inadequate funding, poor administration, political neglect, and the mistaken view that the new Medicare and

Medicaid legislation made municipal hospitals unnecessary.[3] As before the war, the strongest training programs continued to be found at major teaching hospitals deeply rooted in university medicine, while the weakest were at small community hospitals unaffiliated with a medical school.

Students also sought out programs that provided more opportunity to assume responsibility for patient care. They understood that the assumption of responsibility represented the fundamental act of doctoring and that they needed the chance to be in charge of patients to develop more quickly into mature physicians. This factor explained the popularity of hospitals with large ward services as training sites. Some hospitals had two separate house staff programs for a single specialty: one for the ward service, the other for the private service. In every case it was the ward service that carried the prestige and attracted the best applicants. Thus, the great desirability of the Johns Hopkins Hospital as a training site in internal medicine lay in its Osler (ward) service, not its Marburg (private) service, and that of Barnes Hospital in its red (ward) service, not its blue (private) service. "The better men are attracted to the ward teaching service and not to a private teaching service," a report from one medical faculty observed.[4]

No program ever remained the same. Rather, every program in every specialty changed from year to year. Many of these changes were small, as programs continually tinkered with the details, trying to make the next academic year better than the last. Thus, programs regularly removed inadequate attending physicians from the teaching schedule, added new attending physicians, changed the conference format or lecture schedule, and removed or added rotations and responsibilities to the house officers' schedule. Many programs were prodded into making changes by the Residency Review Committees, but even the best programs regularly underwent continuous quality improvement prompted by an internal desire to improve. Typical in this regard was the pediatrics program at the Cleveland Clinic. There the department chair considered the residency "excellent at present." But he added, "We are continuously upgrading our teaching program.... It continues to be modified from year to year."[5]

During this period, there were also more fundamental changes in the experiences of house officers. These larger changes resulted from powerful secular forces such as the growth of medical knowledge, changes in the clinical practice of medicine, the evolving health care delivery system, and changing social mores. A particularly prominent development was the decline of the sense of community in residency programs. The explanation for this was not hard to find. In the 1950s and 1960s, most residency programs became too large to allow house officers the same close sense of personal association. House officers had always lived together in dormitory style in the hospital. With the growth in the number of house officers, hospitals could no longer accommodate them all. Thus, hospitals reluctantly began providing house officers living allowances to reside outside the hospital—at first chief residents, later senior residents, then junior residents, and, ultimately, interns. Camaraderie and commitment to the program generally remained strong, but gone was the easy intimacy of an earlier era that came from living together, knowing everyone, sharing meals, and engaging in regular late-night conversations. As academic medical centers established teaching affiliations with other hospitals, house officers frequently were gone from the mother institution for weeks at a time, further diluting the sense of being part of a closely knit family.

Another cause of the postwar decline in community was that house officers increasingly chose to marry and start families. Before the war, some house officers had spouses and children, but what had once been an unusual occurrence became common. By 1959 the house staff of one major teaching hospital had been so prolific that it required two staff pediatricians working full-time to care for their children.[6] In this behavior, house officers were reflecting general cultural changes in American society of this era: the liberalization of lifestyle, the heightened concern with leisure and personal indulgence, and the growing emphasis on consumerism and consumption.[7] In this climate, house officers rejected the paternalistic rules that hospitals had traditionally imposed on their behavior, insisting instead on having personal lives of their own. Fewer and fewer felt obligated to delay personal gratification for their professional education. They remained dedicated to their work, but the centrality of the hospital to their lives diminished as they made a commitment to their spouse and accepted the personal and familial responsibilities of a more adult stage of life.

A second major change in the experience of house officers was being assigned many more private patients—that is, patients with private physicians of their own. Private patients had always been used in teaching, particularly at community hospitals. As the traditional ward census declined after the war, however, these beds were filled with private patients, who also required the participation of house officers in their care. Most house officers resented this development, in view of the more restricted role they played in managing these patients. These feelings were particularly intense at major teaching hospitals that had always had large, proud ward services. Thus, at Mount Sinai Hospital (New York), Presbyterian Hospital (New York), and other hospitals, the quality of education and clinical care was considered less satisfactory on the private than on the ward services, and house officers exhibited a poor attitude toward their private service rotations.[8] At the Massachusetts General Hospital, virtually all the house officers in internal medicine sought to take their vacations during their rotations on the private service, to lessen their time in attendance there.[9] Tensions between house officers and private physicians frequently erupted, with house officers resentful of the private doctors for usurping the sacrosanct teaching beds, and with private physicians offended by the condescension of many house officers.[10]

For house officers, the growing numbers of private and semiprivate patients carried a silver lining. For the first time they received livable salaries. In the past, house staff stipends had been meager. Now, fueled by growing clinical revenues, competitive pressures to attract interns, and increasingly insistent demands from house officers themselves, hospitals began to provide much higher salaries to their house staffs. For instance, in 1951 the Massachusetts General Hospital for the first time paid interns a salary ($300 per year). Prior to that, interns had received only room and board. By 1967, interns at the hospital received $6,000 per year.[11] After 1965, with the influx of Medicare and Medicaid dollars, house staff salaries grew even more. By the 1970s, house officers received salaries that approximated the median family income in their geographical area. Residents also received raises for each year they were in the program as well as a variety of fringe benefits, such as paid medical, life, and malpractice insurance; free parking; complimentary breakfasts and lunches; uniforms furnished and laundered; and sometimes other perquisites such as free indoor athletic facilities or the opportunity to attend a medical meeting, expenses paid.[12] The growth of house staff salaries is illustrated in Tables 9.1, 9.2, and 9.3.[13]

A third change in the experience of house officers, particularly those at hospitals where medical students were taught, was their expanded role in teaching. House officers had always worn multiple hats: learners, providers of care, and teachers. After World War II, as clinical clerkships for medical students became less didactic and more focused on practical bedside experience, house officers came to have a more important role than ever in

Table 9.1 AVERAGE ANNUAL US INTERN SALARIES

Year	Amount
1955–56	$1,034
1960–61	$2,136
1965–66	$3,797
1970–71	$8,031
1982–83	$18,961

Table 9.2 HOUSE STAFF STIPENDS, NEW YORK HOSPITAL, 1961–62

Postgraduate Year	Amount
Intern	$2,500
1st-year Assistant Resident	$3,000
2nd-year Assistant Resident	$3,200
3rd-year Assistant Resident	$3,400
4th-year Assistant Resident	$3,400
5th-year Assistant Resident	$3,400
1st-year Chief Resident	$3,700
2nd-year Chief Resident	$5,000

the teaching of medical students. Medical students in the third and fourth years spent more time with their interns and residents than anyone else, and medical educators everywhere believed that "the most important variable contributing to success or failure of the clerkship is the house officer."[14] Medical schools began to recognize the role of residents in student teaching by granting them faculty appointments, with titles such as "assistant," "teaching assistant," or "teaching associate." Not all residents were good teachers, but those who taught the best benefited the most because there was no better way to learn a subject than to teach it to someone.

A fourth important difference in the lives of house officers was the more frenetic pace. The number of admissions was rising, the average length of hospital stay was decreasing, and patients tended to be sicker. There was much more that medical practice could do, and accordingly there was more work for interns and residents. Medical house officers used antibiotics, antihypertensive agents, diuretics, and anti-inflammatory drugs to save

Table 9.3 HOUSE STAFF STIPENDS, NEW YORK HOSPITAL, 1975–76

Year	Amount
Postgraduate Year 1	$14,800
Postgraduate Year 2	$16,300
Postgraduate Year 3	$17,100
Postgraduate Year 4	$18,000
Postgraduate Year 5	$18,800
Postgraduate Year 6	$19,500
Postgraduate Year 7	$20,300

the lives of patients who before World War II would have died. Beginning in the early 1960s, they cared for the sickest patients in intensive care units, employing ventilators, dialysis machines, cardiac monitoring, and other new technologies. In surgery, there was an increase in longer, more complex procedures. Simple operations, such as appendectomies and inguinal hernia repairs, provided less of a surgical resident's experience; they were replaced by operations such as gastrectomy (removal of the stomach), colectomy (removal of the colon), pneumonectomy (removal of a lung), and porto-caval anastomosis (a dangerous, complex procedure to relieve portal hypertension in patients with cirrhosis of the liver). Surgical house officers were also busier providing adequate pre- and post-operative care to these often critically ill patients.[15] Voice pages from the overhead speaker system and, beginning in the early 1960s, radio pagers served as constant reminders to house officers that they could never get away. "We came to hate those loudspeakers, to curse at them, to cringe at the sound of our own names," one intern wrote.[16] In 1958 A. McGehee Harvey, chair of the department of medicine at Johns Hopkins, told Russell A. Nelson, director of the hospital, that it was a great mistake to use pre–World War II ratios of house officers to beds in calculating the number of interns and residents needed to cover the internal medicine service because the service had become much busier and more demanding. "This service is different than when you and I were on the house staff. These boys work very hard."[17]

Worries among house officers changed conspicuously in the 1950s and 1960s. One traditional concern that substantially lessened was the fear of being cut from a residency program. Previously, one of the most disheartening aspects of the residency system—for faculty as well as house officers—was the dismissal of capable, dedicated junior residents who had been doing excellent work because the pyramid system did not provide room for them at the higher levels. The pyramid system had made many residency programs unduly competitive because house officers fought against each other to rise to the top. After World War II, the pyramid was converted to a rectangle, allowing house officers who had performed well the opportunity to progress to the level where they were eligible to sit for their specialty board examination. In the medical fields, this happened in the 1950s and 1960s; in the surgical fields, in the 1960s and 1970s. Graduate medical education remained a highly competitive enterprise, as house officers sought to impress the faculty, obtain the prize of a chief residency, or land an especially desirable subspecialty fellowship. However, the fear of being cut from a program despite an excellent performance ultimately ceased to be a troubling issue.

Many house officers in the 1950s and 1960s had new worries, however. The most conspicuous among them was money trouble. Even though house officers were now receiving modest salaries, the financial pressures of having to support a family could be severe. Adding to their money woes were the opportunity costs of spending increasingly long periods of time in training before they could finally enter practice. Some house officers had educational debts as well. In 1968, the average debt of a resident at a major Eastern teaching hospital at the end of three years of residency was $5,300.[18] (This figure was soon to grow much larger, for in the 1970s educational debts began to soar.) Many hospitals established loan funds for the use of their residents, though these funds hardly touched the problem.[19] Some house officers began moonlighting, a practice most programs did not sanction but condoned. A particularly popular vehicle for moonlighting at this time was performing physical examinations for insurance companies because this activity could easily be scheduled around call schedules.[20]

As before the war, great diversity existed in the residency experience. In addition to the notable differences among programs at community and teaching hospitals,[21] the life of a house officer also varied from one field to another. Residents in psychiatry, dermatology, radiology, and pathology had far fewer late-night duties than residents in other specialties. Surgery, despite its heavy workload, tended to be a "happy" field in that successful outcomes were expected and highly apparent when they occurred. Internal medicine had the flavor of a "cerebral" field.[22] Pediatric interns tended to be treated respectfully as physicians who had a great deal of responsibility in the care of patients, whereas surgical interns often felt like "low man on the totem pole" both in and out of the operating room.[23] In surgery and in obstetrics and gynecology, responsibility came to house officers more slowly, and interns in those fields tended to have larger amounts of menial chores. These circumstances caused frustration levels to be higher among interns in those specialties.[24]

Even within the same residency program at the same hospital, no two house officers had identical experiences. The "laissez-faire" method of education continued to be in place. That is, house officers admitted the next patient requiring hospitalization; house officers were not assigned patients according to the dictates of a designed curriculum. Thus, each house officer cared for different patients, the assumption being that all house officers would in the course of their training see a sufficiently broad group of conditions to emerge well prepared for practice. Residents also worked with different students, fellow house officers, and faculty—which once again led to a different experience for each house officer. One intern might get along famously with his resident, while another pair might constantly quarrel.

Some faculty members were kind, supportive, and gentle; others were supercilious, condescending, reluctant to delegate authority, and taught by humiliation. As one intern said of his attending physicians, "Trouble is you can't pick and choose in a residency; you get the sheep with the goats."[25]

Similarly, different house officers worked with different nurses, which also led to varying experiences for each intern and resident. As the same intern put it, "A good nurse can help so damned much and make things easy and save so much time, and a slovenly nurse can kill you by inches."[26] Nurses were subordinate in status to interns and residents, but in certain respects they still held power over neophyte physicians. Their knowledge of many practical details of patient care often trumped that of house officers, and they frequently understood better than house officers how the hospital functioned organizationally. In general, nurses tended to respond to the demeanor of the house officers—particularly the interns, some of whom mistakenly thought that graduation from medical school put them in a position of authority. Wise interns knew to ask, not order.

Though some of the experience of residency changed, much remained the same. As always, the first day of internship, marking the transition from student to doctor, represented the most important day of a physician's life, and there was no other period as critical as the internship year in shaping a doctor's professional identity. Interns in all specialties were focused on "how" questions: how to do the common procedures, how to diagnosis and manage this problem or that, how to assess the severity of a patient's condition, and how to get things done. Virtually all interns experienced a roller-coaster ride of emotions: self-doubts about their worthiness, soaring pride after a clinical triumph, seasoned with hard work and continual fear of sleepless nights. More than a few experienced nausea, diaphoresis, and palpitations when summoned about a new admission. The most feared rotation was the emergency room, where there was the additional challenge of quickly and accurately distinguishing those who were seriously ill from the majority who were not; after 1960 it was the intensive care unit, where the sickest patients were encountered.[27] Self-doubts and fear diminished during the course of the year, confidence grew, and most interns derived considerable satisfaction knowing they were gaining palpably in knowledge, efficiency, and judgment.

Residents also enjoyed the thrill of being on a steep learning curve. During the residency years, the focus of learning shifted to questions of "why," "whether," and "when": why a particular therapeutic approach was used instead of another, whether clinical observation or the initiation of therapy was indicated at a particular point of time, or when to take out the patient's diseased gall bladder. It was also a time to read deeply in the underlying science of a field, to perform procedures of increasing technical complexity, to receive greater responsibility in the care of patients, and to gain experience managing uncertainty. Typically, the work of a resident was less "hands on" than that of an intern. It was the intern who was first called to see a patient, who wrote the orders, and who did the minor procedures. It was the resident's job, however, to supervise the intern closely (or, for senior residents, to supervise more junior residents) and to take charge when the intern was in over his head.[28] By the end of residency, most were well prepared to enter practice.

A lucky few house officers were selected for the exalted position of chief resident. This position carried no formal job description; rather, it was molded as the incumbent saw fit. Chief residents typically rounded with house officers each day, served as consultants for challenging cases, and, in general surgery, the surgical subspecialties, and obstetrics and gynecology, performed large numbers of complex operations. The experience offered them the opportunity to read widely and deeply, and customarily they engaged heavily in teaching house officers and medical students—the specific duty that provided many the greatest joy. Chief residents had numerous administrative chores, such as arranging call schedules and conferences, and they typically had ready access to the department chair. Perhaps their most important function was to help keep the morale of the house staff high. The chief residency was a time of enormous professional growth and maturation; for many, it was an intoxicating experience. "This year has been the best experience and most fun I have ever had," one chief resident in internal medicine at the Massachusetts General Hospital told his successor.[29]

Interns and residents faced many familiar challenges: finding misplaced or sequestered charts and X-rays, interpreting nearly illegible handwriting, remembering to sign for verbal or telephone orders, and keeping current with discharge summaries.[30] At some hospitals, they had to keep their fingers crossed that elevators would work, supplies would not run out, and that their patients would be admitted to one location rather than dispersed throughout the institution. Nursing shortages regularly occurred, as did shortages of phlebotomists, transporters, and other personnel. Full occupancy, leading to admissions late in the day as ill patients waited for a bed to become available, was another common, vexing problem. House officers often endured inconvenient parking, decrepit call rooms, long cafeteria lines, delays in receiving laboratory results, and inadequate support services at nights and on weekends. Health hazards were also present, especially tuberculosis, hepatitis from needle sticks, physical attacks from violent patients, and deconditioning and weight gain from insufficient exercise. On top of all of this, house officers were under the normal pressures of young adulthood, including separating from parents, forming committed relationships, and having children.

As from the beginning, residency training remained primarily an inpatient experience. The director of the Massachusetts General Hospital acknowledged this in 1962: "The OPD [outpatient department] has received short shrift."[31] This situation resulted from the traditional disdain of medical faculties for outpatient instruction, a failure to recognize the growing importance of ambulatory medicine in an era of chronic diseases, and, after the passage of Medicare and Medicaid, reimbursement schemes that promoted inpatient but not outpatient education. The chief value of ambulatory clinics, in the view of many faculty members, was as a feeder to the inpatient services. The major exception was pediatrics, which beginning in the 1950s took far more advantage of ambulatory learning environments than other specialties. Most house officers acquired diversity in their clinical experience not by outpatient work but by rotation through affiliated hospitals, such as Veterans Administration hospitals and selected community hospitals, which offered exposure to different patient populations and diseases.

The most conspicuous continuity of all in the lives of house officers was the hard work. Evenings, weekends, and holidays provided house officers little respite from their duties, for sickness did not take a vacation. Even as the general workforce in the United States was enjoying a progressive shortening of the working week and lengthening of the weekend recess, house officers continued to be consumed by their work because there was work to be done. "There is no inalienable 'right' to time off," Francis A. Moore told his surgical house staff at the Peter Bent Brigham Hospital. "It is the mark of a fine House Officer that his time off is regulated by the pressure of his duties and his willingness to share the load of responsibility with his fellows, and not by a time schedule."[32] Department chairs in every specialty detested laziness and showed little sympathy for interns and residents who failed to put in a full effort. As Stead put it in another famous Steadism, "If you can't get your work done in 24 hours, you'd better work nights."[33]

House officers continued to labor under the long-standing myth that doctors, unlike lay persons, were invulnerable to fatigue, capable of performing well under conditions of prolonged sleep deprivation. Good doctors, it was assumed, had the "right stuff"—the ability to withstand stress and exhaustion. "With our well-motivated house staff," one Massachusetts General Hospital chief resident said of his internal medicine house staff, "the last thing they want to do is to take any extra time off.... They may casually mention to you that they have a fever of 108°, but they think they will be all right."[34] The prevailing attitude was the traditional one: Good house officers were "iron men." Stead declared, "If you're doing what you want to do, you're never tired."[35]

Of course, sleep deprivation took its toll. Severe emotional and physical pressure did bizarre things to caring, intelligent, and mature individuals. Countless house officers said, did, or thought things while exhausted that they found mortifying after a good night's sleep.[36] At the New York Hospital, one frustrated resident ripped the handle off a door, another broke a lock, and many regularly left their hospital-owned apartments in total disorder.[37] At the Johns Hopkins Hospital, two interns engaged in a shouting match (which nearly became a fistfight) at the nursing station over who should work up the patient who arrived on the floor within five minutes of the cut-off time for "short" admissions.[38] (The "short" intern thought the patient should go to the intern on overnight "long" call; the "long" intern thought the "short" intern should take the patient.) One study showed that sleep deprivation among interns could not only impair performance but also cause negative mood swings and transient psychopathology in seemingly the healthiest of individuals.[39] No one was immune to the rigors of the job.

Nevertheless, house officers of this era complained relatively little. To the contrary, as from the beginning of the residency system, house officers found meaning in work. For many, work was still play. A typical example was David C. Sabiston Jr., later the chair of the department of surgery at Duke for three decades and an eminent clinical investigator. Sabiston did his surgical residency in the late 1940s and early 1950s under Alfred Blalock at Johns Hopkins. As a Blalock resident, Sabiston lived in the hospital, was always on call, and was never able to leave the premises for more than one night per week. Yet Sabiston considered himself one of those who could not help doing what he loved and loving what he did. "I was always happiest when I was working," he recalled.[40] As to the rigors of his call schedule, he and his fellow residents hardly gave it a thought. "We thought nothing of it really, because everyone else was doing it."[41]

Few house officers had the gifts of David Sabiston. Many shared his experiences, however, as large numbers continued to find meaning in their work. A chief resident at the Massachusetts General Hospital described the rewards that hard work could bring: "A measure of the purity of a membrane preparation somehow justifies the dull hours of processing that were required, just as a falling fever surely validates the importance of the sputum you smeared and the orders you wrote."[42] Despite episodic exhaustion and frustration, house officers reveled in the knowledge that they were helping their patients and that their many years of dedication were bearing fruit. Residents were deeply engaged with what they were doing, took ownership of their patients, and basked in the freedom to learn and grow. There were often moments of fun or even sheer ecstasy amid the challenges and periodic lows, and many house officers found it difficult at times to distinguish between work and play. The stronger the residency program, the better the house officer, the truer these observations. Thus, at the Massachusetts General Hospital, the country's most prestigious training site, another medical chief resident observed, "Each house officer will strive to reach a standard of performance which approaches perfection."[43]

House staff spirits were usually bolstered by robust camaraderie. House officers came to each other's aid much more frequently than they quarreled. At the Boston City Hospital in the mid-1960s—a demanding program at a hospital often short on supplies and support personnel—the diverse, competitive group of medical interns sustained "a nurturing, supportive relationship." According to one of them, "We never tried to outshine each other; rather, it was a point of pride to help whoever was in greatest need."[44] Morale benefited from a sense of collective pride in the institution and the knowledge that theirs was a shared sacrifice. Camaraderie tended to be the highest at major teaching hospitals, where the prestige of the institution helped foster the loyalty of the house staff and where house officers stayed for several years, in contrast to community hospitals with only freestanding internships, where the house staff changed completely each year.[45]

Good morale and a focus on work were more easily attained in programs where the faculty took their educational duties seriously. The 1950s and 1960s were an era of increasing sophistication in clinical research, and more and more full-time faculty spent considerable time in the laboratory. Nevertheless, most full-time clinical faculty were excellent clinicians, and many managed to maintain a strong clinical presence. A large number retained a deep interest in the well-being of the house staff—if for no other reason than to gain an advantage in recruiting the best residents to their clinical specialty fellowship programs. The result was an educational environment that was highly learner-centered—that is, house officers were a major focus of faculty attention. Robert Ebert, at the time the director of internal medicine at University Hospitals of Cleveland, was one of many who noted the importance of the faculty to maintaining house staff spirits. "The morale of internes and residents is a good index of the quality of the staff and their dedication to teaching."[46]

The most important individual in setting standards and fostering morale was the department chair. As before the war, most department chairs took a deep interest in the education and welfare of their house staffs. They had exacting standards, created nurturing environments, then helped their house officers succeed—and they took joy in the process. Department chairs rounded regularly with the house officers, interacted with the house staff at conferences, and showed up unexpectedly on the wards to find out what was going on or just to talk. Department chairs advised and counseled residents about career decisions, helped residents obtain the fellowship or practice opportunity of their choice, and remained keenly interested in the professional and personal development of the house officers after they left the program. Most important, department chairs often knew and cared about their house officers as people, keeping tabs on spouses, children, or any personal problems. Alfred Blalock, the chair of surgery at Johns Hopkins from 1941 to 1964, once said, "With the exception of my family and close friends of my own vintage, my greatest pleasure in life has come from the resident staff."[47] In short, most department chairs were "personal" chairs whose presence was felt by house officers throughout the program and stayed with them throughout their lifetimes.

Two prototypical examples of "personal" department chairs were Paul Beeson of Yale and Eugene Stead of Duke—internationally renowned internists, close personal friends, with much different personalities but equally powerful impacts on their students and house officers. Beeson did part of his graduate training at the Peter Bent Brigham Hospital, where he, like Stead, came under the spell of Soma Weiss. Beeson became a brilliant investigator in infectious diseases. He established the link between blood transfusion and hepatitis and discovered the first cytokine (intercellular mediator), endogenous pyrogen (now called interleukin-1 or IL-1). Yet, influenced by Weiss, he remained wary of overspecialization and edited a major textbook of internal medicine. The one principle he followed as department chair was that "the success of the department depended on getting good house staff."[48] Thus, Beeson interviewed all the candidates for house staff positions himself. All year long he took residents' report at 8 a.m. in his office, discussing the admissions from the night before, and he attended regularly on the wards as well. He also made rounds at Yale's two affiliated hospitals, the symbolism of which was not lost on students and house officers. The soft-spoken, elegant Beeson exuded warmth and kindness. House officers, however, were the particular focus of his attention, and his concern and interest in them were palpable. The net effect was that he brought out the best in them. One of his former residents recalled, "All of us who worked under him loved him and respected him to the extent that we overachieved greatly in order to meet the standards we thought would please him."[49]

The much more outspoken Stead commanded a room with his presence and carried an air of extreme self-confidence that sometimes bordered on arrogance. He, too, however, loved his house officers. Stead traveled little, often showing reluctance to join national societies or deliver important lectures so he could remain close to the medical service. He rounded on the ward service three days a week, 11 months a year. He lived only a five-minute walk from the hospital; accordingly, he frequently appeared on the wards unexpectedly, including nights and weekends. This created a pervasive sense that Stead was always around the corner, and it generated among the house staff a compulsive level of thoroughness and attention to detail. No one dared trying to get by with only the minimum. "He was almost psychic in knowing what hadn't been done," one former resident recalled.[50] Stead valued all careers in medicine, seeing his role as helping each intern and resident define his interests and realize his potential. Thus, he was exceedingly flexible in providing his residents as much freedom as possible. When the young David M. Kipnis asked Stead if he could deviate from the standard residency program to spend time studying biochemistry, Stead granted permission, but only on the condition that Kipnis met with him regularly to tell him what he had learned.[51] Stead's greatest joy came from working with young physicians and helping them grow. James B. Wyngaarden, a former resident and later Stead's successor as chair of medicine at Duke and then director of the National Institutes of Health, said of him, "He could get students, house officers, fellows, and young faculty to reach heights they did not know they could reach."[52] Stead's high standards and uncompromising commitment to his house staff cast an indelible imprint on them. One former resident recalled: "I, like many of his interns and residents, totally worshipped the man. The group of us talked like him, walked like him, used his figures of speech, and adopted his mannerisms."[53]

Much of the teaching of the department chairs (and the rest of the faculty) was implicit. House officers watched them closely, learning as much from what they did as what they said. Implicit learning was especially important in transmitting the values and attitudes of good patient care—the importance of thoroughness, attention to detail, kindness, respect, and placing the interests of the patient first. Thus, Stead often told his residents (in another "Steadism"), "The word physician equals a willingness to serve."[54] Stead's residents internalized this message, however, when they observed his manner each day on rounds, demonstrating in attitude and performance the dignity of patients, as when he patiently spent an hour and a half at the bedside of an anxious woman, discussing a host of personal problems that the resident had not even elicited. Such behavior "instilled in his house officers a concept of human charity which patterned their lives in the practice of medicine," a former resident wrote.[55] Similarly, Beeson cared deeply about his patients. To his house officers: "He didn't lecture us about it; he just showed it. That struck a cord in all of us who would like to think that doctors should care about their patients and that we should be like that."[56]

Of course, not all house officers had stimulating or enjoyable experiences. In the book *Intern* (1965), the first of what has become a minitorrent of memoirs by house officers and medical students, Dr. X (the pseudonym of the author) described an oppressive internship year. He spoke repeatedly of the exhaustion, discouragement, frustration, depression, and insecurities that he and his fellow interns experienced. The medical staff hardly taught, delegated little responsibility, and imposed too much work. Dr. X recounted working up 10 or 12 patients each call night and managing a service of 20 to 25 patients at a time. "One thing that bothers me is that I seem to be so busy working up new patients all the time that I don't have much chance to dig into the real diagnostic problems and follow them through."[57] What little teaching was provided was often teaching by humiliation, as when one attending physician publicly berated an intern for missing a heart murmur on a patient's physical examination. Particularly discouraging was the lack of responsibility the interns received. One intern was so starved for clinical responsibility that he returned to the hospital on a day off when one of the doctors offered him a rare chance to do a delivery. Although Dr. X described his maturation as a physician during the year and the satisfaction he derived therefrom, his overall portrayal of the experience was dark.

Dr. X and his group of interns clearly had a difficult time. However, his account also illustrated the larger point that the learning environment and conditions of work were what mattered in determining the quality of an internship or residency. Dr. X did a rotating internship at a community hospital that did not fill its allotted number of positions. Thus, five interns did the work planned for 10 or 12. As was typical at some community hospital programs, the staff had few academic qualifications, little interest in teaching, and even less interest in delegating clinical responsibility to house officers. Dr. X's account provided no examples of faculty members who showed intellectual curiosity or had an inspirational effect on the house staff. Interns were regularly exploited to work up patients for the private attending staff but received little of educational value in return. As Dr. X put it, "We end up doing the routine work and miss out on the participation and follow-up."[58]

It is wise not to be overly nostalgic about the past. This is certainly the case for residency training, particularly in view of the fact that memories quickly fade and unhappy feelings of the moment typically attenuate with time.[59] Years or decades later, doctors often wax eloquently about the wonders of their years as house officers. What they are really saying, however, is that they love medicine and are grateful to their residency for having prepared them for their calling—and not that every moment was perfect. Many house officers had unpleasant experiences, including outstanding house officers at elite institutions. Arguments among house officers, excessive workloads, sleep deprivation, a decline in morale and camaraderie, and dismissive attitudes from the faculty occurred everywhere.

Nevertheless, it is also clear that the one great continuity in the evolution of the residency system was the importance of the learning environment. When there were excellent teachers, outstanding house officers, the opportunity to assume responsibility in patient management, an inquisitive atmosphere, the freedom to pursue intellectual interests, time for reflection, a caring faculty and administration, and robust camaraderie, house officers were generally happy, morale was usually high, and interns and residents typically felt they were receiving an educational return for their investment of time, energy, and self. When these factors were less evident, morale was not as strong, house officers were not as happy, and accounts of the experience were more critical. Residency training was never perfect, but the conditions of work always mattered.

QUALITY, SAFETY, AND SUPERVISION

If one assumption characterized American health care in the 1950s and 1960s, that was the continued belief that teaching hospitals provided the best patient care. The superiority of teaching hospitals was presumed, never proven. Few challenged the point, however, so self-apparent did it seem. Teaching hospitals attracted the leaders of their fields to their medical staffs as well as the best interns, residents, and clinical fellows. Teaching hospitals possessed the latest medical technologies, including some that were not available at even the largest community hospitals. Clinical practice at teaching hospitals was characterized by an attitude of questioning and curiosity, which kept doctors at every level at the forefront of knowledge and prevented patient care from deteriorating into perfunctory routine. For these reasons, published lists of the nation's "best" hospitals typically contained teaching institutions exclusively.

Teaching hospitals were considered the best hospitals *because* they were homes to medical education. "One cannot attain the highest quality of care without the best teaching," one educational leader declared.[60] The importance of education to good clinical care was acknowledged by the federal government as it established affiliations with medical schools for dozens of newly constructed Veterans Administration hospitals. The government's reason for these affiliations was simple: to allow veterans to receive "the highest quality of medical care."[61] Medical educators saw their task as creating an environment of patient care as close to perfection as possible, thereby instilling in all learners a model of professional excellence that would last a professional lifetime.

Most direct patient care at teaching hospitals was provided by the house staff. As before, responsibility was graded—that is, the more a house officer progressed, the more responsibilities that individual received. The ophthalmology program at Johns Hopkins provided a typical example. House officers entered the program after completing an internship, typically a one-year surgical or medical internship (though some ophthalmology residents did two or even three preparatory years). First-year residents in ophthalmology did no surgery until the end of the year, when they were allowed to do a few extraocular procedures. Second-year residents did all the muscle operations (generally 25 to 50 cases per resident), covered the emergency room, and managed all nighttime cases of eye trauma. Toward the end of the year they were also permitted to do a few intraocular procedures, such as surgery for cataracts and glaucoma. Third-year residents were freely allowed to do intraocular surgery. The chief resident did all the major surgical procedures.[62] In the surgical fields, where the length of training was the longest, house officers often became impatient to operate. Before performing an operation for the first time, however, they had seen the operation done so many times and had rehearsed each step in their minds time and time again, that the actual act of performing the operation usually occurred seamlessly.

As always, house officers worked under supervision. Most "direct" supervision (that is, someone more experienced being physically present) was performed by house officers a year or two farther along, guiding their juniors through the details of diagnosis and management. This was legally recognized as effective supervision. For example, the hospital code of New York State required the admission history and physical examination of an intern or junior resident to be reviewed and countersigned by the attending physician or by a third-, fourth-, or fifth-year resident with a New York State license.[63] Faculty generally provided "indirect" supervision—that is, they were immediately available if needed but not necessarily physically there. In the surgical fields, chief residents enjoyed great discretion as to whether they operated with the help of an attending surgeon. In most cases, chief residents operated without summoning the attending, though typically the attending surgeon was on the premises. If the case was especially complex, or if the chief resident had not done the operation before, the chief resident might request the attending to serve as first assistant, or on occasion, to do the operation, with the chief resident assisting.

Evidence is strong that house officers, on balance, delivered excellent care. Department chairs in every specialty commonly praised the clinical work of their house staff. In the surgical fields, operative results were indistinguishable between patients operated on by house officers and those by the faculty.[64] Indeed, surgical care was probably better at many teaching hospitals, where fourth- or fifth-year residents performed major operations and provided pre- and postoperative care, than at the community hospitals, where the same operations were often performed by general practitioners or by surgeons trained in an earlier, less rigorous era. The culture of thoroughness and attention to detail that permeated teaching programs contributed to the safety and high quality of care provided by residents. So did the sense of ownership that most house officers felt toward their patients, which led them to make certain that everything that needed to be done for their patients was in fact done. At Presbyterian Hospital (New York), the medical board considered the quality of care on its ward services is the various specialties to be so good that insured patients would find it to their "advantage to be a ward patient here rather than a semi-private patient in some hospital elsewhere."[65]

In many cases, it is likely that house officers provided better care than the faculty. Some subspecialist clinical scientists, spending most of their time in the laboratory, found that their clinical skills were rusty when called to attend on an inpatient service. Sometimes they taught nervously, hoping the house officers would not discover their unfamiliarity with the latest clinical literature. Clinical obsolescence could develop in even the greatest physicians. Thus, at the Peter Bent Brigham Hospital, William Murphy, who had received a Nobel Prize for his work in pernicious anemia, became antiquated at the end of his career. When house officers complained about how often they found themselves covering for Murphy, George Thorn, the chief of internal medicine, told them he did not wish to embarrass Dr. Murphy and that "it was the job of the interns and residents to care for Dr. Murphy's patients because he was no longer capable of managing difficult medical problems."[66] One year at Emory, a large group of house officers in internal medicine did not attend Grady Memorial Hospital's annual summer barbecue, even though faculty members had been assigned to cover for them in the hospital so that they could attend. When the department chair, J. Willis Hurst, investigated, one of the residents, H. Kenneth Walker, later to become a prominent internist, told Hurst, "We didn't want the faculty messing up our wards."[67]

Of course, house officers did make errors. There are no data on the incidence or nature of errors committed by residents, the frequency with which errors resulted in harm to the patient, or the relative frequency with which house officers committed errors compared with faculty or private practitioners in the community. Nevertheless, the risk of committing an error was part of the experience of every house officer. Eugene Stead pointed out that making errors was part of learning medicine.[68] A surgeon remarked, "Any surgeon who says he has never erred has never done surgery."[69]

When problems arose in patient management, they were usually thoroughly analyzed. Morbidity and mortality conferences remained robust throughout this era, as did autopsy rates. For instance, through 1970, the autopsy rate at the New York Hospital varied between 66 and 76 percent of patients who died.[70] Medical educators understood that most adverse events were not the result of error and that many errors caused no harm to the patient. However, the attention faculty gave to any adverse outcome stood as an important indicator of their concern with maximizing quality and safety. The main limitation of their viewpoint was the traditional belief that errors resulted from the actions of individuals. Attention was not yet focused on clumsy hospital systems as a cause of error.

Sometimes an error was catastrophic for the house officer, not just the patient. House officers tended to be extremely hard on themselves, and mistakes at their stage had a tendency to scar. Albert Wu later called doctors who made mistakes the "second victims" of error because they often were emotionally wounded from having made the mistake.[71] Most programs tried to make errors a learning process. They helped residents understand the cause of their mistake, identify their weaknesses, and refine their skills. Using the phrase of Charles L. Bosk, programs employed occupational rituals to help house officers "forgive and remember" their mistakes.[72] Later studies showed that house officers who accepted responsibility for a mistake and discussed it with a faculty member were likely to be able to "move on" emotionally and report constructive changes in practice.[73] Nevertheless, the problem of the "second victim" always lurked, and faculty members knew they needed to use a high grade of kid in their gloves in discussing management mistakes with house officers.

Rarely, certain house officers proved dangerous. Either they were incomplete or inaccurate in their histories and physical examinations, made too many management or judgmental errors, paid insufficient attention to detail in following their patients' day-to-day progress, cared for patients in an insensitive way, or showed an inability to learn from past mistakes. With such individuals, problems occurred more from sloppiness or arrogance than from the lack of knowledge. The American Board of Medical

Specialties considered residents who were "smart but dangerous" a greater problem than those who were "dumb but safe."[74] The worst sin, as always, was dishonesty. At the Cleveland Clinic, one intern was summarily dismissed from the program for reporting in the hospital chart that he had done a pelvic examination when in fact he had not.[75]

Some programs had a disciplinary policy in place to deal with errant individuals. For example, at the Cleveland Clinic,

> if the department or division head believes the performance of a Fellow [the clinic's term for resident] or Intern is substandard, it should be discussed with the Fellow or Intern. Continued substandard performance after discussion will constitute grounds for dismissal, subject to the review of the Faculty Board. Any Fellow or Intern being considered for dismissal, shall have the privilege of appearing before the Faculty Board to present his case.[76]

Most faculties, however, found it difficult to discipline their house officers, given that residents had already invested so much in their education. Even the Cleveland Clinic, with a clear disciplinary policy, acknowledged that it did not counsel residents frequently enough, kept poor written records of counseling sessions, provided inadequate feedback on improvement after counseling, and did not place residents on probation as often as it should.[77] Residency programs experienced mixed results in counseling weak house officers, given that some practicing physicians continued to practice sloppily, make too many avoidable mistakes, or engage in unethical behavior.

Why did errors occur—particularly errors made by competent house officers? Curiously, fatigue seems not to have been an important factor, despite the exhausting schedules and demanding work hours. Archival and published sources of the era revealed virtually no instances of serious error that could be attributed to that cause. An important sociological "participant-observer" study of house officers in both teaching and community hospitals also observed no major error resulting from sleep deprivation over a one-year time period.[78] House officers frequently acted out because of sleep deprivation or made minor mistakes, such as requiring multiple sticks to draw blood from patients who should have been easy "hits." Undoubtedly more serious errors did occur from fatigue, but their frequency seems to have been low. Sleep deprivation took its greatest toll on the house officers who experienced it, not on their patients.

The same sources, however, revealed many incidents of serious error attributable to another factor: inadequate supervision. Problems most commonly occurred when house officers practiced beyond their level of competence. Thus, at Freedmen's Hospital (the teaching hospital of Howard

College of Medicine), unsupervised interns mistakenly sent home several severely ill patients from the emergency room. One was a three-year-old boy with acute nephritis; another was a two-month-old febrile baby who subsequently died of renal failure.[79] On the internal medicine wards of the Johns Hopkins Hospital, serious errors made by inadequately supervised house officers also occurred. A former resident, Thomas Duffy, one of the best in the hospital's history and now a distinguished faculty member at Yale, recounted some of the major mistakes he made during his internship in the 1960s. "I had not forgotten the bungled lumbar puncture that cost a patient's life, the mix-up of potassium chloride for saline that resulted in a cardiac arrest, the suicide of a woman whose anguish I had overlooked."[80] Though Duffy was often tired, he did not attribute his errors to fatigue. For instance, he berated himself for many weeks for his failure to recognize early eclampsia as the cause of a young woman's headaches, but "her arrival near the end of my twenty-four-hour shift was not an acceptable excuse for my diagnostic error."[81] Rather, the problem was inadequate supervision, or in Duffy's words, "a form of training that plunged young physicians into waters far above their heads."[82]

It should be no surprise that such incidents occurred. The supervision that faculty provided house officers, particularly on the ward services, was far less than ideal. The most dangerous area, from a safety perspective, was the emergency room, where interns and first-year residents, and sometimes interns alone, worked in extremely busy, stressful circumstances without anyone more senior physically present. At the Columbia Presbyterian Medical Center, "there is currently no mechanism for assuring the quality of care given" in the emergency room; at the Massachusetts General Hospital, the emergency room was considered "the most traumatic rotation of the entire year"; at Charity Hospital, the emergency room was described as a "war-zone"; and at Johns Hopkins the emergency area was "manned by the house staff with little, if any, faculty input."[83] Part of the problem in the emergency room was the "iron gate syndrome" exhibited by many interns and first-year residents. Trying to make work easier for their friends on the inpatient services, the "iron gates" admitted only the sickest patients, often turning away less severely ill patients who nonetheless merited hospitalization. With no one more senior to override their decisions, the "iron gates" typically got away with such behavior, even though some patients they sent home later had complications.[84]

Inadequate supervision also occurred on the inpatient wards. Consider the Osler Medical Service at the Johns Hopkins Hospital, which was considered neck-and-neck with the internal medicine program at the Massachusetts General Hospital as the nation's best residency program in the field. On admission, all patients were examined by the intern, assistant resident, and chief resident. Thereafter, the intern and assistant resident were on their own. Between 50 and 60 percent of patients were managed without the benefit of faculty consultation. Attending physicians were available, but they rounded three days a week and spent much more time teaching general points than reviewing and discussing the management of the patients on hand. The faculty devoted little effort to evaluating the appropriateness of an admission, the duration of stay, or the diagnostic and therapeutic plan that was implemented. According to the medical board, this approach carried the benefit that "it encourages individual growth and scholarship in medical practice." Quality care, however, was "aimed for, but not necessarily insured."[85]

In theory, help was available. All house officers needed to do was place a telephone call to consult with a faculty member or ask the faculty member to come by. Most programs emphasized to house officers the importance of seeking help when needed. However, the "hidden curriculum" discouraged house officers from doing so. This was because house officers knew they were at risk of being labeled as insecure and indecisive if they did. An intern at one surgical program remarked, "Bill [his resident] and I were lost, but it would never occur to us to call for help. That would be a sign of weakness."[86] At Barnes Hospital, a medical intern in his first month was caring for a complicated patient who went into shock. Because the intern's resident and attending physician had left contradictory instructions and could not be reached, the intern asked the chief resident for help, thinking it the responsible thing to do. The chief resident provided the necessary assistance but recorded in the intern's evaluation for that month that he was "weak," "insecure," and "needed to be watched closely."[87] Supervision could hardly be considered adequate if house officers were intimidated from calling for help.

In some cases house officers did not call for help because they so valued their autonomy that they wished no one, including the faculty, to interfere. For instance, at the Massachusetts General Hospital, residents in internal medicine were known to make major decisions on private patients without consulting the private physician, or even to "steal" private patients for themselves by admitting private patients in the emergency room to the ward service and notifying the private physician only after the patient had gone home.[88] At Charity Hospital, residents in surgery and obstetrics and gynecology often failed to contact faculty in time to scrub for an operation, thus preventing the faculty from taking over the "house staff" cases.[89] Such incidents illustrated the free-wheeling, cowboy mentality that sometimes occurred among residents.

It is doubtful that supervision in the 1950s, 1960s, and 1970s was any different from what it had been before the war. Rather, what changed was that medical care became more potent, and as that happened, the consequences of an error became potentially greater. Consider the treatment of pneumonia. Before the advent of antibiotics, there was little a physician could do but provide supportive care and hope for the best. One physician who did his internship at that time remembered the frustration he and his peers felt about the lack of effective treatment: "Often we stood by helplessly while they recovered or died, because so little could be done."[90] A missed diagnosis or error in judgment mattered little to the patient's ultimate outcome. With antibiotics and ventilators, medical care developed the potential to cure even the most life-threatening cases of pneumonia. However, the challenges of management also became much greater. Good care now required, among other things, not missing the diagnosis, remembering to obtain blood and sputum cultures before administering the first dose of antibiotics, starting antibiotics quickly, selecting the right antibiotic in the proper dose, delivering oxygen in the right concentration through the proper type of oxygen mask, recognizing respiratory failure should it develop, knowing how to intubate, and understanding how to manage a ventilator, including how much oxygen to administer, how to determine the respiratory rate and volume of each breath, and whether to apply positive pressure to each breath, and if so, whether to do so continuously or at the end of expiration. Mistakes of omission or commission at any step could result in serious injury or death.

It would be a mistake to exaggerate the problem of errors by house officers at this time. Many safeguards were in place, and overall, the quality of care provided by house officers was excellent. The public respected academic medical centers and expressed few concerns about the safety or quality of care received there. (Indeed, widespread public worry about safety and errors did not appear until the very end of the century.) Confidence in medicine was high, the prestige of doctors was great, and a patients' rights movement had yet to appear. If there was any disinclination of patients to be treated at teaching hospitals in general or on the ward services in particular, that attitude reflected concerns about comfort, privacy, and impersonal treatment, not about safety.

It would also be a mistake, however, not to recognize that conditions in medical education had changed. The definition of proper supervision is always shifting, as medical and cultural conditions evolve. In the 1950s and 1960s, as medical and surgical care became more powerful, they also became more dangerous. This mandated a change in thinking about how best to supervise house officers. Medical educators of the era rarely discussed this problem, expressing their faith instead in the traditional approach to supervision. Indeed, medical educators were scarcely aware that there was a problem. However, it was clear that they were overlooking a major crack in the system and that more and better supervision had become medically mandated.

EDUCATION AND SERVICE, AGAIN

A major continuity in the lives of house officers was hard work. Throughout the evolution of the residency system, however, much of the work of house officers did not pertain directly to their medical roles of learners, teachers, and providers of care. Rather, graduate medical education, with its roots partly in the apprenticeship system, had always imposed on house officers a vast amount of chores that could easily have been done by individuals without the MD degree. This tradition continued in the 1950s, 1960s, and 1970s. There were few hospitals in the country that did not require house officers to perform a large number of duties that had little educational value. As interns and residents began to receive salaries, it sometimes became unclear whether house officers were students, as medical educators contended, or hospital employees. To one leading surgeon, "The presence of the labor-management relationship [between house officers and hospitals] cannot be denied."[91]

The use of the term "service" to draw a distinction from education was a misnomer. Properly, the word meant doing good things for others. Thus, it evoked the best of medicine—compassion for patients and tending to their needs even if inconvenient to oneself. The term also connoted "clinical service," that is, caring for patients, which is in fact what medical education and practice were all about. Early in the history of graduate medical education, however, the term "service" also came to connote the economic exploitation of house officers—that is, using house officers for a variety of mundane tasks to save hospitals money and doctors time. The use of the term "service" in this fashion appeared in the first report on graduate medical education in 1940[92] and has been regularly used by medical educators in this way ever since. Thus, in deference to convention, the word "service" is used in this context here.

At hospitals everywhere, house officers were required to perform an extraordinary range and amount of service duties. These included drawing blood specimens, starting intravenous lines, carrying blood to and from the blood bank, remaining present throughout a blood transfusion, filling out routine forms and requisitions, labeling specimens and carrying them to the laboratory, transporting patients to and from the X-ray department or procedure rooms, administering medications, changing bandages, holding retractors during surgery on patients they did not know, and performing a variety of chemical, bacteriological, and hematological tests. Such obligations occurred even at the best teaching hospitals. At the Johns Hopkins Hospital, a faculty committee found that house officers engaged in "a large amount of routine work" that "might be more efficiently delegated to clerks or technicians."[93] A study of the internship at 27 hospitals conducted by the Association of American Medical Colleges confirmed that the exploitation of interns regularly occurred, including at outstanding hospitals.[94] Heavy service duties tended to be worse at nights and on weekends, when fewer ancillary staff were present and many support services were unavailable. Service duties also mounted rapidly at hospitals that operated inefficiently. Nursing shortages, excessive patient loads in clinics and emergency departments, late-day admission of patients with elective problems, and other similar problems all added to the workloads of house officers.

The problem with these activities was not that they were unimportant to patient care. Rather, it was that they could be done equally well by ancillary staff. A faculty committee at Johns Hopkins acknowledged, "Many of the chores now performed by interns and assistant residents could be taken over by paramedical personnel."[95] In doing these tasks, house officers were working far below their levels of competence. These chores typically came on top of their medical duties and hence posed a burden on their efforts to learn and care for patients. The work usually got done, but the cost was frequent exhaustion and frustration.

The distribution of chores (called "scut" by interns and residents) did not fall on house officers evenly. In general, interns bore the brunt of the duties, though not all interns to the same degree. Rotating interns typically endured more scut than straight interns. Among straight interns, surgical interns had the most scut, followed by those in obstetrics and gynecology. Interns in pediatrics and internal medicine fared somewhat better, not so much because they had less to do but because their residents tended to help more with the work. House officers at all levels usually encountered more scut work at municipal hospitals, where there were fewer nurses, phlebotomists, orderlies, clerks, and other support personnel. Scut work on the private services of teaching hospitals grated interns much more than the same work on the ward services. This was because they received less teaching and clinical responsibility on the private floors, providing them less of an educational quid pro quo.[96]

Discussion of the tension between education and service required all involved to remember certain points. House officers and faculty alike knew that "education" did not simply mean spending time at conferences and lectures. Rather, they understood that most learning came from the direct care of patients, with discussions, reading, and reflection supplementing the process. They also knew that much clinical work was mundane. The *sine qua non* of a good residency was the opportunity to assume responsibility. This meant, among other things, that the responsible house officer would do anything necessary for his patients' care, even if it was not really in his job description. Thus, the responsible house officer would draw his sick patient's blood at 2 a.m. if no one else were around to do it. Medical education and service to patients were thus inseparable. What distinguished work that was legitimately a part of clinical responsibility from scut work? Common sense. It was one thing for an intern to draw blood at 2 a.m. from his own patient. It was quite another to come in an hour or two early every morning to draw blood from every patient on the floor because the hospital did not wish to spend the money to hire a phlebotomy team.

The line between education and service was thin and frequently transgressed. Sometimes what began as an educational opportunity for house officers turned into a service for the hospital. For instance, when the Psoriasis Unit was established at the Columbia-Presbyterian Medical Center, dermatology residents were made responsible for providing phototherapy to patients on weekends, when no nurse was on duty. Three or four patients a day were in the unit, and the faculty thought this would be a good learning experience for the dermatology residents. The number of patients on the service quickly grew to about 20, however, requiring the resident on call to spend seven or eight hours each Saturday and Sunday providing phototherapy. The residents pleaded for more nursing support, but to no avail.[97]

Few house officers enjoyed the service obligations of residency. Service alone, however, did not lead to feelings of exploitation among house officers. Rather, such feelings typically occurred when house officers felt they were not receiving an educational return for their hard work. The study by the Association of American Medical Colleges found that interns were most likely to feel exploited when they received little teaching, too little clinical responsibility, and assignment to services with excessive numbers of patients.[98] The most important factor influencing the satisfaction of interns in the study was the attitude of the senior staff. Faculty attitudes exerted "a powerful influence" on the interns and were instrumental in determining whether house officers felt their internship was good or only mediocre.[99] Another study found that about 75 percent of interns and residents felt that much of their work lacked educational value but that only "a small minority" felt they were being exploited."[100] Once again, when house officers believed that they were learning and that the faculty cared about them, they were much less likely to feel exploited.

House officers were not without recourse if their service obligations became too great. Given that there were more internship and residency positions than individuals to fill them, house officers could vote with their feet. Word about abusive programs quickly spread, and any program or hospital that too aggressively exploited its house officers stood at risk of attracting too few house officers (or even none) during the next application cycle. In addition, medical students working as clinical clerks often provided their teams assistance with the chores. Care had to be taken, however, that interns not hand over too much work to the students, lest the students be deprived of their own learning opportunities.

Medical faculties were keenly aware that their house officers were saddled with many tasks that carried little educational value. Discussion of this situation appeared regularly in medical board and faculty minutes, departmental reports, and individual correspondence. For instance, a faculty committee at Johns Hopkins concluded that delegating some of the routine work of house officers to clerks and technicians "would improve the quality of the house staff training."[101] An important report in 1953 proclaimed, "Exploitation of interns and residents should be stopped."[102] Another important report in 1966 argued that the conflict between education and service goals "cannot be resolved by contending that service and education are identical, for they are not." According to the report, "The service a house officer renders may be useful to the hospital and its patients, but it will not be maximally useful to him unless it is truly educational, and this it cannot be unless it is consistently planned and thought of as part of his graduate medical education."[103] In these views, medical educators were echoing the same plea to decrease the service duties of residency training that had been made by previous generations of educational leaders.

Despite such pleadings, nothing changed. Hospitals continued to extract huge amounts of work from house officers, much as they did from nurses and student nurses. The reason was that hospitals lacked the money to make the needed changes. For instance, in 1971 the Columbia-Presbyterian Medical Center considered establishing intravenous (IV) teams during weekdays. The projected annual cost was $320,000. Other local teaching hospitals had not yet put such teams into place, and the hospital demurred. A hospital administrator pointed out, "There would be a major problem in getting additional reimbursement for a service that is currently being performed by the house staff."[104] At Los Angeles County Hospital, authorities acknowledged the economic advantages of having the house staff perform much of the routine work. "Without the interns and residents, it would cost the county a fortune to run the hospital."[105]

Doctors, too, had become complicit in the status quo. Having a skilled, reliable house staff made their lives easier. Full-time faculty profited from the system because the presence of a talented house staff allowed them more time for research (or, in more recent times, to see more private patients, thereby increasing their "clinical productivity" and income). Members of the private medical staffs also benefited from having their hospitalized patients overseen by house officers. Such an arrangement made their lives richer and easier, allowing them more time in the office and requiring fewer trips to the hospital on evenings and weekends. It seemed in no one's interest to change the system except for the house officers, and their subjugation was only temporary, for they would soon enter practice, standing ready to benefit from the labors of new generations of house officers.

Thus, exhortations to reduce the service burden of residency accomplished little because no one addressed the underlying financial issue—that is, how to pay for the services rendered by house officers. The residency system represented a huge expense. Not only were house officers now receiving salaries and fringe benefits and medical schools receiving compensation for faculty time and administrative expenses but ancillary personnel also had to be hired to relieve house officers of some of their more onerous service obligations. Medical educators rarely spoke of where this money might come from.

After 1965, needed financial relief arrived, as Medicare began providing hospitals payments for residents' salaries ("direct" graduate medical education [GME] payments) as well as for such items as faculty teaching time and the additional expenses teaching hospitals incurred from having sicker patients ("indirect" GME payments). Nowhere, however, was there provision to improve the learning environment by providing for a larger ancillary staff to reduce the service demands on house officers. House officers saw their salaries rise but their working conditions remain brutal as they strove to care for patients with far too few nurses, orderlies, ward clerks, phlebotomists, and other important aides.

What was lacking was a national discussion about the value of graduate medical education to the health of the public and how to pay for it. Of course, the nation's medical costs were already rising, and after 1965 they hit an inflection point. Doctors and hospitals incurred the obligation of spending money responsibly. In this climate it was easy to continue to delegate so much routine work to residents. Accordingly, the residency system plodded along, its house officers desperately overworked. Many commentators over the years have wondered why graduate medical education has seemingly been so resistant to change, particularly in terms of lessening the workloads of house officers. The reason is that medical staffs and hospitals have been unable or unwilling to provide the necessary funds to do so.

CHAPTER 10
The Weakening of the Educational Community

After World War II American medical schools grew rapidly. From 1945 to 1965, fueled heavily by research funding from the National Institutes of Health (NIH), the number of full-time faculty at US medical schools rose from approximately 5,000 to 17,118, and the budget of a major medical school increased from one or two million dollars a year to 40 or 50 million dollars a year. Even more spectacular growth occurred between 1965 and 1990, following the enactment of Medicare and Medicaid. During this period, the number of full-time faculty grew from 17,118 to 74,621, and the revenue of medical schools increased from $882 million to nearly $21 billion. The main driver of this growth was clinical income, which from 1965 to 1990 rose nearly 200-fold, compared with an 11-fold increase in NIH funding. Accordingly, the largest growth occurred in the clinical departments, where full-time faculty increased from 11,447 to 59,189, compared with the basic science departments, where the full-time faculty grew from 5,671 to 15,432.[1]

As medical schools, together with their affiliated hospitals, grew to gargantuan proportions, they ceased to be close, tightly knit communities. By 1990, academic health centers had grown large and impersonal, continually doing battle with the centrifugal forces that threatened their institutional integrity. Faculty members no longer knew each other, even within their own departments. Rivalries among professors, chairs, divisions, and departments for space, resources, and academic turf became fierce. Medical schools were no longer isolated academic enclaves concentrating on teaching and research but parts of complex medical centers delivering large volumes of patient services and engaging in a variety of community outreach programs. Academic health centers had become one of the largest employers in their cities, one of the major tax-exempt landowners, and home to many complex minisocieties. Academic medicine prospered, but the genteel collegiality that had characterized it at earlier times disappeared. Among the activities that declined in importance in the faculty value system was teaching.[2]

These developments carried great consequences for graduate medical education. Residency programs, not just medical schools and teaching hospitals, lost their sense of being closely knit communities, an important quality that house officers for generations had found nurturing and sustaining. In this more impersonal context, traditional problems of graduate medical education, especially work overload and sleep deprivation, grated on house officers more intensely. In the past, house officers had at least felt appreciated by the medical faculty and hospital administrators. Now, their sense of being appreciated diminished. One consequence was the widespread appearance among house officers of emotions that earlier had been rare: anger, cynicism, and burnout. Such feelings were common particularly during the early and mid-1970s, as militant protests among house officers over conditions of work and pay erupted at residency programs nationwide. To the relief of academic administrators, militancy among house officers was short-lived, unable to survive the normalcy that returned to the country following the end of the Vietnam War. However, the conditions of exhaustion, overwork, and underappreciation that led to house staff militancy persisted. Accordingly, burnout, cynicism, and anger have persisted as a permanent part of the landscape of graduate medical education ever since.

THE MARGINALIZATION OF HOUSE OFFICERS

Traditionally, a critical ingredient of the better residency programs had been their ability to foster a sense of strong communal ties. Even as the size of residency programs after World War II grew larger, and as house officers moved from hospital quarters to outside housing, a strong sense of community persisted. The large number of "personal" department chairs in every specialty helped guarantee that the education and well-being of house officers remained a central concern of their department. Accordingly, most house officers continued to feel that they were important to the faculty. Those who did not tended to be at less prominent programs.

Beginning in the late 1960s, that situation changed. Interns and residents of the 1970s and 1980s felt less important to the institution than did their predecessors. Even at the best programs, house officers frequently experienced a sense of isolation from the faculty and hospital administration. The comfort house officers once derived from belonging to a metaphorical family conspicuously diminished.

Part of this change resulted from the ongoing growth in the size of residency programs. By 1979, for instance, the Columbia-Presbyterian Medical Center had 300 residents and 400 clinical fellows—hardly an intimate group.[3] Collectively, graduate medical education after 1970 became an industry. House staff costs represented nearly one-half of 1 percent of the country's total health care expenditures and 3 to 4 percent of the budget of a typical teaching hospital.[4] In addition, the trend toward marriage, which became prominent after World War II, continued unabated. Large numbers of house officers (and medical students) chose to marry, and many began families. The result was that more and more house officers assumed a broad set of personal and familial responsibilities. After their long, arduous hours were through, they now had personal commitments requiring their attention, and they had to give time and thought to many matters beyond medicine and their own training.[5]

In addition, as residency programs grew larger, they became more diverse. In the late 1960s, in response to the civil rights movement and active minority recruitment, the number of minority students admitted to medical school began to increase. From 1968 to 1974, the proportion of African-Americans in the entering class rose from 2.7 to 7.5 percent, while the number of Latinos increased 11-fold and the numbers of Native Americans and mainland Puerto Ricans, more than 20-fold. Overall, by 1974, underrepresented minority groups represented approximately 10 percent of entering medical students, compared to 3 percent in 1968.[6] Thereafter, the percentage of students from minority groups leveled off, the result of soaring tuition, a decline in the availability of scholarship funds, the temporarily chilling effect on affirmative action of the *Bakke* decision,[7] and the deeply rooted educational, cultural, and economic inequalities that produced insufficient numbers of academically well-prepared minority students applying to medical school.

Even greater increases occurred in the number of women entering medicine. Through the late 1960s, women represented between 6 and 7 percent of the country's doctors.[8] Thereafter, in response to the growing influence of the feminist movement and the enactment in 1972 of Title IX of the Higher Education Act, which banned gender discrimination in educational institutions receiving federal funds, the number of women entering the profession grew sharply. In 1969, 929 women entered medical school, or 9.9 percent of the entering class. A decade later, 4,575 women began medical school, or 27.8 percent of the first-year class. By 1993, 6,851 women enrolled in medical school, or 42 percent of matriculants.[9]

Even after gaining entry, racial minorities and women still encountered large obstacles. These problems became particularly clear during the residency years. Many African-American residents, for instance, faced repeated indignities—women, being mistaken for maids; men, being taken for orderlies; finding racial epithets scrawled on bathroom walls; encountering white patients who refused their care because of race. Minority house officers had few mentors, role models, or heroes from the history of medicine. They often had to overcome the handicap of working with faculty and peers who, thinking they were there only because of the color of their skin, expected them to fail. Minority house officers spoke frequently of their feelings of isolation and alienation from the rest of the professional staff. As one commented, "It's a difficult task to be in such a high-powered position, and no one around looks like you."[10]

Women, too, often experienced a sense of marginalization, despite their rapidly growing numbers. Like minority house officers, they lacked role models and mentors on the faculty, particularly during the 1970s. They were subject to insensitive, condescending remarks by male faculty and residents, and patients often mistook them for nurses. They frequently experienced "microinequities"—that is, small but real slights that are difficult to measure but nonetheless hurtful. Examples include sexual humor disparaging to women, focusing on a woman's appearance while downplaying her professional attributes, attributing a woman's idea to a man, and labeling women as "overly aggressive" for behavior that in a man would be considered "strong" or "forceful."[11] Few programs made accommodations for pregnancy, child care, or women's health. Perhaps most vexing, women physicians did not have the same career opportunities as men. The majority of women selected residencies in internal medicine, pediatrics, psychiatry, obstetrics and gynecology, and family medicine but not in general surgery or the surgical subspecialties. Prejudices against women and sexual stereotypes were unusually strong in the surgical fields, and many women chose not to work in such a hostile environment.[12]

Larger, more diverse house staffs certainly contributed to a decline of communal ties within residency programs. At many hospitals, however, house officers also began to feel that they were not valued by the institution. These feelings resulted in part from the fact that they were often treated in a demeaning fashion by the hospital. House officers regularly endured such indignities as inadequate call rooms, unappetizing food, the lack of complimentary meals while on call, and insufficient parking. Residents often found hospital administrators condescending, unappreciative of their efforts, and insensitive to their welfare. On one internal medicine rotation at Barnes Hospital in 1974, for instance, there were no adequate on-call rooms for the residents. Five house officers each night had to compete for one bunk bed in a converted closet, with a toilet and sink but no shower. Yet two of the hospital's administrative interns also took call every night, each sleeping in a luxury private hospital room. At a meeting, representatives of the house staff asked a hospital vice president why the administrative interns enjoyed such plush rooms while the residents had no call rooms of their own. "Of course the administrative interns deserve their luxury accommodations," the vice president replied without a hint of disingenuousness in his voice. "After all, they're college graduates."[13]

House officers also began to feel that they were unimportant to the faculty. In part, this reflected the extraordinary growth in size of the clinical faculties. With so many instructors, it became much more difficult for house officers to know the faculty well or to enjoy the earlier sense of closeness and collegiality. This shift, however, also reflected changes in the culture of clinical departments: Faculties were less and less interested in teaching. At a major conference on residency training in 1993, the keynote speaker acknowledged this point. "Individuals engaged in GME [graduate medical education] do not spend enough time in GME.... [O]ur trainees have not received from us, in my view, the degree of close consideration that they merit."[14]

Their indifference was understandable, given that faculty members were increasingly diverted into other directions. Many clinical instructors, like faculty members throughout the university, were consumed by the "publish or perish" ethic—securing grants, publishing papers, participating in national organizations and committees, and serving on major editorial boards. Other faculty members with mainly clinical duties were under growing pressure to increase their "clinical productivity"—that is, to generate larger and larger amounts of clinical revenue. In either case, research and clinical care generated income for the department and medical school, whereas teaching did not. Accordingly, faculty members were rewarded for accomplishments in research and patient care much more readily than for teaching. As a report at one major Midwest medical center put it, "Members of the professional staff perceive that their educational activities are neither recognized nor rewarded."[15] Some noted sardonically that the surest way not to receive tenure in a clinical department was to win an award for teaching.[16] In the 1970s and 1980s, excellent clinical instructors regularly worked with house officers. This was by chance, however, and not by design. The system did not encourage teaching, given that educational work received little consideration in determining a faculty member's salary or academic rank.[17]

One who took note of the disappearance of senior faculty from the wards was Lewis Thomas, director of the Memorial Sloan-Kettering Cancer Center and an eminent medical statesman. In 1987 Thomas reviewed a book by Melvin Konner, a physician and anthropologist, recounting his experiences as a student in the early 1980s at Harvard Medical School. What astonished Thomas was the nearly total absence of senior physicians on the wards during Konner's clinical clerkships. "Where on earth were these people in Konner's Harvard?" Thomas asked. When Thomas had been a medical student at Harvard several decades before, senior faculty members "were always near at hand, in and out of the wards, making rounds at all hours." At Konner's Harvard, the senior clinical instructors were not on the wards but "were off somewhere else."[18]

In an era of ever-increasing specialization, some of the interest of faculty in teaching was diverted upward—that is, to clinical subspecialty fellows. With fellows, faculty members engaged in detailed conversations about research problems or the nuances of subspecialty care that once were reserved for house officers. "The best part of my day is the time I spend with my fellows," an eminent cardiologist told this writer. Faculty members retained a strong presence in clinical fellowship programs, even as they began to disappear from residency programs.

It was during this period that house officers lost their greatest champions: the "personal" department chairs. Beginning in the mid-1960s, the "personal" department chairs of the previous generation retired or died. In internal medicine, for instance, Paul Beeson left Yale to go to Oxford in 1965, Eugene Stead retired in 1967, Carl Moore died in 1972, and A. McGehee Harvey retired in 1973. Although their successors were usually exceedingly talented individuals, the new generation of chairs was much less involved with residents. Department chairs of the 1970s, 1980s, and thereafter did not run the residency program themselves but delegated this responsibility to "program directors," often of junior faculty status, who assumed all the administrative duties. This soon became a national movement, as witnessed by the formation of the Association of Program Directors in Surgery (1977), the Association of Program Directors in Internal Medicine (1978), the Association of Pediatric Program Directors (1985), and similar organizations in other specialties. Most department chairs greatly reduced their teaching as well. Typically, department chairs took residents' report a few months a year, rather than year-round as before, and seldom if ever ventured onto the house staff wards. Particularly in the larger programs, they did not know their house officers well, sometimes not even knowing all their names. A few chairs did not even know their chief residents well. Thus, in his autobiography, the chair of one important Midwest program in internal medicine wrote that he could not remember the accomplishments, subsequent careers, or even the names of his last eight chief residents.[19]

The withdrawal of the new generation of department chairs from close involvement with residents did not necessarily represent a lack of interest in their house staff. Rather, it reflected an understandable response to the changing circumstances of academic medicine. In the 1970s and 1980s, clinical departments grew enormously, both in size and complexity. The administrative challenges of managing a modern clinical department became staggering. Department chairs found their time consumed by a host of fiscal and administrative issues pertaining to large budgets, the ever-growing number of faculty and trainees, and the ever-expanding scope of educational, research, and clinical programs. Considerable time was required to deal with third-party payers, hospital and university officials, business and community leaders, government agencies, and local citizen groups. Chairs had to make certain their departments were in compliance with a bewildering set of rules for environmental protection, occupational safety, hiring and firing practices, workers' compensation, and affirmative action. As David E. Rogers and Robert J. Blendon wrote, this new level of managerial effort was "a large order for a collection of doctor scholars."[20] The new generation of department chairs and their successors succeeded—sometimes brilliantly—at running huge departments and promoting broad academic aims. They were not so successful, however, in having a personal impact on the educational and moral growth of their residents.

Nevertheless, the consequences for house officers were the same, no matter why department chairs now worked much more in their offices than on the hospital wards. Increasingly, house officers did not feel supported by the leadership of their department, and often they did not perceive that the leaders even cared about them. On the wards, they saw much of the subspecialty fellows and some junior faculty members. They saw much less of the department chair or the senior faculty, however, and the resident staff was keenly aware of their absence. Studies showed that house officers particularly valued their contact with senior faculty, who typically were the instructors most effective at inspiring learners to see beyond the immediate needs of good medical practice.[21] Many junior faculty members and program directors, of course, were superb teachers and clinicians. Even the best program directors, however, could not by themselves re-create the sense of community the house staff once enjoyed when the department chairs and senior faculty regularly roamed the wards and led the clinical teaching.

Indeed, clinical departments everywhere after 1970 seemed to be evolving in a faculty-oriented, not a learner-oriented, direction. Thus, residency programs in some fields (particularly radiology, surgery, and the surgical subspecialties) insisted that medical students do electives rotations with them if they wished to be considered for an internship. This policy wreaked havoc on the fourth year of medical school, as many students spent one month after another in "audition electives" in the same specialty at various hospitals rather than using the time to complete their general professional education.[22] In internal medicine, subspecialty fellowship programs required applicants to apply during the second year of residency, 18 months before they were scheduled to start work as clinical fellows. This policy was good for subspecialty fellowship programs because they had considerable time to fill their places, but it was extremely difficult for many second-year residents, who had not yet acquired enough experience to make an informed subspecialty choice.[23] As another sign of the faculty-centric evolution of clinical departments, faculty members increasingly inserted their names on papers written by house officers or clinical fellows, even if they had contributed little to the project.[24] This represented a marked departure in faculty behavior, given the generosity that faculty had traditionally shown in making certain that house officers and students received credit for their research work.

The growing marginalization of house officers was illustrated by developments at the Johns Hopkins Hospital. In the 1980s house officers there became increasingly frustrated with what they termed the "loss of an educational community." In 1991, the House Staff Society Council reported on this situation to the faculty. In the Council's view, residency training was threatened "by the declining quality of close working relationships between senior clinicians and housestaff." This occurred because the growing demands of research, the provision of personal clinical services, and subspecialty training left senior faculty with little time for meaningful interactions with house officers. "There is neither time nor incentive [for senior faculty] to mentor or teach housestaff," the Council observed. In the Council's view, this situation contributed "substantially" to low morale among the house staff and impeded the creation of "a humane, nurturing environment that would facilitate and foster establishment of professional mentoring relationships."[25]

It would be a mistake to conclude that house officers had become unimportant to academic medical centers. Quite the contrary: These institutions could not have run without them. Rather, the marginalization of house officers referred to their declining position in the value system of academic medical centers. To many hospital administrators, house officers were a nuisance and distraction, an irritating source of requests and complaints. Administrators knew that their hospital depended on house officers, but their attitudes toward the house staff often reflected disdain, condescension, and a lack of concern. Department chairs had become preoccupied with other issues, particularly the complexities of financing and administering a modern clinical department. They had little time to spend with house officers and even less to spend with students. Senior faculty, too, found their gaze diverted in other directions. They focused on research, patient care, generating income, and their subspecialty fellows rather than on teaching and mentoring interns and residents. Thus, the house staff, the glue of every teaching hospital, became arguably its least appreciated members.

HOUSE STAFF ACTIVISM

The voices of house officers had always been discernible to medical educators. From the beginning house officers had shared their views with their teachers as to what was working in their education and what was not: which rotations were the most successful, which conferences were the most rewarding, which attending physicians provided the most effective teaching, which consulting services offered the most timely and useful help, which nursing and hospital services functioned the most efficiently, and which low-level chores were the most burdensome. Thus, the house staff contributed to the year-by-year improvements that virtually every residency program made. House officers also communicated with fourth-year medical students who were considering applying to their program. This they did directly, through interactions with students appearing for intern interviews, as well as indirectly, by relating their experiences to the dean and personal friends at their medical alma mater. A contented house staff proved instrumental in attracting qualified applicants for the next year, whereas disgruntlement discouraged applicants. In these ways, interns and residents shaped their environment, as their environment shaped them.

Through the mid-1960s, house officers usually expressed their opinions politely. They came largely from middle-class or affluent family backgrounds, and they had little inclination to challenge authority by displaying unconventional attitudes, dress, or behaviors. They felt comfortable in medicine's button-downed, white-coated, conformist, sometimes dictatorial culture. During or after residency, many of them gladly joined the highly conservative American Medical Association, with its strong free-enterprise, antigovernment, and antilabor positions. When house officers objected, they did so courteously and respectfully.[26]

Before the mid-1960s house officers also tended to cast their criticisms toward noncontroversial matters, such as the capabilities of particular teachers of the quality of various conferences. The most emotionally charged issue of the era was salary. For instance, in 1964 house officers at the University of California, Los Angeles, engaged in what for the times was considered a "lengthy and acrid debate" with hospital administrators on the subject of their pay.[27] In a petition with four pages of signatures, house officers said to the administration, "We the undersigned, and our families, would appreciate knowing why we have been denied a living wage."[28] Before 1965, however, house officers did not make the academic medical center the subject of their scrutiny, much less broader political issues of any sort. Indeed, like most Americans, they were enraptured with the hospital's image as a charitable, nonprofit institution that provided invaluable services to the community. It was this view of hospitals that justified the low salaries and benefits they traditionally paid their workers. It was also this view of hospitals that allowed them a specific exemption from the Taft-Hartley Act of 1947, which meant that hospital employees could not unionize.[29]

In the late 1960s, house officers became much more restless. Animated by the fervor of the civil rights movement, the anti–Vietnam War protests, and the in-your-face youth rebelliousness of the period, the voices of house officers, like those of students in general, for the first time became strident, their rhetoric radical, and their methods confrontational. House officers in many programs could be found signing petitions, joining rallies and demonstrations, and participating in marches and teach-ins, particularly against the Vietnam War. Long hair, sideburns, mustaches, and beards became common, as did more informal—some faculty said unkempt—styles of dress. House officers should be "directed to wear a tie and not just simply have a tie in their pocket," a faculty member at one important Midwest medical school proclaimed at a faculty meeting.[30] When another faculty member at the same meeting railed against "beards, bangs and so forth," he received a roaring round of applause.[31] Some academic medical centers enacted dress and behavior codes for house officers and students, though these codes were difficult to enforce, particularly because some of the younger faculty also dressed in a similar fashion.[32]

As house officers became more activist, the issue of pay remained important to them. House officers had good reason to be upset about this matter because they continued to receive low wages, even after their salaries began to rise in the 1950s and 1960s. It was ironic and frustrating that interns and residents, highly educated individuals with great responsibilities for patient care, received less for their services than many unskilled workers. One study in 1968 found that few married house officers could live at any level of middle-class comfort without borrowing money or having their spouses work.[33] In addition, the lengthening time of residency and subspecialty training carried large opportunity costs, delaying by many years the ability of house officers to begin earning a full professional income. Perhaps the most vocal house staff on the issue of pay was the resident staff at the University of Michigan, where in the early and mid-1970s house officers battled bitterly with hospital administrators each year over the issue of pay and fringe benefits, ultimately winning a guarantee that their salary scale would always rank in the top 20 percent of residency programs.[34]

Within a few years, however, concerns about wages generally lessened, and much house staff protest came to be aimed directly at the academic medical center. Here, the key issues to house officers were improving patient care and treating patients with greater dignity. For instance, at Boston City Hospital, 270 interns and residents (over 90 percent of the house staff) signed a petition to the mayor of Boston protesting the deteriorating conditions of patient care that existed there. According to the house officers, the city needed to hire more hospital staff, provide adequate supplies and equipment essential for patient care, and modernize the decaying physical plant.[35] At Los Angeles County Hospital, residents sued the county and the medical center for excessive patient loads, overcrowding of wards, and the practice of placing patients in hallways when rooms or wards were full. Such problems were "forcing us to practice unethical medicine," the lawsuit contended.[36] At Charity Hospital (New Orleans), the Chief Residents' Council documented to the hospital director a wide variety of problems affecting patient care, including inadequate staffing, malfunctioning equipment, and decaying facilities.[37] At Freedmen's Hospital (the teaching hospital of Howard University), house officers filed a list of suggestions to improve patient care, such as staffing emergency rooms with residents (and not just interns alone), hiring more nurses or reducing the hospital census so that the nursing staff could provide adequate care, ensuring that patients' charts be available when they presented to the clinic or the emergency room, and taking steps to make certain that reports of laboratory tests and X-ray procedures were promptly placed in patients' charts.[38] At Presbyterian Hospital (New York), the house staff urged that improvements be made in the outpatient clinics, which are "recognized by almost all to be inefficient, and, on numerous occasions, degrading to the dignity of our patients." The Presbyterian house officers reiterated their main goal: "We desire to provide a higher quality, more rapid, as well as more compassionate medical care than the present system permits us."[39]

Considerable house staff protest was also directed against their own conditions of work, particularly the long hours and the enforced performance of "out-of-title" work, that is, the performance of tasks that could easily be done by nonphysicians. (This term was borrowed from organized labor.) This was a critically important issue to most house officers, not merely because it affected their personal well-being but, more important, because it also affected the quality of patient care. For instance, house officers at Presbyterian Hospital (New York) told the medical board:

> It seems incongruous to us who serve at the patient care level—the House Staff—to see salvageable patients die here because the arrest team could not be reached by the antequated [*sic*] page system we currently exist with.... It seems incongruous to us that a patient should herniate in the Neurological Institute while his physician is traveling across the street, out of reach, to reach the Blood Bank because there is no runner system here. It seems incongruous to us that our present I.V. system still exists when numerous studies have clearly shown that the incidence of phlebitis and sepsis, morbidity and mortality, is clearly reduced in institutions that have I.V. teams.[40]

In making these claims, the residents at Presbyterian made clear that they had no interest in organizing for purposes of collective bargaining; rather, they emphasized their desire to improve patient care at the hospital.[41] Excessive fatigue and the lack of ancillary help, they pointed out, took a toll on patients as well as themselves.

As the protests intensified, house officers organized. The standard vehicle was a hospitalwide house staff association that claimed the right to speak on behalf of all the house officers at the institution. By 1972, house staff associations had been organized at 70 percent of all hospitals with residency programs and 81 percent of all hospitals run by municipal or state governments.[42] At the same time, initial steps toward unionization also occurred. Pioneering this move was the Committee of Interns and Residents (CIR), formed in New York City in 1958. By 1972 the CIR represented nearly 1,200 interns and residents at 18 municipal hospitals, and it also negotiated the contracts for house officers at 7 voluntary (private, nonprofit) hospitals. The CIR developed the groundwork for organizing house staff into unionlike groups, and it encouraged house staff associations to adopt a much more militant approach in their dealings with hospital administrations.[43]

Considerable diversity existed among house staff associations. Some, like the association at the University of Michigan, focused on pay and benefits. The majority, such as the association at Presbyterian Hospital (New York), concentrated on the larger issues of conditions of work and quality of patient care. Some groups were militant and confrontational, while others were much more willing to listen to what hospital administrators had to say. It was never clear to what degree the association leaders spoke for themselves or for the house officers they represented, nor was it ever clear how many rank-and-file members of a house staff association were sympathetic with the radical rhetoric of some of their leaders. Radical house officers often disagreed among themselves. During a three-day meeting in St. Louis in March 1971, for instance, considerable disagreement broke out among more than 200 interns and residents from all parts of the country attempting to lay the groundwork for a national union.[44]

Underlying house staff activism was the fundamental ambiguity of residency training programs: Were house officers students or employees? To medical educators, who had always viewed residency training as part of the continuum of medical education, house officers were students who engaged in patient care as part of their learning. In the educators' view, house officers received an educational stipend, and part of residents' compensation came in the form of their learning. In contrast, house officers of the era called themselves employees who happened to receive on-the-job training as a by-product of delivering patient care. They considered their pay to represent a salary, not an educational stipend. The federal government perpetuated the confusion. Medicare and Medicaid defined house officers as students, thus rendering them unable to bill directly for providing clinical services. The Internal Revenue Service considered house officers to be employees, which meant that their salaries were subject to income tax. In fact, this simplistic dualism was incorrect; house officers were both students and employees. Residents were learning a specialty, and they could not legally practice that specialty outside of the training program. They were also providing important services to patients that had a monetary value. Few individuals, however, acknowledged the complexity of the issue. Most chose to speak of house officers simplistically as either "students" or "employees," depending on which term better fitted their political purposes.

House staff activism reached a new level of intensity in the summer of 1974, following amendments to the National Labor Relations Act that allowed employees of institutions in the health care field to organize for purposes of collective bargaining. Individual house staff associations became more militant, and efforts to establish a national house staff union accelerated, led mainly by house officers from city, county, and state hospitals. By this time, the focus of most house staff associations was not pay but rather conditions of work and quality of care. In March 1975, the CIR went on strike against 21 voluntary and city hospitals in New York City to protest work schedules said to run up to 100 hours per week with stretches of up to 50 hours at a time. This was the first strike of its kind in the country, during which at least 1,000 of the CIR's 3,000 members failed to report to work. The strike was ultimately resolved when the hospitals agreed to an 80-hour workweek.[45]

The CIR strike demonstrated that an enormous generation gap had developed in medicine. Hospital authorities and many senior physicians defended the traditional system on the grounds that the physical and emotional challenges of internship and residency had the positive value of "toughening up" young physicians to deal with the intrinsically stressful and demanding life of a physician. Sickness did not follow the clock, they argued, and physicians needed to be prepared to respond anytime. To them, the CIR demands for an 80-hour workweek smacked of unprofessionalism and a weak backbone. "When I was a boy," one medical director complained after the strike had ended, "we worked two out of three nights, and now they're working only one out of three."[46] To this, house officers retorted that senior physicians had lost touch with the realities of modern hospital practice. The greater number of admissions, the presence of sicker patients, and the use of so many sophisticated procedures had made life on call much more challenging and fatiguing than in the past. One house officer stated succinctly: "Hospitals are complex places. There's a lot more to do now."[47]

The CIR strike also demonstrated the deep frustration of house officers that institutional priorities at many hospitals were endangering patient care. After the passage of Medicare and Medicaid in 1965, as Rosemary Stevens has shown, hospitals entered an era of unprecedented growth and expansion, fueled by ever-growing clinical income from public and private third-party payers. As this occurred, hospitals entered the marketplace—engaging for the first time in advertising, competing intensely with each other for patients, and beginning to act more like businesses than service-oriented charities.[48] "The modern hospital, whether operated by a city, a church, or a group of private investors, is essentially a business," one observer commented in 1978.[49] To the concern of many socially conscious house officers, hospitals seemed to be spending heavily on their physical plants in the hope of attracting more and more paying patients while at the same time shortchanging staffing needs. In one nationwide survey, fewer than 5 percent of surveyed house officers reported any progress toward getting their hospitals to hire more nurses and other paramedical personnel or to improve patient care.[50]

This frustration over institutional priorities was very apparent at Presbyterian Hospital (New York), where the house staff association worked assiduously to improve patient care at the hospital while eschewing demands for higher salaries or shorter working hours. Presbyterian house officers could not understand why deficiencies in nursing staffing, laboratory capabilities, and ancillary support were continuing while the hospital was investing heavily in its physical plant, including a new pediatric facility, library building, and parking lot. The house staff association spoke harshly of

> certain glaring deficiencies [that] exist at our institution: deficiencies that are keeping patient mortality and morbidity above a more acceptable minimum; ... deficiencies whose cost of reduction is minimal when compared to the cost of the unused shell of Babies Hospital, or to the cost of a new high rise tower containing a new library which, though long overdue could be done without for one more year; or to the cost of air conditioning our growing facilities—welcome certainly, but absolutely essential, we're not so sure.

To the house staff, the hospital was placing a greater priority on capturing market share than on improving patient care. "What could be a more important priority in a medical facility than saving lives and reducing morbidity?" the house staff asked. "Certainly not air conditioning! Probably not even a new library in year X rather than X+1. Yet we are told otherwise. Even the candlelight sconces outside each new room on Harkness 1 have been provided while a beeper page system must wait."[51]

Adding to the frustration of house officers was their sense of marginalization described in the previous section. At one hospital after another, house officers felt frustrated and angry that faculty and hospital administrators were not listening to them. At one New York medical center, a faculty leader simply dismissed the CIR's wish to reduce the 100-hour workweek as "outrageous," unwilling to discuss the CIR's concerns about the impact of such hours on house staff well-being or patient care.[52] At another New York medical center, a sympathetic neurologist acknowledged the difficulties house officers were encountering in getting anyone's attention.[53] At the Cleveland Clinic, the house staff association complained that decisions about education and patient care "have heretofore been handled by an unknown force from above, usually without the opinions and feelings of those most directly involved—us."[54] At Presbyterian Hospital (New York), the house staff association's creation was a spontaneous development in 1970 motivated "by a deep concern for the quality of patient care and of medical education in the Medical Center, and by our frustrating inability to influence policies and decisions in areas of vital concern to us."[55] Three years later, despite an active house staff association and the creation of positions for residents on the medical board and some important committees, Presbyterian house officers still felt no one was listening. "We have frequently raised questions and suggestions in the context of improving the quality of patient care and medical education in this University teaching hospital. Such proposals were infrequently answered in either word or action.... We were left feeling quite distant from what seemed to us an unresponsive administration and we were frustrated."[56]

The era of house staff activism did not last long. In 1976, the National Labor Relations Board ruled that interns, residents, and clinical fellows were students rather than employees with regard to their petitions to engage in union organization and collective bargaining. After various appeals the decision was upheld in 1980, when the US Supreme Court refused to review the matter. This decision cast a chill on the unionization movement in graduate medical education. Equally important, the conclusion of the Vietnam War, the resolution of the Watergate affair, and the end of the protest era in American society diminished much of the interest of house officers in radical politics. They had achieved better pay and, in some cases, fewer hours, and most were glad to focus fully on the business of preparing for their life's work. Most house staff associations dissolved or became inactive, faculty-house staff relations were normalized, and academic health centers were spared further threats of strikes or collective bargaining from their resident staffs. In 1999 the National Labor Relations Board reversed its long-standing ruling, redefining residents as employees for purposes of collective bargaining.[57] As of this writing, however, that decision has produced relatively little new movement among interns and residents toward unionization.

Although over, the protest era had contributed to the weakening of the educational community in graduate medical education. The fact that house officers thought to call themselves "employees" represented a shock to senior faculty and hospital administrators, who remembered an earlier era when house officers and faculty were part of a closely knit professional family. Few on the faculty could comprehend what had led to a confrontational "we versus they" attitude or the idea among house officers that they were engaged in labor management rather than educational relationships. In the late 1970s faculty and house officers alike were glad to see the return of a more normal educational environment and the restoration of professional relationships. The aftershocks lingered, however, and they have never quite gone away.

If the protest era ended, the underlying causes of concern had not disappeared. Despite some improvements, the conditions of work remained brutal—both in terms of the hours of work and the lack of ancillary help.

In the 1990s, a generation after the protest era had started, house officers were still seeking relief from menial chores. Few hospitals had yet provided much attention to the learning environment or working conditions,[58] and the president of the Association of American Medical Colleges called once again for the "E" to be honored in graduate medical education.[59] Like their predecessors, house officers of the 1990s and beyond continued to plead with hospitals for less "out-of-title" work so that they could spend more time learning and healing. Hospitals rarely listened.

Similarly, academic medical centers did not listen to pleas from house officers to refocus on their traditional patient-oriented values. Instead, they proceeded farther into the marketplace, focusing more and more on being the biggest rather than the best. Amid the incessant drive to advertise and self-promote, capture a larger market share (of paying patients only), and increase their profitability, teaching hospitals lost much of their traditional identity as charitable institutions. In this new environment it was easy for patient care to be seen as a marketplace commodity rather than a human service and for patients to be viewed as customers buying products rather than as suffering human beings. Some house officers never stopped trying to remind academic medical centers of their mission—including the CIR, which remains today a vibrant organization focusing more on improving patient care than on employee issues. On this point, however, the voices of house officers, as those of many others, were scarcely heard. As hospitals became big businesses, it was easy for house officers, not to mention other employees and even patients, to be marginalized.

THE DISCOVERY OF BURNOUT

The era of house staff militancy was short-lived. The 1970s witnessed another development, however, which was more long-lasting: burnout in residency training. This syndrome appeared most commonly and intensely among interns, though house officers at any level of training were susceptible. Unlike the unionization movement, which faded over time, the phenomenon of burnout became a conspicuous and enduring part of the landscape of graduate medical education. It served as yet another indication that the strong communal bonds that occurred during residency training were weakening.

Burnout is defined as "a state of mental and physical exhaustion related to work or caregiving activities."[60] The term was first used in 1974 by the psychologist Herbert Freudenberger in an article discussing work-related stress.[61] Burnout is different from fatigue or stress (although both fatigue and stress can contribute to the development of burnout). The syndrome of burnout consists of three symptoms: emotional exhaustion, depersonalization (that is, negative, callous, and detached responses to others), and a reduced sense of personal accomplishment and self-worth. Burnout is often associated with a variety of emotional difficulties, including depression, suicidal ideation or attempts, low or irritable mood, cynicism, diminished concentration, and drug and alcohol abuse, as well as with a variety of physical ailments, such as fatigue, insomnia, decreased appetite, headaches, diminished libido, frequent colds or flu, gastrointestinal distress, and cardiovascular disease.[62]

The medical community became widely aware that burnout occurred in house officers following the publication of Samuel Shem's satirical novel, *The House of God*, in 1978.[63] (Samuel Shem was the pen name of Stephen Bergman, a psychiatrist, writer, and former Rhodes Scholar.) The novel, which became a sensation that sold over 2,000,000 copies in 30 languages, did for medical training what Joseph Heller's satirical treatment of the insanity of war, *Catch-22*, did for military life. In a raunchy, hilarious, and at times troubling text, *The House of God* depicted the brutality and inhumanity of residency training through the travails of Roy Basch, a medical intern at the House of God. The book employed scatological medical terms, such as "gomer" ("*g*et *o*ut of *m*y *e*mergency *r*oom," denoting elderly individuals), and it promulgated the Thirteen Laws of the House of God, such as "they can always hurt you more" (Law 8), "the only good admission is a dead admission" (Law 9), and "if you don't take a temperature, you can't find a fever" (Law 10).[64] The novel quickly assumed a life of its own, serving as an underground travel guide to the experiences of interns and residents at major American teaching hospitals. *The Lancet*, a prestigious British medical journal, declared it to be one of the two most important American medical novels of the twentieth century (the other being Sinclair Lewis's Pulitzer Prize–winning *Arrowsmith*, which, unlike *The House of God*, portrayed medicine in a heroic light).[65]

The House of God was a thinly veiled account of the author's own medical internship at the Beth Israel Hospital (now Beth Israel Deaconess Hospital) in 1973–74. Bergman came of age during the era of the protest movements. Like many of his contemporaries, he believed "that if you see an injustice you could hang together and take action to right it."[66] Bergman used fiction as resistance and catharsis, employing mordantly funny black humor to cope with the stresses and indignities of internship that otherwise would have been too painful to bear or discuss. The book was also a cry for help. As Bergman put it, in writing the novel he envisioned "life as it should be in addition to life as it is."[67] Many memorable characters populated its pages, but at its heart the novel was a criticism not of individuals but of the medical system itself. Older physicians often hated the book, and many of them pilloried Bergman for having written it. The novel resonated among younger physicians, however; many saw their own experiences as house officers validated.[68]

The House of God did not catch all physicians by surprise, for some had been studying stress and burnout in house officers for 10 or 15 years prior to the book's publication. Much of this work was summarized in a landmark, though often overlooked, report published in 1979 by the Resident Physician Section of the American Medical Association: *Beyond Survival*.[69] The book described the stressful working situation of house officers, observing that interns and residents frequently experienced periods of intense loneliness, alienation, depression, isolation, and frustration. It also discussed the problems of marital stress, drug and alcohol addiction, and suicide among house officers. The report found that the appearance of burnout depended on both the environment of the residency program and the premorbid personality of the house officer. It also observed that the internship year was the most vulnerable point and that some fields, such as psychiatry, had higher rates of burnout than others. A major concern of the report was that burnout was injurious not only to house officers but potentially to patients as well. That was because the burned-out house officer frequently found it difficult to concentrate on the work at hand. It was also because the pain and hurt of burnout were easily turned into aggressive actions, such as anger toward a newly admitted patient whose mere presence meant more work for the already exhausted resident.

Burnout was also apparent in the new genre of medical memoirs that began appearing with great regularity after 1970. Why these books started appearing at this time is not known, though it is likely that the burnout phenomenon itself contributed to their appearance. It has also been suggested that they also were encouraged by the new discipline of literature and medicine.[70] Undoubtedly it was not an accident that the escalation in publication of critical medical memoirs occurred during an era of fervent social protest, when virtually all established institutions, including medicine, came under attack. There was also a public appetite for such memoirs, for the dramatization of life, death, and doctoring had long been the fodder of short stories, novels, and later movies and television.

In these books, physicians described their experiences as house officers (and, in some cases, medical students), focusing on how their hostile and alienating training environments led to not only physical but also emotional exhaustion. Suzanne Poirier has analyzed 43 of these memoirs from their first appearance in 1965 through 2005. She found that they all had a dark mood, reflecting the dehumanizing effects of medical training. "I do not know of any physician who has written an unquestionably upbeat memoir about her or his internship," she wrote.[71] Poirier analyzed the pain and poignancy contained in these memoirs, observing that they were reactive—"blowing off steam or indulging in self-pity"—as much as reflective.[72] The memoirs consistently demonstrated anger about the overwhelming amounts of work, absence of sleep, and lack of good teaching; the authors also described their loss of connection with other people, themselves, and their ideals. All the writers suffered at one time or another "from a debilitating sense of emotional exhaustion."[73] Poirier found great redundancy in the accounts, for the causes of joy and grief among house officers remained the same over time, even as diseases and treatments changed.

No one was immune from developing burnout—even the brightest, most highly motivated, and most dedicated house officers. Consider the case of David B. Hellmann, a distinguished rheumatologist at Johns Hopkins and a modern icon of clinical excellence. Hellmann's experience as a resident in internal medicine at Johns Hopkins from 1977 to 1980 almost drove him away from clinical medicine. Hellmann was grateful to his residency for imbuing him with the notion that there is nothing finer in life than trying to be a superb physician who always places the needs of patients first. He felt so depleted by the process, however, that he was not certain that he wanted to continue seeing patients. He then did a subspecialty fellowship in rheumatology at the University of California, San Francisco, intending to become a full-time clinical investigator. Likening himself to a marathon runner who at the end of the race vows never to run another, he felt that if he never saw another patient, that would be fine. During his fellowship, however, he realized that he loved clinical medicine and that it was the physical and emotional exhaustion of residency that had temporarily made him think otherwise. His emotional batteries recharged, he returned to Johns Hopkins to join the faculty, where he became a master clinician and teacher and a leader of its internal medicine training program. He did not forget the lessons of his residency, however, keeping them ever in mind as he strove to create an environment for residency training at Johns Hopkins that invigorates rather than depletes.[74]

It would be a mistake to attribute all emotional distress that house officers experienced to burnout. House officers were also transitioning into adulthood—a pressure-ridden process of its own, replete with insecurities, self-doubts, uncertainties about career and goals, worries about money, and concerns about finding a partner. Thus, some of the angst experienced by house officers could have been age-related, not education-related.[75] Burnout in medical education, however, does not have a counterpart in education for other demanding careers, such as law, science, academia, or business. This suggests that there was something in the environment of residency training itself that predisposed to burnout. Moreover, it is clear that the stresses of internship and residency also created tensions in house officers' personal lives. Unmarried house officers, lacking domestic refuge from the pressure and confinement of hospital routine, were vulnerable to loneliness and despair. In turn, many married house officers found that the rigors of residency led to considerable marital discord.[76]

What caused the appearance of burnout in residency training during the late 1960s and 1970s? The level of cynicism, anger, and bitterness that many house officers displayed was new to graduate medical education. So was the fact that so many house officers seemed not to be enjoying themselves. The president of the Association of American Medical Colleges observed, "The fun in residency training appears to have disappeared."[77] The absence of joy in the work contrasted markedly with the experience of so many residents of earlier generations who, despite fatigue, felt the ebullience of being engaged in "good work." Sleep deprivation, work overload, physical exhaustion, and stress were not new to the residency experience. Something else had changed.

Much more study of this question needs to be done, but one change stood out: the physical and emotional abandonment of the house staff by the senior faculty. In the 1970s, as described earlier, house officers lost their best friends and most ardent advocates. Before, house officers worked hard and coped continuously with physical and emotional stress. In doing so, however, they felt that their work was appreciated and valued, particularly by the department chairs and senior professors. This allowed their spirits to be buoyed. Of course, that was in the day when the "personal" department chairs spent many hours each day with their house staff—rounding, teaching, talking—and had a presence that house officers felt even when they were not there. Beginning in the late 1960s and early 1970s, department chairs and senior faculty members were no longer regularly around. Some no longer knew the names or even recognized the faces of their interns and residents. For many house officers this created a void—a sense that no one cared about their work or personal welfare. This was a deflating realization and an important contributing factor to burnout.

The impact of the abandonment by the faculty was clearly apparent in *The House of God*, whose power derived from its success at capturing so perfectly the universal experience of residency training.[78] In the book, Chuck, the sole African-American on the house staff, identified the core problem: "How can we care for our patients, if'n nobody cares for us?"[79] This was a question that house officers from earlier times would not have even thought to ask. Roy, the main protagonist, also concluded that house officers at the House of God were dehumanized by their teachers, who showed no interest in them and provided them little inspiration or support. At the end of the novel Roy told his chief, "What we're saying is that the real problem this year hasn't been the gomers, it's been that we didn't have anyone to look up to."[80] The emotional coldness of the training system at the House of God was underscored by the fact that the only ones who genuinely cared about the house officers were the two cops, Sergeant Gilheeny and Officer Quick. The supervising physicians certainly did not.

The withdrawal of faculty support came precisely at a moment when house officers required their support more than ever. The practice of medicine had changed in ways that made it much more challenging for house officers: As medical care had become more effective, it had become more dangerous. When the residency system began, nihilistic attitudes surrounded medical therapeutics, and house officers were frequently frustrated as to what medical treatment was unable to accomplish. Now the problem had become that medical therapy was sometimes too powerful, as manifested by its ability to do harm as well as good. Thus, powerful new treatments of the 1950s, 1960s, 1970s, and subsequent decades—immunosuppressive treatment, cancer chemotherapy, new antibiotics, and cardiovascular drugs—carried the ability to harm patients, even when used appropriately. Sometimes appropriate treatments produced new diseases of their own, such as toxic hepatitis or steroid psychosis.[81] The advent of cardiopulmonary resuscitation, hemodialysis, and intensive care units in the 1960s intensified the problem. More and more frequently, doing good for patients could not be accomplished without first inflicting pain and suffering—surgery, for instance, or cancer chemotherapy. Patients, once concerned that doctors could not do enough to keep them alive, now began to worry that doctors might do too much—submitting them to unnecessary physical and emotional torture for no tangible clinical purpose. Critics of medicine began charging that doctors were often doing too much, as witnessed by Ivan Illich's famous book, *Medical Nemesis*, and the emergence of the bioethics movement in the late 1960s advocating, among other things, the importance of death with dignity.[82]

Worry over causing harm created no small amount of consternation for many house officers. This was a major motif in *The House of God*. At the House of God, as at hospitals everywhere in the country, there was a powerful institutional culture promoting aggressive treatment, even after it was clear that aggressive management could do no good and after the patient and family had indicated they did not want it. The orthodoxy of the House of God was characterized by this compulsion to cure: House officers were expected to do everything possible in any situation imaginable. Hospital orthodoxy was embodied in Jo, the most ruthless and competitive resident at the House of God, whose credo was "the more you do in medicine, the better care you give."[83] Or, as she said in the intensive care unit, "I want to make one thing perfectly clear: we are going to win this war against death."[84] Roy and a few of his fellow interns were repelled by this philosophy, for the more they did, the worse patients fared. They found solace and guidance in another resident, the unconventional Fatman. As Fats saw it, "The cure is the disease. The main source of illness in this world is the doctor's own illness: his compulsion to try to cure and his fraudulent belief that he can."[85] Thus, Law 13 of the House of God: "The delivery of medical care is to do as much nothing as possible."[86]

House officers also needed help in coming to terms with the limits of medical care. Some modern medical skeptics, such as Thomas McKeown, argued that most improvements in human survival had resulted from public health measures, better nutrition, and improved standards of living rather than modern therapeutics.[87] Others, such as Lewis Thomas, pointed out the relative ineffectiveness of modern therapy in combating the new scourge of chronic diseases.[88] Still others, such as René Dubos, reminded the public that immortality was but a mirage—that as long as humans remained mortal, death was inevitable.[89] This new world of perceived medical limits was reinforced by a broader sense of limits that developed in response to America's defeat in Vietnam, the Watergate affair, environmental deterioration, economic decline, and oil embargoes.

Accordingly, house officers in the 1970s faced a quandary. Doctors had to ask a new set of questions: How much is too much? When should curative care be switched to supportive care? When and how should doctors facilitate a death with comfort and dignity rather than continue with aggressive management? How could they learn to cope with the death of patients and with issues of mortality, including their own? Yet they received little help from the faculty in addressing these complex and trying issues. Nor did house officers receive much help in dealing with the emotional dimensions of medical practice, such as their reactions to death, suffering, the turning off of life support, patients with self-destructive behaviors, hostile patients, or patients from dissimilar backgrounds. Poirier observed that a central concern in nearly every memoir was "how to enter into a positive emotional, caring relationship with patients."[90] Addressing this concern, she wrote, required not formal coursework but caring teachers working individually with house officers. Courses "can never compensate for an educational environment that is inherently hostile."[91]

Much more needs to be known about the burnout that occurred—and still occurs—during residency. What other factors contribute to its appearance, and how do the various factors interact? Is there something that can be learned from studying residents who survived the rigors of training without developing burnout? Do burned-out house officers recover, or do they retain an element of coldness and cynicism for life? What are the long-term consequences of burnout on house officers' moral development and on their relations with future patients and students? Do those who are dominated as house officers become dominators as practicing physicians or faculty members? Do burned-out residents enter practice with the attitude that "the world owes me something"?

Though much is left to learn about burnout, the fact remains that large numbers of interns and residents suffered from it—and still do.[92] Despite repeated cries for help from house officers, the faculty did not respond. Little professional and personal support was forthcoming to aid house officers with their emotions or their work. As long as the system functioned, senior faculty members were content to leave it alone, concentrating instead on their research, clinical productivity, and other important prestige- and income-enhancing activities. A conference on graduate medical education in 1993 observed that despite many pleas to improve working conditions in residency training over the preceding generation, little had been done. Hospitals were still using house officers for menial chores, and faculties were still providing house officers much more work than teaching or supervision. "We have not gone to bat for them [interns and residents]," one speaker at the conference declared.[93] By the 1980s, house staff associations were no longer agitating, but the underlying problems had not been addressed. The concerns of house officers had been marginalized, burnout was a frequent occurrence, and the educational community of academic medical centers was weaker for that.

CHAPTER 11
The Era of High Throughput

From the beginning residency training, as all of medical education, had been shaped by powerful societal forces. Examples included the funding of hospitals and medical schools, the availability of charity patients, the development of private or governmental medical insurance, the position of the consumer, the deference toward the medical profession, and cultural attitudes about work. Still, through the 1980s, movement in residency training seemed to be driven largely by professional considerations. Issues such as the content, duration, and nature of training, the accreditation of residency and subspecialty training programs, and the certification of specialists and subspecialists were negotiated within the house of medicine. To many medical educators, this created the illusion of autonomy.

This illusion was made possible by the abundance of resources that an admiring public bestowed on medical practice and research. Particularly following World War II, with the rise of the National Institutes of Health and the enactment of Medicare and Medicaid, both academic medicine and the profession at large prospered greatly. In such a luxurious and forgiving environment, academic medical centers could grow incessantly, and medical faculty members and private physicians alike could practice as they liked, spend as they wished, and not have to worry about such mundane concerns as money.

In the early 1980s, this situation rapidly changed. The soaring costs of medical care showed no signs of abating, and those who paid for medical care became increasingly concerned with how their money was being used. After years of concern about growing health care costs, in the 1980s third-party payers revolted. Prospective payment, greater administrative regulation, and the managed care movement were among the manifestations of this heightened cost-consciousness. No one expected that the country would spend less on health care in the years ahead. It was clear, however, that resources would no longer be so freely available for the asking. The age of abundance gave way to the age of resource constraints and accountability.

From the perspective of residency education, the critical change in the financing of health care was the implementation of prospective payment of hospitals. Traditionally, both federal and private payers had retroactively reimbursed hospitals for the costs of care incurred by insured individuals. A short, uncomplicated admission resulted in a relatively low bill; a lengthy, complicated hospital stay resulted in a very high charge. Both were fully paid by the insurer (though some insurers were more generous than others). Under the new system, hospitals received a fixed payment per case, depending on which of the 467 "diagnosis-related groups" (DRGs) the patient's condition fell within. If the costs of a patient's care were less than the DRG payment, a hospital kept the difference as a profit. If the costs ran higher than the DRG payment, the hospital suffered a loss. The federal government passed legislation establishing the DRG system in 1983.[1] Private insurers quickly followed, particularly as the "managed care" movement took force—that is, the new movement among insurance companies to try to control costs by limiting the utilization of medical services, in contrast to the "hands-off" style of traditional indemnity (fee-for-service) health insurance.

The new system of prospective payment immediately changed the rules of hospital economics. Traditionally, when insurers paid hospital bills in full, hospitals sought to achieve a high occupancy rate without worrying about the average length of stay for the patients they treated. From a purely financial perspective, lengthy stays were to a hospital's advantage because that helped keep beds full. Under prospective payment, when hospital fees were determined by a patient's diagnosis (technically, the predicted use of resources for the patient's condition calculated by the DRG system) instead of the actual cost of care, financial success depended on caring for a greater number of patients ever more rapidly. Hospitals made money not by maintaining a high occupancy per se but by attracting a large number of insured patients who were admitted and discharged quickly. Speed became the objective of care under the new payment system: larger numbers of admissions, shorter lengths of stay, and much greater turnover of patients. The new financial goal of hospitals became that of maximizing the "throughput" of patients.

Prospective payment represented a rational approach to hospital financing, given the magnitude of hospital costs in America and the failure of the medical profession to provide leadership in controlling those costs.

However, the new system inadvertently aggravated the central fault line in graduate medical education: the tension between education and institutional service. From the beginning of the residency system, house officers had been the glue allowing hospitals to function efficiently, to the benefit of the institution, the full-time faculty, and the part-time faculty alike. In the era of high throughput, as always, the task of keeping hospitals running fell to the house staff. House officers began working up more and more patients who stayed for shorter and shorter periods of time. These efforts paid off, allowing most teaching hospitals to remain profitable, despite the much harsher and less forgiving environment. However, this success came at a cost: namely, the quality of graduate medical education. The availability of time that had benefited previous generations of house officers became scarce. There were simply too many patients for residents to manage, so residents had less time for reading, reflecting, observing patients carefully, pondering a patient's problem, and being attentive to detail. By the early 2000s, it was clear that academic medical centers were institutional survivors in the new competitive medical marketplace. In the process, however, the core principles those institutions had been entrusted to preserve were being compromised.

At the end of the twentieth century, as the reimbursement system for hospitals changed, so did cultural attitudes toward work. These changing societal values affected the outlook of medical students, house officers, and physicians as they did all members of society. In this new climate, William Osler's maxim that in medicine "work is the master-word" seemed suddenly quaint and antiquated. Many medical students and house officers became enraptured with the search for personal fulfillment, not merely the quest for learning, skill, and service to patients. These new attitudes began to shape their selection of careers within medicine and their expectations for what their professional lives would be like. By the early twenty-first century, medical students and house officers were renegotiating the balance between work and personal life in a way that often stunned their elders. Thus, cultural changes as well as changes in the financing of hospitals left their mark on residency training. The illusion of autonomy was shattered.

THE NEW LEARNING ENVIRONMENT

For nearly two centuries, hospitalizations in America had progressively been becoming shorter. Before 1870, patients lingered in hospitals for months at a time, receiving as much moral suasion as direct medical or surgical care.[2] By World War I, the average length of stay at acute care hospitals had dropped to three or four weeks, and by World War II, to two or three weeks. After World War II, it became possible to care for many patients with chronic conditions on an outpatient basis—some of whom had previously kept beds occupied for weeks at a time. By the early 1980s, the average length of stay had fallen to 10 to 12 days.[3] In this context the shortening of the length of stay mandated by prospective payment represented the continuation of a powerful historical trend.

As hospitalizations had been growing shorter, hospitalized patients had been becoming sicker. This represented the growing power of medical and surgical care, which allowed ever-more dramatic interventions in a broadening array of conditions. New medical treatments became more effective (and potentially more hazardous); operative procedures became bolder, longer, and more complex; and both diagnostics and treatment came to employ ever-more sophisticated technologies. Over time, more and more patients who once would have died emerged from their illnesses alive and well.[4] Hospitals became bustling institutions where hope was extended to very sick individuals with increasingly complex conditions. This was a change welcomed by the medical profession and patients alike.

Traditionally, the great strength of residency training, and indeed all of medical education in America, had been its linkage to the patient care system, in contrast to the classroom alone. Through the early 1980s, hospitals continued to provide excellent learning environments for clinical education. A diversity of patients was present (though some believed that in an era of chronic diseases, residents needed more ambulatory opportunities), and house officers assumed increasing responsibility for patient care as they progressed through their residencies and subspecialty fellowships. Most important, time was present for learning and teaching. Even with the shorter hospitalizations of the early 1980s, house officers still had sufficient time to observe the natural history of disease, monitor the results of a diagnostic or therapeutic strategy, learn the nuances of clinical medicine, and explore in depth issues of particular interest. Faculty members—at least those who were willing to teach—found that they, too, still had sufficient time to do that work well.

In the mid-1980s, prospective payment resulted in a dramatic shift in these long-standing trends. Within a decade, the average length of stay fell to five or six days, compared with the 10 or 12 days immediately before DRGs began.[5] In subsequent years the average length of stay at most hospitals decreased another two or three days, to three or four days. In addition, government and private payers mandated, often for economic rather than medical reasons, that many workups, procedures, and treatments be moved from the hospital to the less expensive ambulatory setting. Thus, patients with difficult diagnostic dilemmas who previously would have been admitted to sort things out as quickly as possible now had to have the entire workup done on an outpatient basis. More and more the inpatient units of hospitals came to be populated with two types of patients: one group that was seriously ill, and another that was admitted the day of an elective procedure and discharged as soon as possible thereafter, often with 24 hours. These changes were particularly conspicuous at teaching hospitals, which, as referral centers, continued to receive the sickest and most complex patients and accordingly saw the average acuity of illness of their patients increase markedly. Thus, a five-day hospitalization at a teaching hospital often required much more work than one of similar length at a community hospital. As the governing board of one major teaching hospital wryly noted in 1989, the hospital's average length of stay "is remarkably low given the acuity of the patients admitted."[6]

Much of the shortened length of stay under prospective payment occurred for important, justifiable reasons. In many cases advances in medical care made possible briefer hospital stays. For instance, as late as 1980 standard practice dictated that patients recovering from an uncomplicated myocardial infarction required three weeks of bed rest and hospital observation. The discovery that early ambulation promoted recovery enabled much shorter hospitalizations and faster healing. The development of intravenous catheters suitable for long-term use, together with improved home health services, allowed a dramatic shortening of hospital stays for certain conditions as well. For example, osteomyelitis and subacute bacterial endocarditis, both life-threatening infections, required six weeks of intravenous antibiotic treatment. Previously, patients with these illnesses had no choice but to remain in the hospital for the duration of treatment. Now, once stable, these patients could be discharged, to receive most of their therapy at home.[7]

Similar trends occurred elsewhere in medicine. The introduction of new anesthetic agents allowed many procedures that formerly had required hospitalization, such as colonoscopy, to be safely performed in outpatient settings. The development of laparoscopic (minimally invasive) surgery allowed many operations that formerly had required several days in the hospital to be performed safely on an outpatient basis or during a 24-hour admission. Examples included arthroscopic surgery on joints, laparoscopic inguinal hernia repair, and laparoscopic cholecystectomy. Advances in the speed and accuracy of diagnosis, such as those made possible by computed tomographic (CT) scanning and magnetic resonance imaging (MRI), also contributed to the shortening of hospital stays.

Prospective payment also placed a much-needed emphasis on responsible, skilled management. Accordingly, hospitals improved their purchasing procedures, accounting and billing practices, and methods for managing inventories. In addition, hospitals began to make patient care much more efficient. Thus, hospitals worked to achieve a better flow of patients from the emergency room or admitting office to their rooms and to make more efficient use of patients' time once in the hospital. For instance, hospitals purchased additional scanners to decrease waiting time for CT or MRI scans. The introduction of computer terminals at nursing stations in the early 1980s allowed a level of coordination between the laboratories and clinical units that had never before been possible. Delays in receiving laboratory information became much less common, and physicians could find out 24 hours a day the status of a test, such as whether the specimen had been received or the test performed. The growing use of electronic medical records in the 1990s and early 2000s greatly reduced time wasted looking for a chart, hunting down an X-ray image in the radiology department, or trying to decipher an illegible handwritten note. These and many other organizational changes helped speed patient flow and shorten length of stay. Hospitals were aided in these efforts by the ideas for enhancing the quality of production processes pioneered by W. Edwards Deming and others, which were being widely adopted in many industries in the 1980s and 1990s.

At many hospitals house officers contributed to this process. Thus, at one teaching hospital the house officers brought to the administration's attention the scarcity of intravenous pumps on the floor, the need for revision of the list of drugs and solutions that could be mixed and administered by nurses, and the need for improved monitoring of personnel on the new blood-drawing teams.[8] During the protest era, hospital administrators often rebuffed any suggestions from house officers for improving patient care. Now, administrators usually welcomed their suggestions under the new guise of efficiency and quality improvement.

Prospective payment immediately altered the institutional contour of residency training. In the new, competitive environment, not all hospitals succeeded in admitting a large-enough volume of patients to remain profitable. Between 1986 and 1996, as hospital profit margins contracted, the number of hospitals fell by 20 percent.[9] The main victims were small and midsized community hospitals, some of which had graduate training programs. Accordingly, the trend for residency training to concentrate in large, highly specialized "tertiary care" medical centers, already under way, accelerated.[10]

In addition, the growing workload, as always, prompted most hospitals to increase the size of their house staffs. For instance, by 1995, the internal medicine program at the Massachusetts General Hospital had reached 104 house officers, triple the number in 1965.[11] The top programs continued to attract mainly US medical graduates; less competitive programs hired more international medical graduates or did not fill positions. House officers represented a good value to financially beleaguered hospitals. For instance, in 1982 the Johns Hopkins Hospital had to pay $35,000 a year for a nurse anesthetist working a 40-hour week, whereas the cost of an anesthesiology resident working far longer hours was less than $20,000.[12]

The expansion in program size continued until the passage of the Balanced Budget Act of 1997, which included financial disincentives for adding new residency positions. The bill slashed the Medicare budget, in part by reducing funds that had gone directly to teaching hospitals to support their residency training programs. The bill also capped at 1996 levels the number of residency positions for which hospitals could receive direct and indirect graduate medical education payments from Medicare. Thereafter, hospitals could have additional residents if they wished but received no additional Medicare support if they did so. As a result, programs grew much more slowly in size after that date.[13]

As prospective payment spread, coupled with lower reimbursement rates from managed care companies, hospitals everywhere responded by increasing their volume of admissions and shortening the average length of stay. Teaching hospitals were under especially intense financial pressures because few private payers covered their additional costs of education, research, and the larger amount of charity care they provided. As a result, academic medical centers worked especially hard to increase throughput, and the ambience within them changed.[14] "It is remarkable what that impact [more admissions and shorter length of stays] has upon an institution," one hospital administrator noted.[15] All emphasis was on industrial speed and efficiency—"Taylorized medicine," one observer called it, referring to the pioneering efficiency expert Frederick Winslow Taylor.[16] Hospital administrators, even with an average length of stay that had fallen to four days, worked assiduously to squeeze out another 0.2 or 0.3 days.[17] Administrators, who once had asked doctors how their patients were doing, now more typically asked when their patients were going home. Physicians at many academic medical centers complained that staff morale had been lowered, and the atmosphere at most teaching hospitals became more corporate, less personal, and exquisitely focused on limiting the length of stay as much as possible.

This new environment profoundly affected the residency experience. As always, most of the increased burden fell to the house staff, who found themselves deluged with far more admissions than ever before. Despite the fact that many residency programs had grown in size, house officers struggled to keep up with the incoming tide. This increased workload was intensified by the fact that low reimbursement rates from managed care organizations forced many hospitals to reduce the number of nurses and other support personnel, thereby creating additional work for house officers.[18] The critical ingredient of a strong learning environment had always been, in the words of one notable surgical educator, "a manageable number of patients."[19] Now, this fundamental educational principle was violated.

All specialties were affected by the institutional goal of increasing throughput, but none more so than internal medicine, which received some of the sickest and most complex patients. Consider a typical example: the internal medicine service at Barnes Hospital (which, after its merger with Jewish Hospital in 1996, became Barnes-Jewish Hospital). Before prospective payment, the service was covered by teams consisting of a resident, intern, and medical students. Depending on the specific rotation, teams were on call every third or fourth night. A typical call day resulted in three new admissions (a fourth admission made the day unusually heavy), and the average length of stay was around 10 days.[20] Within a decade under the new system, "long" call was still every four days, but the average length of stay had fallen to around four days, and each team was consistently working up 14 patients per call day. A second intern had been added to the teams, so each intern regularly worked up seven patients. The supervising resident looked over the new patients to guard against a flagrant error or oversight. However, the resident no longer worked up the patients himself as before.

The increased workload facing house officers was actually greater than might be surmised from the number of admissions alone. This was because no part of a patient's hospitalization, particularly in the nonsurgical fields, required more time, thought, and effort from the house officer than the admission evaluation. Thereafter, even with very sick patients, house officers typically had some respite in terms of the work required to care for the patient. In the era of high throughput, this natural rhythm was broken. House officers seemed reduced to being workup machines and disposition arrangers. A chief resident in internal medicine described how the intense throughput pressures affected his house officers: "The residents are doing their usual thorough evaluations one night, and working like dogs the next day to get the work-up done only to see the patient transferred to a rehab facility [or discharged]... almost immediately, so that the whole process begins again for them."[21]

In the era of high throughput, house officers finally obtained relief from some of their traditional chores. Interns at most hospitals no longer had to draw routine blood specimens, insert as many intravenous lines, examine urine specimens, prepare and examine slides of blood smears and sputum, or perform as many bedside procedures. Phlebotomists, IV teams, laboratory technicians, and procedure teams were hired instead to do much of this work.[22] However, house officers found themselves buried under a new set of administrative chores: scheduling tests, arranging for procedures, calling for consultations, handling discharge arrangements, preparing discharge summaries, and making certain that all the required chart documentation had been completed. Much of this work could have been done by ward secretaries. In the era of high throughput, "scut work" did not disappear. Rather, it changed in form.

The effects of prospective payment on the quality of patient care were controversial and unclear.[23] However, one consequence was quickly apparent: the erosive effects of the new system on the learning environment of hospital wards. House officers desperately tried to keep up with one tidal wave of patients after another. They had little time to reflect, be mindful (the process of actively noticing new things, relinquishing preconceived mindsets, and then acting on the new observations), or establish meaningful relations with patients and families. Attendance at formal educational conferences became more difficult, as did participation in the even more important informal learning processes, such as carefully observing patients through the course of an illness, talking with consultants or one another, reading about a subject in depth, teaching students, or wondering.

The effects of the new system varied somewhat by field. In surgery, residents increasingly met patients with known diagnoses under the drapes of the operating table. This approach allowed them to learn surgical techniques, but it made it much more difficult to acquire diagnostic skill and clinical judgment. The new approach thus violated the fundamental principle of teaching surgery espoused by William Halsted, Harvey Cushing, Francis Moore, and other surgical masters that the most important quality that must be inculcated into a good surgeon is the judgment to know when not to operate. In internal medicine and other nonsurgical fields, the experience of residents suffered from the loss of quality control in medical education. In the past, house officers had received the results of diagnostic tests and observed the effects of therapy while their patients were still in the hospital. This opportunity greatly sharpened their clinical skill and acumen. Now, patients were routinely discharged with important test results still pending, the effects of therapy still unclear, and sometimes with a diagnosis still unestablished. Residents no longer learned whether their initial impressions had been right or wrong, their diagnosis or treatment plan on target or not. Unlike previous generations of house officers, they could not so readily learn from their mistakes or acquire the same level of clinical experience to sharpen their judgment.

In all specialties, residency training came to be dominated by an overriding goal: discharging patients as quickly as possible. House officers were instructed to begin discharge planning on day one of a hospitalization, sometimes even before meeting the patient. They focused on what absolutely needed to be accomplished in the hospital, then sent patients home, often with much more diagnostic work or treatment remaining to be completed. The imperative to discharge was noticed by David M. Kipnis and Eugene A. Stead Jr., both of whom continued to teach house officers on inpatient wards until the 1990s. Kipnis lost interest in serving as an attending physician when it became clear to him that "house officers want to talk only about discharge and not about disease."[24] Stead stopped rounding on the medical wards at Duke for similar reasons, claiming that it was "no longer fun."[25] Molly Cooke, David M. Irby, and Bridget C. O'Brien made similar observations in a major study of medical education they conducted for the Carnegie Foundation for the Advancement of Teaching. In contemporary graduate medical education, they noted, "Discharge becomes the highest goal."[26]

No program was immune from the educational challenges imposed by high throughput. Consider the two most prestigious residencies in internal medicine: the programs at the Johns Hopkins Hospital and Massachusetts General Hospital. At Johns Hopkins, the average length of stay on the medicine service fell from 11 days in 1980 to 7 days in 1985, during which time the yearly discharges from the service increased from 7,700 to 9,000. By 1988, 40 percent of the patients on the medical service were in the hospital for three days or fewer. This "turnstile effect," as the department's official history called it, significantly affected residency training since "less time was available to consider the problem and the patient at hand."[27] At Massachusetts General Hospital, the internal medicine program also grappled with the problem of how to allow adequate time for teaching and learning as patient volume continued to increase and the average length of stay fell. One chief resident noted that "a disproportionate amount of this increased workload was being borne by the residents," and as a result, "the challenge to provide competent care became the goal and teaching was secondary."[28] Another chief resident observed that a "siege mentality" had arisen among the house staff to combat the pressure imposed by economy and volume.[29] The faculty at the hospital also noted that the educational component of the residency program had suffered because of higher patient volume, and they urged that residents be relieved of some of their workload so that they could have more time to learn.[30]

Medical educators knew that something was amiss. Many programs made constructive changes to help cope with the rising volume of patients and frenetic pace, such as initiating "night float" rotations to provide more house officers at night, establishing "caps" on the number of admissions per intern (often seven patients per "long call"), creating services staffed by moonlighting residents and fellows to help spread the workload, and achieving better geographical localization of patients so house officers would not have to spend as much time running from one part of the hospital to another. These approaches, however, were akin to Band-Aids. One house officer called them "shell games" because the workload as measured by the number of admissions per intern per year continued to grow.[31]

Many professional organizations were also concerned about the problem. In its program standards, the Accreditation Council for Graduate Medical Education (ACGME) clearly stated that residency education should not be driven by service needs. The ACGME required "an adequate level of resident staff to prevent excessive patient loads, excessive new admission work-ups, [and] inappropriate intensity of service or case mix."[32] The organization knew that this requirement was frequently ignored, however, and that service needs too often unduly influenced educational programs.[33] In 2006 the Association of American Medical Colleges (AAMC) published a document, "Compact Between Resident Physicians and Their Teachers," to help graduate medical education focus on its primary educational mission. Over thirty important professional organizations endorsed the compact.[34] This document, too, however, made little difference. Pontification from up high, no matter how well intended, could do little to affect the ground-level problems resulting from increased patient volume and accelerated throughput.

Lara Goitein, a former resident in internal medicine at Massachusetts General Hospital (1998–2001) and now a practicing pulmonary and critical care physician and thought leader in medical education, provided a first-hand account of how the pressures of high throughput affected her during her internship. She and her fellow interns found the job "overwhelming." There was one overriding reason for this: "the sheer volume and acuity of the patients." In this environment, she found her receptiveness to teaching plummet. "I was unable to concentrate [on teaching during attending rounds] because I was constantly reviewing in my mind the work that needed to be done, or being called away to take care of patients." As a result, "I had no interest in learning about the mechanisms or finer points of disease. I just wanted to be told what to do so I could get the job done; to get 'the answer.' I was very much aware of the inadequacies of this kind of learning, and it greatly troubled me."[35]

Deborah Villa, a chief resident in internal medicine at Northwestern, told a similar story about her experiences as a house officer there in the early 1990s. She described a hospital environment where time was a precious but scarce commodity. Trainees experienced "a sense of never having enough time to provide optimum patient care, learn all that is necessary, and get the work done."[36] She recalled a sleepless night on call with 15 admissions and considerable cross-coverage work:

> I remember at 5:00 a.m. walking the halls, thinking I hate my job! And I'm not one to say that. *It's not that I hated my job; it's just that I hated not being able to do my job well.* [Italics added] Why? I couldn't spend the appropriate time with the patients and I couldn't read and learn more. The issue was not just lack of sleep, but lack of time.[37]

Villa's words, like those of Goitein, spoke for countless house officers of the era: There were too many patients to see and too little time with which to see them.

The consequences of this new environment on the learning of house officers were difficult to measure, but a number of changes became clearly apparent. First, it was increasingly difficult for residency training to maintain a scholarly approach to patient care. Time constraints and patient volume were too great; residents understandably focused on getting the clinical work done and not on their education. Faculty members at programs everywhere commented on this development. At the University of Iowa, the faculty noted a decline in the intellectual quality of attending rounds in response to the overarching pressures on residents and attending physicians for speed and efficiency.[38] At Massachusetts General Hospital, the chair of internal medicine observed that house officers had exhibited a "complete suspension of intellectual curiosity" because of the heavy clinical service requirements.[39] One noted medical educator asked, "Is Scholarship Declining in Medical Education?";[40] another described the syndrome of "eurekapenia" (scarcity of "eureka" moments) among contemporary house officers;[41] still another wrote of "the demise of reflective doctoring";[42] and yet another lamented the fact that teaching hospitals had become "too busy for curiosity."[43]

In their important study of medical education, Cooke, Irby, and O'Brien confirmed that this was a national trend. They found that the imperative of efficiency on teaching rounds at every program they visited was inhospitable to exploring scientific ideas or analyzing clinical problems. As a result, they found a less questioning attitude among residents, a greater tendency not to challenge authority, an overemphasis on learning current facts, a diminished focus on acquiring fundamental principles and problem-solving skills, and little contemplation of the larger purposes of medicine or the moral meaning of being a doctor. At one teaching hospital after another, knowing what to do was deemed more important than knowing why, and acquiring wisdom, insight, and understanding became subordinate to learning specific facts. In addition, teaching was moving from the bedside to the classroom ("Socratic Dialogue Gives Way to PowerPoint,"[44] in Lawrence K. Altman's words), even though great teachers had traditionally believed that the goal was to stimulate the student to think and talk rather than listen to the teacher speak. They found that house officers now did the majority of their reading in the online resource UptoDate, which offered authoritative factual information and clinical protocols, to the sacrifice of more extensive reading in journals or textbooks, whether online or in print, to acquire a deeper fundamental understanding of subjects of interest. They concluded that graduate medical education in the current era "overemphasizes current factual knowledge and underemphasizes knowledge seeking and skill building."[45]

A second change was that there was a notable decline in the ability of house officers to take a clinical history and perform an accurate physical examination. This development did not begin at this time. Throughout the century many senior clinicians had criticized the younger generation for inadequate examination skills.[46] In the early 1970s, a documented decline in bedside skills began, as the advent of CT scans and other imaging technologies captured the excitement of physicians and seemed to make many examination techniques less important. Apathy toward the physical examination greatly increased during the era of high throughput, however, as time constraints made it easier to order a chest or abdominal CT than to examine the chest or abdomen. House officers began to show much less interest in the physical examination, and they were rarely embarrassed when they made a mistake. Missing a heart murmur or large liver once would have caused house officers to feel deep chagrin; now such errors barely caused a shrug.[47]

No one was arguing for house officers to do as detailed an examination as in the distant past—percussing the full configuration of the heart, or having patients get on their hands and knees to check for a "puddle sign." However, many senior physicians were deeply concerned over the loss of basic skills, the missing of obvious findings, and the misinterpretation of other physical findings. They knew that many important physical findings were undetectable by imaging studies—a pleural or pericardial friction rub, for instance, of a rash. They considered advanced technology to be best used for verifying rather than formulating clinical impressions since that approach led to less testing, less radiation exposure, and lower costs.[48] They also recognized the ritualistic importance of a good physical examination as well as the power of touch.[49] Yet, in the era of high throughput, that message was lost from residency education.[50]

A third change was that the residency years became less fulfilling. This is not to romanticize the past, which was never blissful, stress-free, or bereft of exhausting work and sleep deprivation. Indeed, as noted previously, the phenomenon of "burnout" had already been described. As the volume and acuity of patients increased, however, satisfaction with the work markedly diminished. Fewer and fewer house officers spoke of the joy they derived from their residency, the fun they were having, or the fact that they were pursuing a calling. One prominent medical educator spoke of the IDD (inspiration deficit disease) that had afflicted modern house officers.[51] In 1999, following a ruling of the National Labor Relations Board that reversed its earlier decision that house officers could not engage in collective bargaining, the unionization movement among residents was reborn—in large part in response to the conditions of work that evolved during the era of high throughput.[52] Jordan Cohen, president of the Association of American Medical Colleges and a vigorous champion of professionalism, deplored the idea that residents might form labor unions. He acknowledged, however, the conditions that led to a recrudescence of the movement: "I am also profoundly troubled that many residents continue to face realities in their training programs that are distressing enough to warrant their even considering union representation."[53]

Goitein provided insight into the mechanisms of what afflicted house officers' mood. During her internship, she became mentally exhausted and frustrated, which she attributed directly to "the high volume and turnover of patients and the high intensity of service."[54] As a result, she felt deprived of the opportunity to do the work as well as she desired:

> I came to residency expecting to work as hard as I could possibly work, to get very little sleep, and to make very little money. These were prices I was fully aware of and willing to pay. What I did not expect was that I would work as hard as I could possibly work, and still do a bad job for my patients and my own education.[55]

Goitein, the daughter of one former editor of the *New England Journal of Medicine* (Marcia Angell) and stepdaughter of another (Arnold "Bud" Relman), contrasted her own emotional exhaustion as a resident with the joy her parents derived. "It seems that the doctors of Bud's and my mother's generations were *energized* by their patient contact, and their dedication was also their pleasure."[56] In short, fatigue and hard work during residency training were not new. Rather, what was new was the loss of the sense of completion, the joy derived from the pursuit of excellence, the pride in a job well done. In the past, many house officers felt they were engaged in doing "good work." Now, house officers increasingly felt that residency was just a job, and they were struggling just to get by. More and more, they were frustrated, as Goitein was, by an environment that did not let them heal and let them learn as they had hoped.

A fourth change during the era of high throughput was that the role of the attending physician or surgeon became more difficult. Traditionally, teaching rounds were highly ritualized to accomplish the goal of patient care while simultaneously providing instruction to learners at different levels of knowledge and experience. On rounds the attending physician met with the patients, clarified points in the history, checked certain physical findings, talked with the patients and their families, and discussed the case with the house officers and medical students. Now, time constraints impeded that process. With so many patients to care for, there was much less time to teach. As the editor-in-chief of the *Journal of the American College of Cardiology* pointed out, "When you are presented with eight or more new admissions in addition to all of the old patients, there is no time for a prolonged and scholarly discussion of each patient."[57] Sometimes faculty members encountered house officers resistant to teaching because educational exercises took them away from their patient-care duties. Thus, an intern at St. Luke's-Roosevelt Hospital Center admitted her dread of a certain attending physician because that individual taught too much, thereby putting her behind schedule for the day.[58]

Other factors also made the teaching role more difficult. In particular, after 1997, faculty members were required to provide much more extensive documentation of their role in patient care in the charts. This requirement was imposed by a reinterpretation of intermediary letter 372 (IL-372) rules governing Medicare Part B billing by teaching physicians. Under the new ruling, physicians had to write extensive daily notes on each patient if they wished to receive payment from Medicare for their clinical services as attending physicians; countersigning a house officer's signature no longer sufficed. This represented welcome accountability, the faculty certainly enjoyed the stream of government dollars, and skilled teachers could perform the documentation without diminishing the role of the house staff. However, this represented a time-consuming diversion of faculty time away from teaching and, to many faculty members, made the role of teaching that much more frustrating.[59]

Some hoped that outpatient instruction could be used to greater advantage to compensate for the growing difficulties of inpatient education. The arguments for more ambulatory experiences were compelling: the broader range of conditions encountered, the opportunity to make fresh diagnoses and observe the earlier stages of disease, and the opportunity to gain experience managing many chronic conditions. The ambulatory setting also seemed like a desirable site to teach about disease prevention, health promotion, psychosocial medicine, and many of the social and economic issues pertaining to medical practice. Family practice residencies since the late 1960s had been using ambulatory sites extensively, as had many pediatrics programs. The first primary care track in internal medicine, pioneered by Allan H. Goroll and John D. Stoeckle at Massachusetts General Hospital in 1973, placed house officers in ambulatory settings for 50 percent of their time.[60] Ambulatory education was "an idea whose time may have finally come," Gerald T. Perkoff wrote in an influential article in 1986.[61]

However, ambulatory experience did not gain much traction in residency education. In part the problem was the traditional one: Medicare reimbursement formulas locked residents into inpatient training. Teaching hospitals did not receive direct or indirect graduate medical education payments for the time that house officers spent offsite, and they had to bear the financial burden of providing additional medical coverage for inpatients while residents were seeing outpatients.[62] Equally important, in the era of high throughput, the same pressures to see more patients more quickly affected outpatient as well as inpatient care. In ambulatory sites, as in inpatient rotations, the imperative for speed and high volume often compromised the quality of education. Some faculty members resented having residents in ambulatory clinics or private offices because the presence of residents and the time required for teaching slowed down the pace of care (and with that, the number of patients seen and the clinical revenues generated).[63] In general, into the 2010s the promise of ambulatory education remained largely unrealized.

Ironically, there was little evidence that prospective payment accomplished its goal of limiting health care costs. In the three decades following the implementation of the new system, health care costs continued to soar, both in absolute dollars and as a percentage of the gross domestic product. In many cases, prospective payment did not save money but shifted costs. For instance, a trial of early discharge after coronary artery bypass surgery reduced the costs of the initial hospitalization, but these savings were offset by the increased use of outpatient nursing services, discharges to extended care facilities, and increased hospital readmissions.[64] More important, many doctors and hospitals compensated in volume for what they lost in price. A large literature on overtesting and overtreatment arose, suggesting that more than 30 percent of tests, procedures, and treatments obtained in the United States were unnecessary.[65] In teaching settings, the prospective payment system itself fostered this process. With little time to care for their patients, house officers ordered a large number of tests to make certain they did not miss anything. Goitein described the process:

> My residency certainly cultivated the tendency to over-test and over-treat. With so little time to think about patients, we would order batteries of tests roughly corresponding to whatever anatomic area was brought to our attention. Chest pain bought orders for cardiac enzymes, EKG, ECHO, holter monitor, stress test, etc. before we'd even seen the patient. At our frantic pace, this was the only way to make sure (we hoped) that we wouldn't "miss anything." The tendency to over-treat began as a survival technique, but—with little attending guidance to offer correction—by the end of residency it was ingrained as our style of practicing medicine. I'm sure this style makes us easy pawns for a medical industry bent on expansion.[66]

Although the new payment system did not succeed in controlling health care costs, it certainly left its imprint on residency training. Its net effect was to shift the gaze of learners from understanding principles to mastering facts. Residents focused on knowing what to do (and, in surgical programs, knowing how to do things) rather than on why things were done. There was much more emphasis on following clinical algorithms than on understanding the evidence that justified current practices, the circumstances that required exceptions to the protocols to be made, and the scientific approaches that might improve medical and surgical care in the future. The net effect was unmistakable: a shift from professional education toward vocationalism. Graduate medical education continued to possess considerable strengths, and it would be a mistake to make too much of this shift. It would be an even greater mistake, however, to minimize it—both the shift that had already occurred and, more important, the future direction residency training was indicating it could go.

Did this matter? Knowledgeable medical educators knew that it did. Strong professional training was what provided doctors with the ability to manage uncertainty, balance multiple competing problems in the same individual, solve unknowns, and incorporate new discoveries into their thinking and practice. Protocol medicine usually worked, but it required professional judgment to know when exceptions needed to be made and then to figure out what to do. As Cooke, Irby, and O'Brien pointed out, "It is not enough to have time-proven and reliable approaches to routine problems: every physician requires a depth of understanding that allows him or her to respond to unusual clinical problems with original rather than habitual approaches."[67] It was precisely this ability that had always been the defining intellectual characteristic of physicians. Now, the strong professional foundation of medical education was being eroded, to the jeopardy of patients and physicians alike.

It was hardly a surprise that this development occurred, given the long-standing fault lines in graduate medical education. Teaching hospitals had always experienced tension between their dual roles as healing and educational institutions. Throughout most of their history, however, when the average length of stay was longer, patient care and education were usually maintained in reasonable balance. Now, under prospective payment, intense financial pressures tilted all teaching hospitals, including the most revered institutions, toward patient care. Indeed, some prominent academic leaders began to worry that the term "academic medical center" was "becoming an oxymoron" and that the "the bond between A and MC (in the A—MC)" was being stretched to the breaking point.[68] When teaching hospitals were in trouble, who better to call on than the house officers, who since the origins of the residency system had borne a disproportionate share of the work of the institution? Ultimately, teaching hospitals survived—indeed, prospered. However, much of the cost of this success was borne by their house staffs, who became responsible for an unwieldy proportion of the growing number of admissions. Under the powerful economic pressures of prospective payment, the ongoing tension in graduate medical education between education and institutional service erupted again, and, once more, service trumped education.

From the perspective of the residency system, the core issue was that graduate medical education was expensive. This had always been true but in the era of high throughput, the costs of graduate medical education grew conspicuously. This was because prospective payment exposed the opportunity costs of medical education. Time spent learning or teaching detracted from the throughput of patients. Fewer patients were seen, and less clinical revenue was generated. In 2009, the Institute of Medicine estimated that $1.7 billion was required to place residency training on a firmer educational footing, primarily by providing for nurse practitioners, physician assistants, or more physicians to assume some of the current patient load of house officers, thereby allowing house officers more time to reflect, study, and learn.[69] However, during a severe recession that proposal generated little enthusiasm. Indeed, as this book went to press, with a stuttering economy, rising federal deficit, and still-growing health care costs, the prevailing economic concern in educational circles was that federal support of graduate medical education might be reduced.

It is important to recognize that there were no villains. The great majority of faculty members, residents, and administrators were good people with high ethical values, working as hard and conscientiously as they could amid difficult circumstances. The villain, if any, was the dysfunctional, highly commercialized health care system, which, in its understandable efforts to control costs, failed to consider the needs of the future of medicine, namely, education and research. The forces that drove super-efficient, fast-paced, high-throughput care also drove an imbalance between service and education at teaching institutions and an atrophy of the academic mission. The system made no provision for the special needs of medical education or academic medical centers.

Yet medical leaders could not be absolved from their share of the responsibility. As the pressures to increase the throughput of patients grew stronger, professional leaders did little to counteract the tide. One distinguished medical educator wrote, "Almost all the [academic medicine] king's men and king's horses did nothing, said nothing, protested nothing, and raised no money to prevent the tarnishing of one of the greatest jewels the world has ever known [the residency system]."[70] As I have discussed elsewhere, academic leaders, faculty members, clinical departments, medical schools, and teaching hospitals behaved in this way for a reason: They benefited too much from the enhanced revenues they received for succumbing to the forces to increase throughput.[71] They followed the money, resting content with the status quo as long as clinical revenues and their own pay continued to grow, even if graduate medical education and patient care might have suffered in the process.

Could strong words or actions from academic leaders have lessened the emphasis on maximizing throughput? Perhaps not. Charles S. Bryan, a noted infectious diseases specialist and medical humanist, wrote of how difficult it was "to honor professionalism in an environment that doesn't value professionalism."[72] Powerful political, economic, and cultural forces were rapidly transforming the health care system. These societal factors enveloped the medical profession; they could not be easily controlled or influenced, even by leading physicians and academics. However, medical leaders made little effort to try. Instead, they chose to serve as willing accomplices of the system. This refusal to resist represented a great failing of medicine's leadership and raised embarrassing questions about the "professionalism" of doctors that have continued to afflict the profession ever since.

THE SUBVERSION OF THE MORAL MISSION

The residency system, as seen in this book, had never been perfect. From the beginning institutional service had always challenged educational goals, even at the best teaching hospitals. House officers continually coped with stress, exhaustion, and self-doubt. This was true of even the most enthusiastic residents who insisted that work was play. Faculty members were sometimes aloof and authoritarian, engaging in what Daniel M. Fox, a noted historian of medicine and foundation officer, has called the "I am" method of proof—"I am the professor, hence what I say goes."[73] Cost-effective practicing habits were rarely emphasized. Hospital administrators often appeared callous to house officers, unconcerned with their needs or even with those of patients. Such problems increased during the protest era of the 1970s, as patients became sicker, the power of medical and surgical care to do good or harm became greater, senior faculty and administrators became more distant, house officers became more outspoken, the cultural challenges to the medical profession grew stronger, and the phenomenon of "burnout" was discovered.

However imperfect, the residency system through the early 1980s, on balance, remained a success. Medical graduates from other countries regularly sought residency training opportunities in the United States; American medical graduates rarely sought such opportunities abroad. This was a reflection of the talent and dedication of faculty and trainees, the strength of the learning environment, and the firm commitment of the residency system to serving the patients' needs. This explains why, for instance, the Harvard medical service at the Boston City Hospital remained a premier training site for so long despite the many horrible physical deficiencies of the hospital, the major inadequacies in its professional and nonprofessional services, and the unusually demanding work schedules of the house staff. The attending physicians and house officers alike were superb, and above all, the program fostered a service tradition that emphasized "concern for the patient and his welfare, no matter what the problem or the hour."[74] This is not to deny the racial and ethnic discrimination that occurred at teaching hospitals, the condescension toward the poor, or the lack of creature amenities for ward patients. Rather, it is to point out that house officers were charged with addressing all of their patients' medical problems, and they were expected to do this by being thorough, responsive, and attentive to detail. This represented the moral dimension of residency training—and of medical practice.

In the late years of the twentieth century and the early years of the twenty-first, prominent medical educators and physicians affirmed the moral principles of medicine as vigorously as ever. Deans (or associate deans, if the dean was not available) and other august individuals spoke eloquently to medical students about the primacy of the patient at introductory lectures to medical school, white-coat ceremonies, patient-doctor courses, and commencement addresses. Residents heard similar messages at various ceremonial occasions. The medical literature was replete with articles and essays on the importance of altruism, thoroughness, good communication, and serving the needs of patients. In 2002 the ABIM (American Board of Internal Medicine) Foundation, ACP (American College of Physicians) Foundation, and European Federation of Internal Medicine jointly published a widely cited statement of professionalism, "A Physician Charter." Within five years the charter had been published in 30 additional professional journals, translated into 10 languages, and endorsed by more than 120 medical organizations.[75]

In the era of high throughput, however, house officers found it increasingly difficult to act in accord with the traditional expectations of professionalism. In particular, it became extremely difficult for them to be thorough and attentive to detail and to make certain that their patients' problems were recognized and addressed. The problem was not the lack of desire. Rather, it was the lack of opportunity. The patient volume was too high, the turnover of patients too great, and time simply in too short supply. Interns and residents in every specialty often experienced panic and anxiety as they struggled to care for far more patients than time reasonably permitted. The only way that they could cope with the high patient load was by cutting corners.

Consider training programs in internal medicine. Traditionally, house officers in no specialty examined patients more carefully than those in this field. Beginning in the mid-1980s, however, internal medicine interns and residents performed increasingly cursory examinations. Ear drums and eye grounds were no longer routinely examined, nor were pelvic, rectal, and genitourinary examinations regularly conducted—even in patients complaining of abdominal pain, where examination of these organs was essential. The lungs and heart were often casually approached, sometimes through layers of clothing, and arterial pulses in the feet, if they were examined at all, were often palpated over socks. One distinguished gastroenterologist related that in patients referred to him for screening colonoscopy, he found much more prostate cancer than colon cancer—the irony being, of course, that prostate cancer is typically in reach of an examining finger and should not have required a colonoscopy for detection.[76]

In addition, with such rapid throughput of patients, house officers had less time to address patients' problems. This was mandated by the pressure toward early discharge, even if important diagnostic tests had not returned, the response to therapy was still uncertain, or important aspects of the clinical presentation remained a puzzle.[77] If major problems were incidentally discovered, they were typically "turfed" to someone else. "A new anemia? That's an outpatient workup—refer to hematology clinic." It thus became easy and common for house officers to hand off patients to someone else rather than to address patients' problems themselves. Often it seemed as if house officers were processing patients rather than attempting to identify and solve patients' medical issues.

The declining focus on solving patients' problems was illustrated by the example of a middle-aged woman admitted one night in the early 2000s to the internal medicine service at Barnes-Jewish Hospital for chest pain. By 7:30 a.m. the next morning she had "ruled out" for a myocardial infarction—that is, serial electrocardiograms and two sets of heart enzymes were normal. The house staff, who wanted to discharge her, even suggested to the attending physician that he need not see her—she was "stable," had "ruled out," and there were 13 other new patients to see (covered by two interns and one resident) in addition to the old patients. The attending physician did examine her, however, and while doing so, noticed that her pain, which was still present, was highly suggestive of gastroesophageal reflux disease (GERD). He suggested keeping her in the hospital that day to perform an upper endoscopic examination to try to make the diagnosis and, if positive, to begin patient education and treatment. "But, Doctor," the resident asked, "isn't GERD an outpatient workup?" "Yes," the attending physician replied—"ordinarily." "However," he continued, "she is with us now. She did not come here asking if she were having a heart attack. She came asking for our help with her chest pain. If we discharge her now, we will have done nothing to have helped her." The attending physician also pointed out an additional consideration: "If we discharge her now, she will endure discomfort and anxiety while waiting for her procedure, and since you won't learn the results, you won't receive any educational return on the considerable investment of time you have already made in working her up." The house officers agreed, she had her endoscopy, a diagnosis of GERD was made, and that evening she was happily discharged. The house officers read about GERD, and soon they knew more about the condition than their attending physician. To all involved with her care, however, the greatest lesson was the illustration of the distinction between processing patients and addressing their problems.[78]

No patient was immune from being ignored in the era of high throughput. Consider the case of Jonathan Epstein, a distinguished cardiologist at the University of Pennsylvania. In his presidential address in 2010 to the

American Society for Clinical Investigation, Epstein related his own experience as a patient at the Hospital of the University of Pennsylvania after the discovery that he had stage III colon cancer. He acknowledged that he was the fortunate beneficiary of wondrous advances in multimodality therapy for colon cancer. "I am alive, and I am grateful." However, the lack of attention he received from the medical staff, particularly the house officers, gave him "a new appreciation for the anger and disappointment of the American public that is a powerful backdrop to the critical health care debate that has dominated public discourse." During several hospitalizations, he was frightened and extremely ill, but not a single physician asked if he understood the prognosis or if he was scared. On one occasion, after a week on the ward, he paged the junior resident, who eventually appeared, asking in an annoyed fashion what was so pressing that he called her directly. He replied that he simply wanted to meet her before he was discharged later that day. When he asked another medical resident if there was genetic testing that might help to predict the likelihood that his children would be at risk for a similar disease, he was told that there probably was and that his outpatient physician would surely fill him in. From a patient's perspective, Epstein observed, "It has become maddeningly and dangerously easy to pass the buck to the next shift worker, the next consultant, or to the outpatient caregiver." He added: "I had no sense that I was on a teaching service or part of an academic mission. I was a cog in a high-throughput industry."[79]

Diminished thoroughness became apparent in many ways in residency programs. In internal medicine, for instance, an important part of the house officers' daily routine traditionally had been afternoon chart rounds. The entire team of house officers and medical students assembled late each afternoon, reviewing the charts of every patient on the service. This provided the opportunity to make certain that all ordered procedures had been done, ascertain the results, make certain that there were no overlooked abnormalities documented in the chart, and review nursing records and consultant notes. These rounds disappeared in the late 1980s and early 1990s, a casualty of time pressures. Similarly, on many internal medicine services, house officer teams had regularly made rounds with the nursing staff. These rounds, too, disappeared, a victim of the fact that many nursing services themselves were understaffed and that doctors and nurses alike had too much work to do for the time allotted. Communication between nurses and house officers, formerly done in person, became largely a matter of reading each others' notes in the charts, at least when there was time to read the notes. Even the best chart correspondence proved an inadequate substitute for face-to-face conversations, however, and miscommunications about patients often resulted.[80] Ironically, the diminishing communication between nurses and house officers occurred at a time when a growing number of voices were calling for "teamwork" to be made a more prominent part of medical education.

The conditions under which house officers worked were not unique to teaching hospitals. Extreme time constraints on patient care characterized all hospitals in the era of high throughput. As Abigail Zuger wrote, "The hospital [in America] thrums to a simple bottom line: get 'em in, get 'em out."[81] Neither was the imperative to maximize throughput confined to inpatient medicine. It was equally present in ambulatory settings, where financial incentives also encouraged physicians to maximize the number of patients seen. In outpatient practice, "The 'hand on the doorknob' phenomenon is well known," Danielle Ofri observed.[82] Such circumstances made it much more convenient for even highly experienced doctors to order tests or write prescriptions rather than to listen to patients or figure out clinical problems.

Of course, time in itself did not ensure good medical care. The availability of time did not guarantee that a doctor cared about his patients or could communicate with them satisfactorily. There were skills involved in communicating effectively with patients—skills that could be taught and learned.[83] In addition, good rapport with patients did not guarantee a physician's technical competence. There were innumerable instances in which appropriate care could be delivered quickly. For instance, otherwise healthy patients with minor complaints could usually be satisfactorily cared for in a brief office visit.[84] Sometimes, particularly in cases of critical illness, time was the enemy, and in those instances good care demanded speed and efficiency. The quicker the patient in the emergency room with a heart attack was diagnosed and sent for coronary angiography, the better.

However, it was increasingly clear that not all patients were served by speed and efficiency. The ones who suffered the most from this type of care tended to be the most complicated patients: individuals posing difficult diagnostic or therapeutic dilemmas, elderly individuals, patients of any age with serious problems or multiple problems where the treatment of one might adversely affect another (and where the risk of adverse drug interactions was especially great), and patients with significant psychological or social issues. In these situations longer amounts of time were typically required for physicians to understand patients' problems, provide reassurance, and determine a sound course of action. Many physicians valued spending time with patients for their less severe problems because it helped them provide better care (and care that was more aligned with patients' values and wishes) should serious situations arise.[85] Wise clinicians also knew that many patients required time to become comfortable before they could discuss their symptoms or health concerns. Not all patients immediately revealed their worry about having cancer or a sexually transmitted disease; many needed to grow comfortable in the conversation before being able to do so. To Leighton E. Cluff, the president of the Robert Wood Johnson Foundation and former chair of internal medicine at the University of Florida, the emphasis on seeing patients quickly represented part of "the lost art of caring" in America.[86]

The dilemma of modern medical care in America was characterized by what Daniel Munoz, then an internal medicine resident at Johns Hopkins, now a cardiologist at Vanderbilt, called the "fast/slow paradox." Sometimes speed was desirable in patient care, and other times, not. It took wisdom and judgment to recognize whether "fast" or "slow" medicine was required for the patient at hand. Munoz, like many others, admired the technological prowess of contemporary medicine. He regretted, however, the fact that "too often, patients, administrators, doctors, and outside observers identify 'quality care' via tragically flawed proxies like speed of care."[87] The great frustration to many residents and practicing physicians was that the system was not designed to let them heal patients who required "slow medicine." As Munoz put it: "Asking physicians to both 'ensure the hospital's profitability/viability' and 'to do the right thing for patients' are often, though admittedly not always, contradictory directives. Somehow the incentives should be better aligned."[88]

Thus, the factors that led to the declining thoroughness exhibited by house officers had little to do with any conscious desires of residency leaders. Indeed, prominent medical educators often deplored this trend. Rather, the decline of thoroughness reflected economic incentives in American health care that encouraged "fast medicine" and discouraged "slow medicine." Teaching hospitals, like all hospitals, were vulnerable to these powerful economic forces. What made the situation poignant from the perspective of medical education was that the traditional goal of residency training was to immerse trainees in settings that embodied medical care at its best. Now, trainees were learning medicine in patient-care environments that medical educators themselves recognized were far from ideal.

Given the importance of academic medical centers to the health of the nation and the adaptability of their leadership, it should be no surprise that they survived—indeed, prospered—during the era of high throughput. In the process, however, they were transformed. Previously, they had defined their success by the quality of their clinical and academic work, and they typically considered a budget deficit as an indicator that they were doing abundant amounts of good work. Now, like voluntary hospitals in general, they became highly commercialized, manifesting an ethos that was more akin to that of a business than a social service. Business titles and practices pervaded the organizations, as hospital administrators became chief executive officers, complete with corporate-sized salaries. Academic medical centers cut expenses by reducing staff sizes to the minimum, sometimes shut down unprofitable "product lines" (clinical services) even if those services were valuable to the community, engaged in aggressive marketing to attract paying patients (whether patients needed medical services or not), and defined success on financial rather than professional criteria. To strengthen the "bottom line," many academic medical centers acquired ownership of for-profit businesses and developed joint for-profit ventures with physicians on their staff. Arnold S. Relman, who famously coined the term "medical-industrial complex" in 1980,[89] 11 years later expressed his astonishment with how far nonprofit hospitals, especially teaching institutions, had come to resemble their for-profit brethren. "Many if not most of our voluntary hospitals now view themselves as businesses competing for paying patients in the health care marketplace. They have, in effect, become part of the medical-industrial complex."[90]

From the perspective of medical education, the unanswered question was how the commercialization of the learning environment was affecting the value system of the next generation of doctors. As students of the "hidden curriculum" understood, house officers and medical students responded to actions, not just words. They watched their teachers carefully for signals as to what behaviors were really valued. To many observers, there was now cause for concern, for faculty protestations of the primacy of the patient carried much less force when the same instructors were striving to maximize the throughput of patients in their own care of patients and encouraging house officers to do the same. The goal of residency training had always been not just to instill knowledge and techniques but also "a professional identity with a moral and ethical core of service and responsibility around which the habits of mind and practice can be organized."[91] In the era of high throughput, the ambience of residency training changed, and house officers were now learning their specialty in settings where institutional leaders spoke more of maximizing market share and profitability than of caring and the relief of suffering. Herein lay the great challenge to the moral mission of residency training in the early years of the twenty-first century: internalizing thoroughness and service to patients as core values of doctors who learned medicine in settings of care where those values were often not honored.

CHANGING ATTITUDES TOWARD WORK AND LIFE

For many generations, doctors seemingly had little choice: Work came first. Doctors were expected to live and breathe medicine, spend long hours at the office or hospital, and, when necessary, neglect their families for the sake of their patients. Thus, witness the physician who boasted to colleagues in the doctors' lounge, "I never attended the graduation ceremonies of any of my children."[92] Such behavior was in accordance with cultural mores of the broader society. Leisure time and material goals were traditionally seen by society as unbecoming of a person dedicated to service.[93]

Physicians' workaholic ways were buoyed by the traditional family structure in America. Anecdotal evidence had long suggested this, but in 1980 Martha R. Fowlkes empirically documented the phenomenon.[94] Most doctors delayed marriage and deferred personal gratifications. When doctors did marry, they tended to select wives less accomplished than spouses of other academic or professional men. During marriage, medical wives customarily subordinated themselves to their husbands' careers. Fowlkes observed, "The kind of man who is attracted to a particular professional role married the kind of woman who shares the values associated with that role and who is prepared to reinforce and uphold that role in her own role as wife."[95] The doctors in her study almost universally indicated that career success was more important to them than satisfaction in other areas of life, and they typically played only secondary roles in child-rearing and family life. To them, as to the majority of Americans for most of the twentieth century, marriage and child-rearing represented "women's work." Men in other demanding occupations also benefited from the contributions of their wives, but none more so than doctors. As Fowlkes put it, "Male professional participation is propped up at every turn by the role that women play as wives of professional men."[96]

Physicians' professional success did not come without cost—particularly for their wives. Spouses had to endure considerable loneliness and solitude. As one put it, "I deal with loneliness all day long, every day," or in the words of another, "I never came first, never."[97] Many medical wives accepted a position of second-class citizenship in relation to both the status and time demands of their husbands' work. Fowlkes wrote, "Doctors who devote unusually long hours to their practice earn the admiration of their patients, but their wives react more ambivalently as they are made to feel guilty and petty if they make demands on their husbands' time that detract from the lofty imperatives of medical practice."[98] Effects on the children of physicians are unknown, although anecdotal evidence suggests that some children also felt ignored, particularly by unusually high-achieving fathers.[99]

In the 1970s, traditional attitudes toward work and family life among young physicians began to change. A major reason for this was the entry of much larger numbers of women into the profession. As Ellen More and others have shown, women physicians had traditionally sought a more harmonious balance between work and family life than their male counterparts.[100] In this sense the entry of large numbers of women into the profession likely represented a leavening influence. (Still unknown was how the feminization of the profession affected patient care, health care systems, or the profession itself.)[101] The effects of the women's movement ran deeper, however. The feminist movement enabled more women to enter virtually every area of the workforce, not just medicine. As a result, there was a rise in two-career families and a corresponding decline in traditional families, where the stay-at-home wives had long enabled the workaholic ways of their husbands. As the traditional family became less common, an important prop for many generations of doctors became weaker.[102]

A decade later, generational changes also began contributing to new attitudes toward work and personal life among house officers. The term "generation" refers to a peer group defined both by its demographics and key life events. Generations are shaped by a common history, influenced by common icons, and affected by common events and conditions; thus, generational changes reflect chances in society. Through the 1980s, the profession of medicine had consisted of members of the "silent generation" (born 1925–44) and "Baby Boomers" (born 1945–62). In the late 1980s, members of "Generation X" or "Gen X" (born 1963–81) began entering medicine, and in the twenty-first century, "Millennials" (born 1982–2000). There were many differences among each of these groups, but of importance here, Generation X and Millennials did not share their elders' preoccupation with work. Younger physicians were not so eager to delay gratification or neglect their families for the sake of a career. They were less career-driven than their parents and grandparents, and they tended to seek jobs that would enable them to attend their children's soccer games—or even to coach—rather than to provide a high income or big house. Compared with the silent generation and Baby Boomers, they focused on achieving meaning in life, not just meaning in work.[103]

In the late twentieth century, the result was a decided shift in interest among many young physicians toward specialties that allowed greater time for personal and family activities. Fields that became especially popular included dermatology, ophthalmology, anesthesiology, plastic and reconstructive surgery, radiology, radiation oncology, and emergency medicine. Medical students often spoke of the "ROAD to happiness"—*r*adiology, *o*phthalmology, *a*nesthesiology, and *d*ermatology, all prestigious, high-paying fields with comfortable lifestyles. These so-called lifestyle fields all had in common fewer work hours, less night call, more predictable schedules, greater flexibility, and more free time for family, leisure, and avocational pursuits. In 2008, 40 percent of the graduating class at Johns Hopkins chose one of these fields, compared with 11 percent in 1988.[104] One widely cited study, which examined medical school graduating classes from 1996 to 2002, demonstrated that the most important factor in specialty choice had become the perception of controllable lifestyle.[105] "I don't want to be a 24-hour doctor," one Gen X member told the *New York Times*.[106] This appeared to be a generational, not just a gender, phenomenon because male graduates sought "lifestyle" specialties even more fervidly than women did.[107]

As Gen X and Millennial students entered medicine, residency programs themselves changed to accommodate the preferences of incoming house officers. Programs granted more vacation time and, in some instances, less onerous on-call schedules. "Split" residencies, wherein two house officers, usually women, shared one residency position, appeared. The granting of maternal leave became a standard benefit, as did paternal leave at some programs. Some house officers participated in nontraditional marriages—for instance, a female resident working full-time while her stay-at-home husband tended to the children and household, or medical couples combining their single surnames into a new blended surname.

At the turn of the century, the emergence of "lifestyle" considerations among house officers created considerable consternation among older doctors. Some felt that contemporary house officers exhibited less intensity, determination, and devotion. One senior clinician wrote, "Doctors do not want to work as hard as their predecessors. Osler's claim that the master-word in medicine is WORK is being challenged by a new generation who finds difficulty in accepting it as a way of life."[108] To the older generation, the lack of complete immersion in medicine was indicative of a less-than-full commitment to being a doctor. They tended to view the desire of many younger doctors to work fewer hours and avoid around-the-clock demands on their time as smacking of unprofessionalism.

That senior doctors frequently complained about the attitudes of contemporary house officers should not be a surprise. Traditionally, older doctors had often belittled the qualities of the younger generation. David E. Rogers, the president of the Robert Wood Johnson Foundation, once pointed this out: "Whenever physicians of middle age and beyond gather together, particularly distinguished physicians such as those who grace our membership, one topic inevitably receives much hand-wringing attention. This is the sorry state of today's house staff."[109] Thus, much of the criticism of Gen X and Millennial house officers reflected the age-old tendency of late-career doctors to speak disparagingly of those who were replacing them. Indeed, there was a certain hypocrisy in the complaints of senior physicians. They, too, valued leisure time much more than they sometimes let on. In the 1960s and 1970s, the desire on the part of both physicians and spouses for more personal time was a major factor in the shift from solo to group practice and, a generation later, in the shift from private group practice to salaried positions with large organizations.[110] Studies of physicians in practice in the 1990s and 2000s showed older doctors just as dissatisfied with long hours as younger doctors.[111]

Thus, the rise of lifestyle considerations among students and house officers did not represent the "decline and fall" of professionalism in medicine, as some older doctors were wont to maintain. Rather, it represented a natural evolution of the profession, another chapter in the ongoing story of generational change. Indeed, studies demonstrated a strong work ethic and firm commitment to their medical careers among Gen X and Millennial doctors. Despite perceptions of a generational shift, young doctors reported similar attitudes toward patient care as senior physicians, and those who had entered practice worked about as long as Baby Boomer doctors did in their respective fields.[112] There were also new forms of idealism among younger doctors, such as their interest in global health and medical humanitarian activities. Thus, the older and younger generations were more alike than sometimes assumed, undoubtedly reflecting the socialization that occurred throughout medical training. The main difference seemed to be that younger doctors defined success by their total life, not just by their work, and thus they strove much harder to keep the two in balance.

The early twenty-first-century controversy over the dedication and commitment of young doctors cast into sharp relief the ongoing dilemmas of professionalism in medicine. At the core of professionalism was the ethic that the needs of patients came first. Illness did not follow a clock; service to patients frequently caused inconvenience for their doctors. No one wanted doctors who did not believe that they had a moral obligation to place patients first. But no one wanted to be attended by exhausted or burned-out physicians, either. For medicine, these observations raised profoundly important questions. How far could and should doctors go to be available to patients who needed their services at odd hours? When was it appropriate to be with a patient, and when was it better to hand off care to someone else? As the average work week in America continued to shorten, were not doctors, like anyone else, entitled to respite? Does being an effective doctor require the family to be neglected, or can fair compromises be reached? What is the relation between professional success and personal fulfillment? Can one truly have one without the other? Of course, each generation ultimately must decide these matters for itself, as must each individual physician of any generation. These tensions are intrinsic to the practice of medicine, however, and accordingly they will never vanish with time.

CHAPTER 12
The Era of Accountability, Patient Safety, and Work-Hour Regulation

Since the end of World War II, as Arnold Relman first observed, the health care system in America experienced three tectonic shifts.[1] The first of these was "the Era of Expansion," occupying the period from the late 1940s to the late 1960s. With the inception of the National Institutes of Health Extramural Program in 1946, the subsequent creation of new institutes, and increased state funding for professional education, medical research and academic medical centers grew and prospered. With the spread of private medical insurance, Medicare, and Medicaid, nearly 85 percent of Americans acquired some form of health insurance. These developments, however, led to the second tectonic shift, "the Era of Cost Containment," or "the Revolt of the Payers." Within two decades after the enactment of Medicare and Medicaid in 1965, the cost of medical care in the United States had risen from about 4 percent to more than 11 percent of the gross domestic product, and the trajectory of health care costs showed no signs of slowing. The results were diagnosis-related groups, prospective payment, managed care, and what I have called in this book "the Era of High Throughput." This era, which began in the 1980s, has continued ever since.

Toward the end of the twentieth century it became increasingly apparent that not all expenditures on health care could be readily justified. John Wennberg, a physician and epidemiologist at Dartmouth, documented the existence of widely divergent practice styles from one geographic region to another with no apparent differences in outcomes. He showed, for instance, that physicians in one Vermont town performed tonsillectomies three times as often as physicians in nearby towns, even though there was no evidence that the children in that one town were any sicker.[2] Other investigators demonstrated that many common procedures were greatly overused. For instance, one study of coronary angiography and coronary bypass surgery in community hospitals found that only about one-half were performed for clearly apparent medical indications.[3] In addition, some unscrupulous hospitals and doctors engaged in abusive billing practices, including billing for services not rendered.[4] Such developments did much to shatter the traditional professional view that rising health care costs were inevitably the product of a rising quality of care. Reflecting the sentiments of many, Relman noted, "It is bad enough, the payers say, to be confronted with uncontrollable medical costs, but the situation becomes intolerable if in addition no one knows what benefits accrue from the services we pay for or the quality of those services."[5] As a result, the "outcomes movement" emerged in medical research, and the public began to clamor for greater transparency and accountability from hospitals and doctors. In 1991, Relman observed that a third tectonic shift in health care, "the Era of Assessment and Accountability," had begun.

The growing accountability demanded of the medical profession by the public arose only in part from economic concerns. It also reflected the rising power of the consumer. Since the 1960s an emerging consumer culture had been demanding greater accountability from both individuals and institutions traditionally vested with power. This was apparent in such developments as the aggressive consumer advocacy led by Ralph Nader, the rise of the environmentalist and feminist movements, and the public disillusionment with the federal government in the wake of the Vietnam War, the Watergate affair, and the 1971 release of the Pentagon Papers, which documented a systematic pattern of public deception by the government concerning events in Vietnam. Not surprisingly, consumerism began to pervade health care, where critics of the medical profession such as Ivan Illich and Thomas McKeown had been challenging the authority of doctors since the 1960s. Among the manifestations were the "patients' rights" movement, much greater attention to informed consent in both medical practice and clinical research, the replacement of the paternalistic model of the doctor-patient relationship by a shared decision-making model, greater attention to the creature comforts provided to patients and visitors in hospitals, public "report cards" for hospitals and doctors, and an unprecedented arming of patients with information, questions, and demands made possible by the appearance of the Internet. Common to all of these developments, the physicians' pedestal no longer seemed so high or their authority so unassailable.[6]

The era of accountability carried great moment for residency training. All of a sudden, the public became worried about the long, arduous hours worked by house officers. The primary concern of the public was not for the well-being of the interns and residents, however. Rather, it was the growing worry that tired house officers might endanger the safety of patients under their care. These concerns gave rise to regulations enacted by the Accreditation Council for Graduate Medical Education (ACGME) in 2003, revised in 2011, that strictly limited the number of hours that house officers could spend on duty. Ironically, the stresses of residency had long been known within the profession. It required external forces—the voices of consumer advocates—for action finally to be taken.

The regulation of resident work hours created the fiercest controversy in medical education since the Flexner report. Many physicians—including many house officers—chafed over the rigidity of the regulations, which brought with them unforeseen consequences that ran counter to the goals of improving patient safety and resident education. Others, particularly among the public, argued that the new regulations did not go far enough. Worried about errors that might be made by tired house officers, they continued to advocate for further reductions of the total hours that house officers worked and the length of individual shifts.

The controversy over work hours placed into sharp relief the fundamental fault line of the residency system: the tension between educational goals and the economic exploitation of house officers. The controversy also placed into relief the perennial dilemmas of medical education: the need for continuity of care versus the need for physicians to rest and recharge, and the tensions between medical education and patient safety. Ultimately, there was room to make the system safer and better, but never was it possible to eliminate risk or dissipate all stress and fatigue.

The controversy over work hours illustrated a fundamental feature of America's evolving health care system: Societal forces were more powerful than professional wishes. The bureaucracy in medical education responded slowly to the public's concerns that the long work hours of residents would endanger patient safety. Accordingly, the initiative for reform shifted to forces outside of medicine—consumers, the federal government, labor, and unions. It became clear that a profession that ignored the public's demand for transparency and accountability did so at its own risk.

WORK-HOUR RESTRICTIONS

There had always been much to admire about the long hours put in by house officers. Beyond the educational benefits that accrued from observing the natural history of disease and therapy, long hours helped instill a sense of commitment to the patient. House officers learned that becoming a doctor meant learning to meet the needs of others. This message was not lost on them. Thus, at the Massachusetts General Hospital, the medical house staff voted in 1968 against switching from every other night to every third night on call because they "would not know their patients well."[7] House officers on Johns Hopkins's Osler Medical Service—commonly known as "Osler's marines" for the legendary self-denial imposed—believed that the experience fostered a sense of "higher purpose."[8] Surgical house officers everywhere believed that operating on a patient created what one called a "sacred contract." "You don't abdicate your responsibility to your patients because it's inconvenient," he admonished.[9] Intense training experiences contributed to the view that medicine represented a calling. House officers never got used to the sleep deprivation, but seeing their patients get better often created an incredible high that helped justify the sacrifices. Nevertheless, the system had developed many characteristics of hazing, of forcing residents to undergo a rites-of-passage experience. Myths arose concerning the "toughness" of doctors and of their ability to withstand levels of fatigue that would lay ordinary mortals low. Some surgeons denied they were vulnerable to fatigue; doctors of every specialty maintained that the rigors of residency training provided a necessary preparation for the rigors of practice. Those who survived often became true believers in a system that they themselves might have once cursed. Within a few years of their residency, they seemingly remembered only the positive features, insisting now that those who followed endure the same ordeal.

It had long been recognized that house officers were routinely overworked. This point was emphasized in the first systematic study of graduate medical education, published in 1940.[10] In the 1950s and 1960s, the hazards of sleep deprivation became known, including mood changes, depression, impaired cognition, diminished psychomotor functioning, difficulty with interpersonal relationships, and an increased risk of driving accidents.[11] In the 1970s the phenomenon of burnout was recognized. House officers understood they were in a dilemma where their high standards of professionalism were used by others to justify sometimes inhumane levels of work. Thus, in 1965 the House Staff Council at Johns Hopkins reaffirmed that "our duty as physicians is to serve the sick no matter what the conditions." The Council continued, however: "We strongly urge the hospital and political leaders not to take advantage of this adherence to professional responsibility" by imposing unreasonable amounts of work.[12]

In the mid-1980s these stresses became more severe. In the era of high throughput, as noted in the last chapter, there were many more patients to see, the patients were sicker, the level of care was more complex, and there was less time with which to care for patients. In addition, since the increase in work outpaced the increase in support staff, house officers (especially interns and junior residents) were also left with considerable nonmedical work. House officers had fewer traditional chores to do—drawing blood samples, examining urine specimens, starting intravenous lines—but they had many additional duties such as filling out insurance forms, completing admission and discharge papers, transporting patients, and searching for X-rays. (The digitalization of X-rays around the end of the century eliminated the task of hunting down X-rays at those hospitals that had adopted electronic medical records.) Work that could be done by nonphysicians comprised as much as 35 percent of a house officer's time, according to one estimate in 2003.[13] In addition, as noted earlier, routinely requiring house officers to be involved in the care of all patients, no matter how many or how skewed the disease spectrum, was itself a form of institutional service: It kept hospital throughput high but did not necessarily add educational value.

In the 1980s a new stress began to beset large numbers of house officers: a staggering educational debt. Low levels of debt had always afflicted many house officers, but in the late 1970s and early 1980s, as medical school tuition rates soared, so did the amount of debt incurred by the majority of students. The average debt carried by graduates of public medical schools in 1984 was $22,000 and private medical schools, $26,500. Such levels of educational debt were unknown only a few years before. Yet the debt loads of medical graduates continued to escalate. By 2004, the average debt had increased to $105,000 for public school and $140,000 for private school graduates, and only 20 percent of students graduated debt-free. The huge debt burden incurred by medical students was unique to the United States. The massive debt load threatened to make medical careers beyond the reach of students from middle-class and working-class families, and it may have influenced some students to eschew low-paying for high-paying specialties.[14] The escalating debt load also helped explain the rising proclivity of house officers to moonlight, usually in the emergency rooms or intensive care units of community hospitals. Medical educators debated the educational merits of moonlighting, and the prevalence of this activity was unknown, but one thing was certain: Moonlighting did not produce more rested house officers.[15]

Despite the long hours, hard work, and considerable stress, house officers, so the public generally believed, continued to provide outstanding medical and surgical care. Through the 1980s, the traditional view that medical education enhanced patient care remained intact. So did the long-standing belief that teaching hospitals provided the best patient care—in large part *because* they were teaching hospitals. Empirical evidence supported this viewpoint. For instance, a comprehensive review in *The Milbank Quarterly* concluded, "The balance of evidence from the most rigorous studies demonstrated a moderately to substantially better overall quality of care in major teaching hospitals than in nonteaching hospitals."[16] The reluctance of some insured patients to be cared for at teaching hospitals related mainly to stereotypes of cold, impersonal institutional care, long waits for procedures, and ungracious treatment by attendants rather than from concern for quality and safety.[17]

In 1984, the traditional belief that medical education leads to better patient care received a sharp rebuke after 18-year old Libby Zion died at the New York Hospital. Ms. Zion, a college freshman, had presented to the hospital with several days of a fever and an earache. In the emergency room she had a temperature of 103.5°F with no obvious source, was highly agitated, and had mysterious jerking movements. She had a history of depression, for which she was taking the antidepressant phenelzine. The physicians who evaluated her thought she had a viral syndrome but admitted her to the floor for observation. The intern and assistant resident who received her administered fluids and meperidine, an opiate drug, to stop the shaking movements. They consulted by telephone with her private physician, who agreed with the plan. The intern and assistant resident had started their shift at 8 a.m.; at that point, it was then around 3 a.m. the following morning. They had just returned from vacation; though tired, they were not combating chronic fatigue as house officers so commonly do. Soon thereafter, Ms. Zion became more agitated. On notification of this change, the intern ordered physical restraints and a shot of haloperidol, another sedating medication. With many other patients to see, however, the intern did not personally evaluate Ms. Zion again, nor did the resident, who by then was trying to get a few hours of sleep. Initially, Ms. Zion calmed down, but at 6 a.m. she was found to have a temperature of 107°F. Shortly thereafter, she arrested and died.[18]

Ordinarily, little would have become of such a tragic event. However, Libby Zion's father, Sydney Zion, an influential lawyer and journalist, hired a lawyer to investigate. Because of Mr. Zion's personal connections, the case immediately became the center of intense media interest. The family alleged that her death resulted from inadequate care provided by overworked, undersupervised house officers. Mr. Zion persuaded Robert Morgenthau, the district attorney of Manhattan, to convene a grand jury to investigate the circumstances surrounding her death.

Despite years of review by the grand jury and later by other medical and legal groups, the cause of Ms. Zion's death was never determined. It was speculated that her death might have resulted from her dose of meperidine, which is contraindicated in patients taking phenelzine. It was also speculated that Ms. Zion's use of cocaine might have contributed to an adverse drug reaction. (She had denied the use of cocaine when asked, but traces were found in her system at autopsy.) The grand jury concluded that the house officers in the main had acted appropriately. Accordingly, the grand jury refused to indict the doctors caring for her on criminal charges, and the state medical board did not revoke their licenses.

The grand jury did indict the residency system, however, and the case came to symbolize the need for major reform. The grand jury ruled that "the most serious deficiencies [in the Zion case and at other Level One hospitals] can be traced to the practice of permitting inexperienced physicians to staff emergency rooms and allowing interns and junior residents to practice medicine without supervision." The grand jury called for interns and junior residents admitting patients to have "contemporaneous, in person consultation with senior physicians before they initiate a course of treatment." The grand jury elaborated:

> A hospital is not the place for recently graduated doctors to grow and develop in isolation; rather it is a place where the learning process should continue under strict supervision. Thus, medical decisions, whether in an emergency room or on a hospital floor should NOT be made by inexperienced interns and junior residents without in-person consultations with more senior physicians.

Almost as an afterthought, the grand jury noted: "We recognize that the number of hours that interns and residents are required to work is counterproductive to medical care. This practice may be cost-efficient for hospital budgets, but its corresponding cost is a diminished quality of health care."[19]

In the wake of the grand jury report, David Axelrod, the commissioner of the New York State Department of Health, appointed a special committee consisting of nine distinguished New York physicians to review the findings of the grand jury. The committee, known as the Ad Hoc Advisory Committee on Emergency Services, was chaired by Bertrand M. Bell, professor of medicine at the Albert Einstein College of Medicine. After 18 months of deliberation, the committee made extensive recommendations, including the on-site supervision of busy emergency rooms by attending physicians and the 24-hour supervision of acute care inpatient wards by experienced doctors. The committee also called for improved working conditions for house officers as well as greater ancillary support. One recommendation called for a limitation of work hours to 80 hours per week averaged over a four-week period and one day off per week.[20]

To many, the idea of an 80-hour week for house officers, once pronounced, seemed like a law of nature, and it quickly became the consensual standard. In fact, the number had no empirical support and was developed serendipitously. In 1993 Bell recounted the process that led to the recommendation of 80 hours.

> For the past 31 years, I have been very fortunate and have rented a beach house on a dune overlooking the ocean on Cape Cod. In the summer of 1986, I was sitting on the beautiful porch of that home with two friends of mine (both Einstein graduates), Dr. Roger Platt and Dr. Shelby Jacobson. I was reviewing with them the draft of the proposed regulations. Roger, one of the most extraordinary people I know, in his very quiet way can solve everything! I was fishing with my non-mathematical mind for defining a number of work hours for residents which might be acceptable to the establishment and provide some relief for residents. He in his very mathematical and precise fashion thought about the week, the scheduling of internal medicine house staff, and came up with the following. There are 168 hours in a week. It is reasonable for residents to work a 10-day week for 5 days a week. It is humane for people to work every fourth night. If you subtract the 50-hour week (10 hours/day x five days) from 168 hours, you end of with 118 hours. If you then divide 118 by 4 (every fourth night), it equals 30. If you then add 50 to 30, eureka that equals an 80-hour work week. So in honor of Roger, we should redub the 80-hour work week as the "Roger Platt 80-hour work week!"[21]

The Bell committee's recommendations on the supervision and working conditions of residents were incorporated into the New York State Health Code. The new law, known as the "Bell Regulations" (also, the "405 Regulations" or the "Libby Zion Regulations"), took effect in July 1989. New York was the only state to pass such legislation, but similar recommendations were voluntarily enacted by most of the Residency Review Committees (RRCs) that governed residency training in the various specialties. Specifics varied from one field to another, but in general the new regulations called for a restriction of the resident work week to 80 hours averaged over four weeks, overnight call no more frequently than every third night, the mandatory provision of one day off per week, limitations on the length of shifts in the emergency room, similar limitations on the frequency of nights on call in the hospital, and the requirement of greater direct supervision by attending physicians. Only the RRCs in surgery and the surgical specialties did not pass such regulations. Unlike the Bell Regulations, the RRC rules focused mainly on work hours, not on the larger issues of supervision or work environment.

As a result of the Libby Zion case, the attention of both the profession and the public became fixated on the subject of resident work hours. In this, the Zion case was widely misunderstood. The intern and junior resident who provided Libby Zion's care had just returned from vacation. Though tired, they were relatively fresh, not suffering from chronic fatigue as so many house officers do, and no evidence that excessive working hours or fatigue contributed to her death was ever found.[22] That is why the Bell committee identified the primary problem in her care as inadequate supervision, not overly long work hours. Of the 17 recommendations for reform in the committee's report, only one concerned the work-hour issue. This point seemed lost on the RRCs, which focused on hours rather than on supervision, as well as on the medical profession and public at large, which likewise focused thereafter on the hours issue. Bell, of course, recognized the need to reduce work hours. In 1993 he spoke of the imperative to "rethink the practice of making sleep deprivation a tradition of graduate medical education."[23] The basic message of the Bell Regulations, however, was that "supervision, not regulation of hours, is the key to improving the quality of patient care."[24] For the next two decades Bell remained upset that the reforms made in his name distorted his primary purpose.[25]

There was little doubt that the residency system needed reform. House officers were simply too tired and overworked, and too many emerged from the experience cynical and convinced that the world owed them something for what they had been through. To many medical educators, it represented a great misfortune that the profession had not acted earlier on its own to address these issues. Robert G. Petersdorf, president of the Association of American Medical Colleges, expressed his regret that "long-overdue changes in structuring residency training were not initiated within our community prior to the serendipitous stimulus of the Zion case." My wish, he said, would be "that the profession had been more perceptive in recognizing the issue and making appropriate changes in training prior to its becoming a cause célèbre."[26]

The Bell Regulations and new RRC rules were not enacted without fierce opposition from within the profession. All 13 medical schools in the state of New York opposed the Bell Regulations.[27] Many medical educators worried that with shorter hours, house officers would acquire less clinical experience, receive fewer opportunities to observe the natural history of disease, and develop less satisfying relationships with patients. A major concern, particularly in New York, where the supervision requirements were stricter, was that the regulations would undermine the principle that house officers should receive graded levels of responsibility. For this reason, one survey found that only 27 percent of chief residents in New York felt that the educational experience of residents would be improved under the Bell Regulations.[28] Many physicians also worried that the new rules would endanger patient care, a consequence of the increased number of patient handoffs and greater discontinuity of care that would occur. Another strong objection, especially among the medical faculties and teaching hospitals, was that an inordinate amount of time and expense would be required to relieve house officers of some of their duties. Behind closed doors, hospital administrators fretted about finding the money that would be needed, and medical faculties worried that some of the work done by residents would shift to the attending staff, thereby interfering with their own research or clinical practice.[29] The teaching hospitals and medical faculties were clearly vested in the status quo.

In the 1990s, the furor over resident hours temporarily abated, for both the Bell Regulations and the new RRC rules had little immediate impact. In New York, teaching hospitals ignored the law, mainly because the mandated changes were expensive to implement, and the state did not vigorously enforce the regulations. In 1995, Bell observed that New York's new regulations were "being widely flouted" because interns and residents were still "too frequently exploited as cheap labor."[30] A widely reported survey by the New York State Health Department in 1998 found gross noncompliance with the law.[31] Nationwide, compliance with the RRC rules was also poor, and for the same reasons—the expense of implementation and ongoing concerns that the quality of education and patient care might paradoxically be worsened. The RRCs did not enforce their written rules, and many house officers still found themselves working more hours than officially permitted. Jordan J. Cohen, president of the Association of American Medical Colleges, in 2001 deplored "our blatant disregard for our own standards."[32]

Although the issue of resident work hours quieted down in the 1990s, the public's concern about the safety of hospital care continued to increase. In 1995, a seeming epidemic of errors, including wrong-site surgery and medication mistakes, erupted at US hospitals. These high-profile tragedies received an enormous amount of media attention. The most highly publicized incident involved the death of 39-year-old Betsy Lehman, a health columnist at the *Boston Globe*, from a massive chemotherapy overdose while being treated for breast cancer at the renowned Dana-Farber Cancer Institute. The American Medical Association (AMA) at first launched a public relations counteroffensive, calling these events isolated mistakes. However, under pressure from the media, the AMA reversed its position, acknowledging that mistakes were common, often resulting from system problems at highly complex institutions. In 1996 the AMA established its National Patient Safety Foundation. In this, the AMA joined forces with physicians such as Donald Berwick and Lucian Leape, who had been leading efforts to improve the quality and safety of care for years.

Public concern for patient safety reached a crescendo in 1999, following the release of the Institute of Medicine's (IOM) highly publicized report *To Err Is Human*. The report concluded that 48,000 to 98,000 Americans died in US hospitals every year because of preventable medical errors.[33] No one was surprised that errors in hospital care occurred; it was the magnitude of the problem that made the report so shocking. A poll taken a few weeks after the report's publication found that 51 percent of the public was aware of its conclusions—an exceedingly high level of awareness for this type of report.[34] The report said very little about the residency system or the work hours of interns and residents. However, it reignited the public's fear that tired residents might endanger the safety of patients. Accordingly, public attention refocused on resident work hours, this time with even greater intensity, anger, and fear than after the Libby Zion case. Vigorous attention from the media, which no longer placed the medical profession on a pedestal, helped stoke public concerns.[35]

How hard were house officers working? It was clear that the stresses of the job were much greater than they were 15 or 20 years earlier, a consequence of caring for larger numbers of much sicker patients as well as of ever-rising educational debt. One study of internal medicine house officers in 2002 showed that depression, cynicism, and burnout had increased conspicuously since 1990, despite many efforts to reform the residency curriculum.[36] How many hours were house officers working? Since the 1960s, the work schedule had been shortening, as many programs went from every other night on call to every third or every fourth, and as vacation time was increased from two weeks a year to three or four. At the end of the century, however, the typical work week of residents remained long and grueling. DeWitt C. Baldwin Jr., who has contributed significantly to our understanding of this subject, found that during the 1998–99 training year, interns (first postgraduate year, or PGY-1) reported working an average of 83 hours a week and first-year residents (second postgraduate year, or PGY-2), an average of 76.2 hours a week. What was particularly notable was the wide variation that existed across specialties. For instance, PGY-2s in general surgery averaged 105.7 hours a week; neurosurgery, 110.6 hours a week; and urology, 98.5 hours a week. PGY-2s in pathology averaged 56.7 hours a week; psychiatry, 59.2 hours a week; and dermatology, 59.9 hours a week. Interns and first-year residents in the primary care specialties (internal medicine, pediatrics, family practice) averaged close to 80 hours a week. Overall, 49.7 percent of PGY-1s averaged more than 80 hours per week, including 28.1 percent over 90 hours per week and 12.4 percent over 100 hours per week. The corresponding figures for PGY-2s were 35.1 percent, 20.8 percent, and 10.9 percent, respectively. Baldwin also found that house officers averaging more than 80 work hours a week were more likely to be involved in a personal accident or injury, become engaged in a serious interpersonal conflict with staff members, or make a significant medical error.[37]

Consideration of the subject of resident work hours proved surprisingly difficult. What, precisely, constituted an hour of work? Time in the hospital sleeping? Time at home while officially on duty (many subspecialties, such as orthopedics, dermatology, and otolaryngology, allowed residents after the first or second year to take evening and weekend call from home)? Time in the hospital after patient-care duties had been completed, perhaps to attend a conference or read in the library? Not all hours of work exacted the same physical toll. Should work on weekends or holidays, or more important from the perspective of fatigue, night duty, count differently than ordinary daytime hours? Individuals differed markedly in their sleep requirements; could or should the particular biological needs of each person receive consideration?[38] In addition, as Baldwin pointed out, house officers had more to their lives than work and sleep. Residents engaged in numerous activities outside the hospital—spending time with spouses, caring for young children, performing household chores, developing friendships and romantic relationships, reading, attending parties, engaging in hobbies, exercising, or moonlighting—many of which affected their degree of energy and alertness when back on duty. Thus, additional hours off the job did not necessarily translate to an equivalent amount of more sleep. For all these reasons, Baldwin and other experts warned against simple approaches or one-size-fits-all solutions to the problem of work hours.[39]

However, after the release of the IOM report, the public showed little interest in the nuances of the debate. To many consumers, long resident work hours represented still another factor threatening patient safety. The general public knew that there were mandated continuous-hour restrictions on truck drivers and pilots; why should these requirements not apply to physicians-in-training as well? As Jeffrey M. Drazen and Arnold M. Epstein wrote in the *New England Journal of Medicine*, "It is very hard to convince the person in the street that there is any rational reason to have residents work more than 80 hours a week."[40] Society had always granted physicians considerable autonomy in determining the conditions of medical education, but never total freedom. Medical education had to meet the burden of proof of reasonableness, and now, in an age of consumerism and accountability, residency training was failing to pass that test.

In the early 2000s, the contentious debate concerning resident work hours re-erupted. Many within the profession argued for not making further changes. They correctly pointed out that little evidence existed that patients had actually suffered at the hands of overly tired residents, and they also claimed that resident education would suffer if held hostage to a time clock. The strongest voices came from the surgical community, where leaders spoke of the importance of developing "a keen sense of personal responsibility for patient care that is not automatically discharged at any given hour."[41] With overly rigid restrictions on work hours, they feared that the inculcation of professionalism and accountability would become more difficult. They also worried about the loss of continuity of care that might result, particularly if residents were unable to participate in the preoperative and postoperative care of patients on whom they had operated.[42] Powerful contrary opinions came from outside the profession, however, particularly from consumer groups and unions. Critics pointed to valid physiological evidence that fatigue causes deterioration of high-level functioning; they also argued that high-quality education cannot occur when residents are too tired to absorb the lessons being taught. It was clear in the debate that the profession's perception of resident work hours was at odds with that of the public. All parties sought the same goals: safe patient care and quality residency training. They were remarkably polarized, however, on how to achieve those goals. It was a classic case, as Jordan Cohen observed, "where everyone is partially right."[43]

As the debate proceeded, the public's voice could not be ignored. In January 2000, the Office of the Inspector General requested a meeting with the Accreditation Council for Graduate Medical Education (ACGME), the organization that governed the RRCs, to investigate the issue of resident work hours as it pertained to patient safety.[44] In April 2001, Public Citizen (a consumer and health advocacy group), the Committee of Interns and Residents, and the American Medical Student Association, along with Bertrand M. Bell and Kingman P. Strohl, a sleep disorder expert at Case Western University, petitioned the Occupational Safety and Health Administration (OSHA) of the US Department of Labor to establish and enforce a federal work-hour standard for house officers. In November 2001, Representative John Conyers Jr. (D-Mich.), introduced legislation in the House of Representatives that would limit residents to 80 hours of work per week, with no averaging among weeks, and provide for federal enforcement of that limit. In June 2002, Senator Jon Corzine (D-N.J.) introduced similar legislation in the Senate. OSHA rejected the petition on the grounds that this matter was much more appropriately handled by the profession. Similarly, in meetings in Washington, D.C., between key members of the House, including Representative Conyers, and leaders of the ACGME, congressional leaders indicated their preference that the ACGME, rather than Congress, act on this issue.[45] It was clear that the federal government was watching closely, however, poised to intervene if the ACGME did not act on its own.

As public pressures to restrict resident working hours increased, the ACGME was in an excellent position to respond, for it had become a much different organization from what it had been at its inception. After World War II, residency programs had been governed by the various RRCs in the individual specialties and subspecialties. The RRCs functioned as autonomous fiefdoms. Each had its own standards and policies, and there was little coordination among them. Recognizing the need for more focused oversight of residency training, five organizations (the AMA, Association of American Medical Colleges, American Board of Medical Specialties, American Hospital Association, and Council of Medical Specialty Societies) came together in 1972 to create the Liaison Committee for Graduate Medical Education (LCGME) to oversee the RRCs. The LCGME proved overly cumbersome; in 1981 it was reorganized as the ACGME, still under the five original sponsoring organizations. The RRCs remained responsible for the specific curricula, rules, and monitoring of programs in their specialties. The ACGME, however, reviewed and governed the RRCs, monitoring them for fairness and effectiveness. In addition, the ACGME established general program requirements that applied to all specialties and subspecialties, to be enforced by the RRCs.

In its early years, the ACGME was an understated, low-profile organization that quietly went about the business of overseeing the RRCs. Its work and that of the RRCs manifested the public-spiritedness of many physicians, for the organizations were dependent on the time and expertise provided by volunteers. In the late 1980s, physicians contributed approximately 30,000 hours of unpaid service each year to the RRCs or the ACGME.[46] In 1997 David C. Leach, an internist and endocrinologist with a strong social conscience and deep philosophical bent, became executive director. Under Leach's leadership, the ACGME became a separately incorporated organization in 2000, independent of the original five sponsoring organizations.[47] Many risks came with independence, but independence allowed the ACGME to go in new directions. The ACGME wished to be transparent and to receive input from all the stakeholders in graduate medical education, including the public. Accordingly, it appointed resident and public members to its board. It began to view itself as an agent of progress and as a center for discourse in graduate medical education, not just as an enforcer of standards. Thus, it began sponsoring educational conferences, collected data pertaining to residency training, established a journal (the *Journal of Graduate Medical Education*, which published its first issue in 2010), and expanded into international graduate medical education accreditation. Under Leach, the ACGME became a "learning organization," engaged in continuous quality improvement, regularly undergoing critical reviews of its activities and effectiveness.[48] It was Leach's desire to have the ACGME become "the best accrediting body in the world."[49]

Thus, the ACGME in the early 2000s had become a much more progressive organization than it historically had been. When public pressure to restrict resident work hours intensified, the ACGME found itself sympathetic. In September 2001, it established a work group to develop common duty-hour standards for all ACGME-accredited programs, recommend enhancements to the compliance process, communicate these changes to the residency educational community and the public at large, and suggest ways for the ACGME to collaborate with other organizations to foster learning, safe patient care, and resident well-being. The ACGME, like the rest of the profession, strongly desired that the federal government not become the regulator of graduate medical education. Beyond its concern for government intrusion, however, the ACGME felt that work-hour restriction was the right thing to do. As Leach put it, "It is our professional obligation as a community to fix the problem, not throw up our hands and turn it over to others."[50]

In June 2002, the ACGME approved new duty-hour standards for residency programs in all specialties. At the time the ACGME accredited 7,800 residency programs in the United States in 118 specialties and subspecialties. The new rules were as follows:

- Residents should not be scheduled for more than 80 duty hours per week, averaged over a four-week period, with the provision that individual programs may apply for an increase in this limit of up to 10 percent, if they can provide a sound educational rationale.
- One day in seven free of patient-care responsibilities, averaged over a four-week period.
- Call no more frequently than every third night, averaged over a four-week period.
- A 24-hour limit on on-call duty, with an added period of up to six hours for continuity and transfer of care, educational debriefing, and didactic activities; no new patients may be accepted after 24 hours.
- A 10-hour minimum rest period between duty periods.
- Call periods from home are counted toward the weekly duty hour limit, if the nature of the call requires residents to return to the hospital.[51]

The ACGME also imposed the requirement of stricter institutional oversight to ensure that the rules be followed. This was important because the ACGME rules were similar to the law already in effect in New York State, which was regularly violated; a critical question was whether the new rules would in fact be enforced.[52] The ACGME requirements were more lenient than those imposed on residents in other Western countries: for instance, Australia, maximum of 75 work hours per week; Denmark, 45 hours per week; United Kingdom, 72 hours per week; European Union, 48 hours per week; Germany, 56 hours per week; and the Netherlands, 60 hours per week.[53] The new US rules took effect in July 2003.

Ironically, as the ACGME passed its new rules, there was little evidence that resident fatigue posed a danger to patients. The pioneering safety expert David Gaba wrote in 2002, "Despite many anecdotes about errors that were attributed to fatigue, no study has proved that fatigue on the part of health care personnel causes errors that harm patients."[54] However, there was abundant and growing evidence that acute and chronic sleep deprivation was harmful to the functioning and well-being of house officers. The strongest argument to restrict work hours was the ethical and educational one: Long hours were potentially exploitive and inhumane, they fostered cynicism and burnout, and they often interfered with residents' ability to learn. As one writer put it, "Overwork interferes with the development of professional values and attitudes that are an essential part of the moral curriculum of residency."[55] In its deliberations, the ACGME's work group took into account new physiological information on the impact of sleep loss and fatigue,[56] and in its final recommendations the ACGME acknowledged that long hours impaired the health, functioning, and attitudes of residents.[57] Thus, resident well-being, not just patient safety, finally became a consideration in the conversation.

Of note, as attention from both the profession and public focused on work hours, little concern was expressed for the quality of the broader learning environment. Throughout the history of graduate medical education, as seen in this book, work hours were but one part of the larger issue of work conditions. Both from the perspective of patient safety and resident learning, the quality of residency training depended on such issues as the volume of patients, the intensity of illness, the sophistication and complexity of care, the burden of nonprofessional chores, the level of supervision, the quality of teaching, and the degree of support and inspiration the house staff received from the faculty and hospital administration. A few at the turn of the century pointed this out. Baldwin in 1998 observed, "The real issue . . . is not merely the time that residents put in, but what they gain from that time."[58] In 1999 I wrote, "The issue of working hours must be seen as part of the larger issue of working conditions."[59] In the mad rush to limit resident work hours, however, the importance of the learning environment was generally overlooked, as if nothing else mattered but the amount of time at work.

PERPETUAL DILEMMAS

In the early 2000s, it was clear that the age of accountability in medicine was fully under way. The profession (and the entire health care system) experienced strong societal pressure to reduce costs, improve quality, maximize safety, and increase transparency. Much of the pressure to do so came from outside of medicine. For instance, the Leapfrog Group, a consortium of large US companies organized in 1998 to wield their enormous purchasing power to promote safety and value in health care, became a powerful force in these matters.[60] However, large segments of the medical profession internalized the message. Leaders of safety and quality in medical care, such as Lucian Leape and Donald Berwick, found more and more doctors listening to their message. The IOM promoted quality, safety, and value in health care through a number of highly publicized reports.[61] By the 2010s, much work remained to be done, but significant movement in this direction had unquestionably occurred.

The shift toward safety, quality, and public accountability could be seen in every aspect of graduate medical education. For instance, the American Board of Medical Specialties (ABMS) and its constituent specialty boards implemented a policy of compulsory recertification (later called maintenance of certification) to ensure that board-certified doctors stayed up-to-date throughout their practicing careers. Recertification had been available in many specialties for decades, but typically on a voluntary basis. In 2004, the ABMS announced that all 24 member boards would make board certification time-limited.[62] Doctors in every field were now required to pass a maintenance of certification examination every six to ten years, depending on the specialty, in order to retain their board certification. In the past, the ABMS had been an inwardly looking organization, but the maintenance of certification program resulted in a "visible external role" for the organization, allowing it to become "a leader in the quest to improve the safety and quality of medical care."[63]

Similarly, the ACGME moved from a "process" to an "outcomes" method of accreditation. Previously, residency programs were accredited on the basis of various structural features—the credentials of the faculty, the quality of the clinical laboratories, the completeness and usability of the library, the amount and variety of "patient material," and so forth. In July 2002, the ACGME began accrediting programs in part on the ability of their residents to acquire six specific "competencies" (patient care, medical knowledge, interpersonal and communication skills, professionalism, systems-based practice, and practice-based learning and improvement) that had been identified and defined in a collaborative effort with several other medical organizations. By focusing on what residents could do, not just on what they knew, the accreditation process found a potential way to help document a linkage between educational quality and the quality of care delivered by program graduates. The net effect was movement toward greater public accountability.[64]

In the early 2000s safety concerns also influenced the actual teaching and learning of medicine and surgery through the impetus they gave to the simulation movement. Simulation technologies allowed house officers and medical students to learn and practice various techniques, from simple blood draws to complex surgeries, on lifelike mannequins. The simulation movement dated to the 1960s, and in the 1990s a few medical schools opened simulation laboratories. The movement was nearly moribund, however, until resuscitated by the public fallout from the IOM report on medical errors. Suddenly, conferences in the field became well attended, new technologies were developed more rapidly, publications in the field increased, and the undergraduate and graduate curricula took greater advantage of these approaches.[65] With simulation laboratories available, it became increasingly unjustifiable for trainees to learn procedures on live patients or on the immediately deceased. They now could learn and practice many procedures in simulated settings, thereby sparing live individuals from many avoidable learning errors.

In the early 2000s, however, the professional and public focus remained fixed on resident work hours. The issue did not go away after the ACGME announced its new work-hour regulations in 2003. Quite the contrary: The controversy intensified as both supporters and opponents awaited the outcomes of the uncontrolled experiment. During this time the ACGME remained under intense criticism—from some, for going too far; from others, for not going far enough.

The acrimonious controversy intensified still further in 2007 when Congress asked the IOM to investigate the matter. The ensuing report,[66] written by a largely nonphysician committee, endorsed the 80-hour maximum work week, averaged over four weeks. Drawing heavily on new data from sleep physiology, the report recommended that each intern and resident not be permitted to work a shift longer than 16 hours and that a mandatory five-hour nap be required of each house officer working overnight. It recommended five days off per month, in contrast to the current four days, as well as limits on how many night rotations (the so-called night float rotation) house officers could work per week. There was also much in the report about the working conditions of house officers—so much so that the committee recommended that the report be entitled "Beyond Duty Hours."[67] This title was unacceptable to IOM leadership, however, so the title "Resident Duty Hours: Enhancing Sleep, Supervision, and Safety" was substituted. Accordingly, all attention after the report's release focused on the specific duty-hour recommendations, and once again the larger issue of the learning environment was forgotten amid the preoccupation with work hours.

The IOM report, released in January 2009, added to the pressure on the ACGME to revisit its work-hour regulations. As before, unions and consumer groups lobbied for more changes. For instance, on one day in June 2010, the ACGME heard from 10,000 individuals who had hit a link on the Consumers Union website to email the ACGME to urge adoption of the IOM recommendations.[68] The ACGME responded, forming a special committee that held public hearings, received written position statements from more than 100 organizations, solicited opinions nationwide, reviewed the published literature, and issued a revised set of recommendations that took effect in July 2011.[69]

The new regulations were similar to the old but were influenced by the studies in sleep physiology. There were two major changes in the new regulations. First, the six hours after overnight call duty that previously had been allowed for residents to care for their patients the next day and participate in educational activities (the "+6" rule) was reduced to four hours (the "+4" rule). Second, an intern was prohibited from working a shift longer than 16 hours, which meant no overnight call duty. The ACGME rejected the IOM recommendation of compulsory naps as too unwieldy but encouraged house officers to take "power naps" whenever possible. This, of course, had always been done by house officers whenever they were on call. The revised ACGME regulations, unlike the old, stated that moonlighting hours should be counted toward the 80-hour limit. (Both sets of regulations prohibited moonlighting by interns.) As with the military's "don't ask, don't tell" policy for gays, however, few house officers volunteered their moonlighting activities, and few program directors asked, so it is unlikely that the regulations had a significant impact on moonlighting. Indeed, there were anecdotal observations of house officers using many of their newly freed hours to increase their amount of moonlighting.

The revised ACGME regulations of 2011 did not end the controversy. Indeed, attention to the issue continued to grow, as emotions soared, tempers sometimes erupted, and predictions of both the end and the salvation of the profession could be regularly heard. Both in 2003 and 2011, supporters of work-hour regulations anticipated that their implementation would result in significant gains in patient safety. Critics, on the other hand, predicted that patient safety would suffer and that house officers would leave training less well prepared for medical practice.

The greatest hostility to the 2011 regulations, as to the 2003 regulations, came from within the medical profession. One chair of internal medicine, who specialized in patient safety and quality improvement, stated, "I don't know of any department chair in any specialty who supports the regulations. The disruptions in the continuity of care jeopardize both safety and education. It's insane."[70] Strong objections came from the surgical community, which considered seceding from the ACGME.[71] Residents themselves held a generally negative attitude toward the regulations. They believed work-hour restrictions improved their quality of life, and for that they were grateful. However, they believed the changes weakened their education, increased the emphasis on institutional service over education, and diminished the quality of patient care.[72] Most residency program directors also viewed the regulations unfavorably, and for much the same reasons as the residents.[73] Even harsh critics of the residency system, such as Robert Press, a psychiatrist in Denver and the inspiration for the character "Runt" in *The House of God*, worried that the recent changes in resident work hours "have created a whole new set of medical problems."[74] The opposition from within the profession was so intense that the ACGME probably would not have enacted the 2011 regulations had it not been for the pressure from the IOM report to do so.[75]

What led to such hostility toward work-hour reform among those most directly involved? It was not the idea of limiting the work week to 80 hours. Indeed, by now even the harshest critics acknowledged that the residency system needed to become more humane, and the once controversial 80-hour limit had become a nonissue. Although they scathingly criticized the new system, for instance, the editors of the *American Journal of Medicine* called the 100-plus-hour weeks of the past a form of "cruel and unusual punishment" and made clear that they were not calling for a return to that system.[76] Rather, skepticism and criticism continued because of the unintended consequences of the rules: The regulations represented an unfunded mandate, the strict restrictions on work following a night on call proved highly disruptive of education and patient care, and it was exceedingly difficult to apply a one-size-fits-all package to all programs in all specialties.

The first problem, the unfunded mandate, became immediately apparent with the 2003 regulations and continued after the 2011 revisions. It was understood by everyone, including the ACGME, that limiting resident work hours would be expensive. Someone would have to see the patients previously cared for by the residents. In certain cases, teaching hospitals did shift some patient care to nonresident services, hired more residents, or made greater use of physician assistants and nurse practitioners. However, this was difficult for most teaching hospitals to do. It typically took two or three nurse practitioners or physician assistants to do the work of one resident. Nurse practitioners and physician assistants received higher salaries than residents, and they brought the hospital no Medicare graduate medical education reimbursements.[77] Accordingly, the bulk of the work continued to be done by the residents, and the phenomenon of "work compression" arose—that is, house officers scrambling to do the same amount of work in fewer hours, with even less time than before for reflective decision making, adopting a mindful approach to patient care, and engaging in educational activities.[78] Residents now spent fewer hours at work, but the time they did spend had become more intense and pressure-packed. The long-standing tradition in graduate medical education of maximizing the use of house officers for institutional service lived on.

Jason Ryan, whose internal medicine residency at the Beth Israel Deaconess Medical Center spanned both the old (pre-work-hour regulation) and new (post-regulation) systems, provided a firsthand account of the effects of work compression. Under the new system, he found that he worked harder than ever. In his words, "A frantic mentality engulfed the ward, with residents and interns rushing from task to task and then out of the hospital." As a result, "the pace at which I worked under the new rules was faster than ever," and he worried that his haste might lead to medical errors—"a potentially malicious irony for a system designed to protect patients." A primary casualty of the new system was learning, which had become marginalized. Education about the diagnosis and management of disease felt "like a hindrance." He elaborated:

> In the new ward environment, we are constantly tempted to sidestep for the sake of expediency decisions that require careful thought. Why look up the differential diagnosis of hematuria when a renal consultant will be called anyway and it's getting late in the night? Why pause to analyze an electrocardiogram when the emergency department has already documented a lack of acute changes and the floor is awaiting orders? Under the new system, the intern who admits 6 patients and discharges 3 others, all the while calling 2 consults, is a champion of the wards. But I still wonder, where does learning fit in?

Ryan acknowledged that having begun his residency during the era of high throughput, the hectic pace and de-emphasis of education were present before work-hour regulations were introduced. However, "The ACGME regulations rapidly accelerated this process so that learning, at all levels, from medical students to senior residents, has been diluted, drowned by a sea of discharge planning, case management, and pressure to get done and get out."[79]

The second problem, the disruptions created by the new system, resulted largely from the rigidity imposed by the "+6" (and, in 2011, the "+4") rule. Traditionally, the several hours following a 24-hour admitting day were invaluable to house officers both for providing patient care and for learning. House officers managed the problems of the patients they had admitted the day or night before, creating continuity that was important for patients as well as for learners. In the medical fields, residents made many "second-level" decisions vital to management. For instance, the patient admitted the night before with chest pain might have been scheduled for a stress test the next day. In the early afternoon the results would be ready, and the resident who admitted the patient and ordered the test could review the findings and make the next decision. In the surgical fields, depending on the level of experience, the resident could perform the operation or assist with it on the patient he had evaluated the night before, as well as be available to attend to any immediate postoperative issues that might occur. The next day's work also involved participating in teaching rounds, attending conferences of particular interest, spending more time with patients and families, and making certain that patients were reasonably stable before signing out to the on-call team. The time a house officer left for the night varied, but it was generally in the late afternoon. This provided the resident enough opportunity for a relaxed evening and a good night's sleep. Of note, this routine was consistent with the ACGME regulation that there should be at least 10 hours off between work periods. This routine also kept the work week to around 80 hours, assuming an overnight call frequency of every third night (the maximum permitted) and one day off per week. For house officers with less frequent overnight duty, the hours worked per week were much fewer than 80.

The institution of the "+6" rule (meaning house officers had to be out of the hospital by roughly 1 p.m. on a post-call day) and the revised "+4" rule (meaning a roughly 11 a.m. deadline for departure) interrupted the natural patient care and educational flow of the workday. Surgical residents frequently had to leave in the middle of an operation or before they could render postoperative care. Medical residents often had to go home before the results of important tests had returned, so the stress test ordered on last night's patient had to be interpreted and acted on by someone unfamiliar with the patient. House officers frequently had to hand off critically ill patients—with diabetic ketoacidosis or hypertensive emergencies, for example—to someone who did not know the patient before the patient had been adequately stabilized. Opportunities to talk with patients and families were truncated. In short, house officers were prevented from doing many of the things central to the practice of good medicine, as patient care and education both took a backseat to the calculus of a shift-work schedule.

Many critics of the new system complained of the increased number of handoffs of patients from one house officer to another that were required by the new system. Handoffs had long been known to be a major source of error, delays, and increased costs in the delivery of care.[80] However, it was not just the absolute increase in the number of handoffs but also the fact that handoffs now regularly occurred at inopportune times that worried so many medical educators. House officers were required to leave, even if the operation was not yet done or the critically ill patient still not stabilized. Many supporters of rigid shift limitations argued for more and better training in handoffs—using computers, formalizing the protocol, or trying to achieve the choreographed efficiency of a Ferrari pit stop.[81] Though better handoffs were much needed, this point of view held certain limitations. Good handoffs always required time, which already was in short supply. More important, it begged the question of whether it was wise to require handoffs of patients who were not yet at reasonable clinical punctuation points in the first place.

The rigidity of the "+6" and "+4" rules created an unprecedented level of fragmentation on the floors of virtually every specialty. Patients wondered who their doctors were or to whom they could reach out for information and comfort.[82] Conversely, it became more difficult for house officers to develop a sense of ownership of their patients. To meet the 1 p.m. or 11 a.m. deadline, corners regularly had to be cut, leading to potentially unsafe care. "Errors are made when people are focused on 'getting out' since the focus is not safe care," one highly regarded educational leader wrote.[83] Formerly, residents in internal medicine customarily reviewed the important X-rays of their patients with a radiologist. They always learned from those conversations and often left with a modified plan of management. Now, they rarely did this. Nor did they often check on the progress of their patients whom they had sent to surgery or another service, something they also had earlier done with regularity. The system also became fragmented for attending physicians trying to teach and supervise. All too often, the intern or resident responsible for a patient was not present on rounds but rather was off to clinic, dismissed early because of shift limits, or at home because the mandatory day off fell on a weekday.[84]

The dilemma imposed by the combination of rigid shift limits and work compression was illustrated by an exchange in 2009 between a program director and faculty member. The program director wrote:

> I have a favor to ask of you. Due to the relatively large number of patients on our medical teams, a number of residents have been having difficulties leaving the hospital in time to fulfill resident work hour rules. I appreciate your attending efforts and all the time you spend with residents and students. However, I am

requesting that, if at all possible, residents finish rounds by 9:30–10 am. This will enable them to get some of their essential work done earlier in the day so they can still attend required conferences and leave on time [1 p.m.] at the end of the day.

The faculty member replied:

> Thanks for your message. We all, of course, want to see our residents go home as early as possible and need to do everything possible to expedite that. At the same time, as I know you know, we have a real dilemma because the work load has not been decreased to accommodate the new work-hour regulations, and, at least with my team, the number of patients and the complexity of their problems have been unusually high the past few weeks. So those who would rigorously enforce the rules are placed in the position of advocating significant corner-cutting in patient care or resident education, which are hardly admirable goals.[85]

In this case the faculty member held his ground. He did not allow his house officers to cut important corners in the care of their patients, and the team had some highly engaging educational discussions. The house officers did, however, leave the hospital an hour or two later than the shift rules permitted.

Most concerning from an educational perspective, the inflexible limitations on shifts squelched initiative. A faculty member in obstetrics and gynecology at the George Washington Hospital invited a resident to observe a sophisticated laparoscopic procedure on a uterine tumor by one of the world's premier experts—a man from whom even senior faculty regularly learned. The resident wanted to do so but declined—this would be violating work-hour regulations.[86] House officers were prohibited from 2 p.m. seminars, 3 p.m. lectures, or 4 p.m. meetings with mentors if their shifts had ended. Traditionally, the residency system had encouraged curiosity and learning. The best residents were those who followed their clinical or scientific passion, taking advantage of any opportunity to go beyond the minimum. Now, like schoolchildren, residents were being told when and where they should be, and efforts to excel were frowned on if a shift rule was violated. Ceilings on performance were being imposed.

As initiative was undermined, house officers derived less joy and meaning from their work. Molly Cooke, David M. Irby, and Bridget C. O'Brien described this as one of the major unintended and deleterious consequences of formal work-hour restrictions. In their study of medical education for the Carnegie Foundation, they found that residents had less curiosity, less interest in studying their patients in detail, and less interest in learning the scientific principles underlying patient care. Many residents now regarded patient care as a burden, and some were heard to say that once they were off duty they should not have to invest personal time in reading or study.[87]

The third problem, the application of a one-size-fits-all model, was less significant but still irksome to program directors. Residency programs represented a heterogeneous group, varying not only in size but in specialty, each of which had its own routines and demands. In general, smaller programs and disciplines encountered more difficulty in adhering to work-hour regulations than larger ones. Programs in radiology, pathology, and laboratory medicine could more easily accommodate to the new rules than programs in most clinical disciplines. Among clinical fields, some, such as emergency medicine, lent themselves more readily to shift scheduling than others. No distinction was made between the needs and abilities of beginners and upper-level trainees. The same rules applied to the surgical intern as to the surgical chief resident, who might be in the eighth to tenth post-graduate year and denied the opportunity to participate in an especially educational case. This type of rigidity caused considerable consternation among many program directors.

By the mid-2010s, the controversy over work-hour restrictions was still raging and the ultimate resolution, unclear. Charges and countercharges abounded. Yet, with over a decade's experience, much had been learned. An important review of the literature on work hours by Ingrid Philibert and colleagues at the ACGME in 2013 found 1,515 published articles of varying quality on the subject.[88] Though the last word on the subject had clearly not yet been spoken, the evidence base had grown considerably from a decade before. In the effort to separate fact from opinion, what had been learned regarding the restriction of work hours?

First, it was clear that the ACGME meant business in its enforcement of the rules. Arguably the greatest problem with earlier rules—both the New York State law and the various RRC regulations—was that they were rarely enforced. Now, the ACGME made clear that it was no longer prepared to tolerate violation of the rules. The Yale surgical residency discovered this in 2001 when it was disaccredited for egregious violation of the surgery RRC work-hour rules, as did the prestigious Johns Hopkins internal medicine residency in 2003 for violation of the new ACGME regulations.[89] Withdrawal of accreditation from a program represented the ACGME's most potent weapon, for then a program could not receive graduate medical education payments from Medicare, roughly $100,000 per resident. A few continued to criticize the ACGME for lax enforcement. For instance, a study in 2006 found that more than 80 percent of interns reported that they had worked hours that were not in compliance with the

ACGME standards.[90] However, the underlying philosophy of the study was that of a zero-tolerance regulatory model, whereas the ACGME followed a substantial compliance, continuous improvement model that carried a range of penalties and that reserved its most severe penalty, the withdrawal of accreditation, for programs that remained in egregious violation of the rules.[91] Most residency program directors appreciated the ACGME's substantial compliance approach; few labored under the illusion that the ACGME still did not take work-hour regulation seriously.

It was also clear that house officers were more rested and alert. Thus, an important objective of the regulations was being met. Only some of the freed-up hours were used for additional sleep—hardly a surprise, given that residents had other things in their lives besides work and sleep. However, on balance, chronic fatigue and burnout were less, and mood and quality of life were improved.[92] Grumblings could still be heard from some corners, where senior physicians echoed the age-old charge that the younger generation was not as tough or devoted as their elders. "They're softies," complained one surgeon at the Massachusetts General Hospital.[93] "They just don't make 'em like they used to," senior faculty at Duke were heard to say.[94] However, the majority of the profession took pride in the more humane treatment that was now being afforded residents.

Work-hour regulations, however, were found to have had no significant effect on patient safety. This was a disturbing finding in that improved patient safety had been the primary justification for their implementation. It was also a surprising finding, given the results of a 2004 study led by Christopher Landrigan, a faculty member at Harvard and a major contributor to work-hour reform. He ran a yearlong study of interns in the intensive care unit at Brigham and Women's Hospital. Interns on the traditional schedule—a 30-hour shift every third night—committed 36 percent more errors than interns on a staggered schedule of shifts, none of which exceeded 16 hours.[95] This study was instrumental in motivating Congress to ask the IOM to study work hours, and it was considered the single strongest argument for limiting doctors' work hours. The study was widely criticized, however, including by interns who were part of the study group: They pointed out that extra interns were added to the intervention group in the ICU, that residents and attending physicians working with the interns on the intervention schedule were hypervigilant in their supervision, that the study counted as "errors" mistakes that were caught by the system without reaching the patient, and that the ability to generalize from the study's findings was highly limited. In addition, they felt that learning had been compromised by the intervention schedule.[96] Subsequently, numerous studies, including a large study of 14,000,000 veterans and Medicare patients published in 2009, found no major improvement in safety after the 2003 reforms.[97] Some studies actually showed an increase in errors and a decrease in safety because of diminished continuity of care.[98] Philibert concluded in her review of duty-hours studies, "It is not possible to make an unqualified statement that patient care has been improved by the implementation of duty-hour limits."[99]

The reasons why the implementation of work-hour reforms had little discernible effect on patient safety were not certain. Perhaps it had to do with the redundancies in the hospital system—the fact that an error by one person was usually picked up by someone else or a computer before harm to a patient occurred. Perhaps it was because the beneficial effects of shift limits on fatigue-induced error were offset by problems caused by increased handoffs, too large a work load, or inadequate supervision. This latter possibility was suggested by one of the era's most highly publicized safety catastrophes—the forced closure of the prestigious liver transplantation program at the Mount Sinai Medical Center (New York) after the death of a donor. The night of the event, one intern was alone with 37 sick patients.[100] On surveys, residents considered the lack of supervision and handoff problems as more serious causes of error than fatigue,[101] and a study of closed malpractice claims found the most important contributing factors to be inadequate supervision and handoff mistakes.[102] In any event, hospitals were complex systems—as the IOM report *To Err Is Human* pointed out—and to some it was not too great a surprise that change of a single variable had little observable effect on overall safety.

Although patient safety seemed unaffected by work-hour reform, there was a negative effect on the educational quality of residency. This occurred because of the increased workload, the work compression, and the reduced clinical and educational continuity of care that resulted from the new system. Philibert found that duty-hour reform was associated with, among other things, reduced empathy in medical interns, lower patient satisfaction, increased risk for mortality and readmission, greater use of diagnostic tests, and reduced educational participation.[103] Residents in the surgical fields were particularly affected. Surgical trainees successfully maintained a sufficient operative volume to develop operative skill. With less perioperative continuity, however, they had less time to develop clinical judgment and patient-management skills, and surgical board scores and pass rates fell.[104] House officers in both the surgical and medical fields finished their residencies less confident about their readiness for independent practice.[105] These were disturbing findings because graduate medical education had always had a dual role in patient safety: the safety of patients cared for by residents today, and the safety of patients cared for in the future by those trained today. In this latter regard, future (or "indirect") safety seemed to be endangered, and by the mid-2010s, some medical educators were beginning to consider the possibility that residency training would have to be prolonged.[106]

Early observations from the European Working Time Directive also pointed toward a negative impact of duty-hour reform on education. In 1998, the Council of Europe in Brussels enacted legislation mandating shorter working weeks for all public workers, including physicians and physicians-in-training. This law took full effect in 2009. In the mid-2010s data were still limited, but available results confirmed the trends observed in the United States. The greatest effect of work-hour restrictions in Europe was observed in the surgical fields. As in the United States, the detrimental effects were less on the acquisition of surgical technique than on the development of surgical judgment and clinical management skills.[107] Expert opinion in Europe was hostile to the reforms. One study found that 80 percent of consultant surgeons and 66 percent of surgical trainees in the United Kingdom felt that patient care and education had suffered under the directive.[108] The president of the Royal College of Surgeons declared, "To say the European Working Time Regulations has failed spectacularly would be a massive understatement."[109]

What about the development of professionalism among residents trained under the new system? Many critics of work-hour reform feared that house officers would become shift workers, with their gaze focused more closely on the clock than on their patients. In this, fears of the demise of professionalism among trainees appeared premature. Data were limited, but several studies showed that residents made explicit decisions about working longer than officially permitted based on their patients' clinical needs. House officers did not stay late for trivial reasons, but they often remained after hours to tend to their patients' important medical problems. The rule that was by far the most frequently violated was the "+6" limitation of work on post-call days. In one survey, 66 percent of residents encountered circumstances in which they considered breaking this rule at least once during the preceding two-week period in order to ensure continuity of care.[110]

In the most important study, the sociologist Charles C. Bosk and colleagues followed medical and surgical residents for three months at two Philadelphia hospitals. The investigators found that the residents did not exhibit a "shift work" mentality in relation to their work. Rather, when patient circumstances demanded, house officers regularly stayed in the hospital to complete the work of caring for their patients, even when, according to the clock, they were required to leave. They did so not because of a desire to work to exhaustion or a lack of confidence in those who would be covering for them. Rather, they did so because of an organizational culture that stressed thoroughness and placing patients first. As one intern put it, describing a fellow intern who regularly stayed late when his patients needed him, "People call him inefficient. It's really because he's doing what we all should be doing.... [He is doing] the kind of things that people wanna believe their doctors would do for them." Of note, residents in Bosk's study who worked late lied when recording their hours because they did not want their program to be penalized for work-hour violations. Clearly, the new system had placed house officers in an untenable position: They had to choose between obeying the rules or caring for their patients and lying about it afterward. In falsifying their records, they did not view themselves as acting unethically. Rather, they were protesting a system that did not let them heal.[111]

Ironically, for all the discussion of safety in graduate medical education circles, the strict limitation of work hours was not foremost on the minds of safety experts in their own conversations about instilling safety into residency training. Rather, safety experts urged medical educators to undertake the task of producing safety-competent physicians who grasped the multiple dimensions of patient safety and who could help develop a culture of safety within their own medical organizations. An important report from the Lucian Leape Institute pointed out that medical education should pay attention to the shaping of "skills, attitudes, and behaviors that will permit them [trainees] to function safely and as architects of safety improvement in the future."[112] This involved learning about systems thinking, problem analysis, the application of human factors science, communication skills, patient-centered care, team concepts and skills, and dealing with feelings of doubt, fear, and uncertainty with respect to medical errors. It required the perfusion of graduate medical education with a culture and ethic of safety. In these regards, residency training—and all of medical education—still had much to do.

It was also ironic that, despite the efforts to reduce errors, the new work-hour system, like the pre-work-hour system, did little to help individuals who had committed an error. Fortunately, most errors were caught before reaching patients, and even more fortunately, most errors that did reach patients caused no permanent harm. However, some errors did result in serious injury or even death. For the physician involved, the commission of an error could be psychologically devastating, with isolation, guilt, and loss of self-esteem as sequelae. This sometimes made it more difficult for the physician to practice good medicine in the future. Despite the ubiquity of error, medical culture continued to provide little support to doctors in that situation. What was needed was a nonjudgmental culture that encouraged physicians to discuss their errors with colleagues without fear of recrimination or shame. In the mid-2010s, such a culture had still not become widespread in medical education or practice.[113]

The ACGME had little choice but to take action limiting work hours, given the compelling arguments for doing so, the profession's failure for many decades to act on its own, and the public's demands that something be done. Some critics faulted the ACGME for the lack of an evidence base justifying the new system or for not insisting that controlled educational trials first be done before changing venerable, time-honored traditions. Such criticism, however, misunderstood the nature of educational reform: New educational systems at all levels and in all countries invariably came about because of the perception that the old system had outlived its usefulness. New systems were created through following best practices at home and abroad, employing tools from educational psychology, and making discerning judgments, but not through controlled, scientific experimentation.

The problems with work-hour restrictions resulted less from the absence of controlled educational studies than from the narrow gaze of the profession and public on work hours alone rather than on the totality of the learning environment. There was little consideration of the number and complexity of cases, supervision, continuity of care, the burden of nonmedical chores, learning objectives, the quality of teaching, or the degree to which programs infused their residents with excitement and inspiration. There was also little discussion of how educational needs might vary from one specialty to another or among house officers in the same specialty of different levels of experience. Ironically, the ACGME was aware that there was more to residency education than work hours, and its Committee on Duty Hours later became the Committee on Innovation and the Learning Environment.[114] These discussions, however, did not reach the level of policy, which focused instead on work hours to the exclusion of other considerations. The results were work compression and a rigid system that made both patient care and learning more difficult. A much-needed comprehensive redesign of graduate medical education had not been produced.

It should hardly have been a surprise that the broader learning environment received little consideration, given the trajectory of graduate medical education for 125 years. The residency system arose in part from the apprenticeship system; accordingly, the service needs of hospitals had always driven the system. Residents prospered enormously from their work, but so did the hospitals that employed them and the faculty that taught them. For this reason, comprehensive educational redesign was more easily talked about than achieved. To reduce work compression and work overload, someone would have to pay for additional workers to do many of the tasks that house officers had traditionally done, and other caregivers—perhaps faculty—would have to see some of the patients residents had been seeing. Without the additional funds and personnel, the economic exploitation of house officers continued.

However, even with ample resources, there is little evidence that the ethical tensions between medical education and patient safety will go away. Ultimately, an elusive balance must be achieved. House officers need to work long hours to learn and to provide continuity of care. Yet, overly long duty hours and onerous on-call schedules can interfere with education and safe patient care. Sound bites—"do you want to be treated by a tired doctor?" "what's better: a tired doctor who knows you or a fresh doctor who doesn't?"—do not help. Such platitudes are devoid of context and ignore the many competing factors that need to be taken into account. Wisdom, judgment, and flexibility are needed as well as the humility to recognize that what is perceived as an appropriate balance in one era is likely to change as scientific and cultural circumstances change. In short, these are perpetual dilemmas intrinsic to medical education and practice. They will always be present, as long as house officers learn by caring for patients.

CHAPTER 13

Preserving Excellence in Residency Training and Medical Care

By the 2010s, the residency system would have been scarcely recognizable to the small "happy band" of faculty and residents at the Johns Hopkins Hospital who had started the enterprise in 1889. The residency system had grown to enormous proportions, with 8,875 specialty and subspecialty training programs educating 109,840 residents and clinical fellows in 2010.[1] Originally intended as scientific training for aspiring clinical investigators, the residency system had evolved into professional education for practicing medical specialists. In 2010, the American Board of Medical Specialties recognized 24 specialties and 121 subspecialties.[2] Over the course of a century, the length of training had become much longer, but the experience of being a resident had become kinder and gentler, as work hours had been restricted, the element of humiliation in the teaching process had diminished, and programs paid more attention to residents' personal well-being. The entry of large numbers of women and Asian-Americans and smaller numbers of underrepresented minorities into medicine had led to a more diverse workforce, although there was still much to be done in that regard.

From the beginning older doctors often became nostalgic when reminiscing about their residency. The fact is, however, that the residency system had never experienced a "golden era." Each generation coped with the medical and cultural challenges of its own age. In addition, medical educators could never avoid the perpetual tensions of graduate medical education (GME): establishing a proper balance between supervision and autonomy, between patient safety and education, and between the needs of physicians for rest and the equally compelling needs of patients for continuity of care. Most important, there was never a time when residency training was not physically and emotionally exhausting. The tension between the educational needs of residents and the tendency of hospitals to use their house officers as a source of inexpensive labor had all along shaped the experiences and conditions of graduate medical education.

Although these fault lines had always been present in residency training, recent changes in the American health care system placed them under greater stress. The traditional tension between autonomy and supervision had been intensified by the growing potency and complexity of medical and surgical care and the increasingly hectic pace. The tension between the need for rest and the provision of continuity of care had been placed into sharp relief by the patients' rights movement, the quest for greater patient autonomy, the appearance of consumerism in medicine, and the Institute of Medicine (IOM) report on medical errors. Most important, the economic exploitation of house officers and the subordination of education to institutional service had been aggravated by the new imperative in American health care to maximize patient throughput. The patient loads of house officers became so large that careful, reflective care was often not possible. This problem was further accentuated by the work compression that came with the restriction of resident work hours. The regulations left house officers with the same number of patients but even less time with which to see them.

In the 2010s, the residency system faced numerous challenges—some new, others old. However, the most important challenge was the traditional one: creating a stimulating learning environment that brought the best out in house officers and fostered the delivery of patient care of the highest quality. The need, as always, was for residents to receive their training in settings that maximized learning, promoted rigorous thinking, fostered curiosity, instilled the highest values and standards, and allowed house officers to once again have the thrill of feeling engaged in "good work." Recent changes in health care delivery merely pointed to the fragility of the learning environment and underscored the imperative for its strengthening.

For medical educators and concerned citizens, there were many opportunities to improve and preserve the learning environment, and these are discussed in the pages that follow. However, for residency training to be at its finest, it was necessary to improve medical care in America. The best learning could occur only in settings where the best patient care was provided. What was needed, both for learners and patients, was a patient-centered system of health care that provided "slow medicine" to those who required it and emphasized the quality, not the quantity, of care. Doctors trained in such a system had a greater potential to deliver high-quality, cost-effective care to their future patients. This integral relationship between residency training and the delivery of medical care—and the multifaceted way by which they influenced each other—was at the core of health care renewal in the United States. Ultimately, the fate of graduate medical education depended on that of the health care delivery system. But there was also much that graduate medical education could do to make medical care in America better and more affordable.

CHALLENGES, NEW AND OLD

Since graduate medical education, as all of medical education, has continuously evolved, it was no surprise to observe powerful forces for change operating in the 2010s. The most conspicuous development was the continued movement from a "process-based" system toward an "outcomes-based" system. The traditional "process-based" model was time-based. That is, residents were steeped in an educational program for a historically determined period of time in order to become competent specialists. This model, which Brian Hodges called the "tea-steeping" model,[3] focused attention on the processes of education, such as the number of faculty and curriculum design. The new, competing "outcomes-based" model emphasized the functional capabilities of the end product, regardless of the time spent in training. Hodges called this the "i-Doc" model, a name suggested by the Apple iPod. This model implied that residency programs, by focusing on specific learning objectives, can produce highly desirable products adapted to user needs and desires.[4]

Explicit movement to an "outcomes-based" model began in 1999, when the Accreditation Council for Graduate Medical Education (ACGME) introduced the Outcomes Project, which occurred in the larger context of the move to competency-based education in other segments of medical education and education. As noted in the last chapter, this project required training programs to assess trainee accomplishment of learning objectives across six general domains of competence: patient care, medical knowledge, systems-based practice, practice-based learning and improvement, professionalism, and interpersonal and communication skills. To facilitate the evaluation of "outcomes," the ACGME in 2009 launched the Milestones Project, in which it charged each specialty with the responsibility of identifying specialty-specific "milestones" of competency development.

Milestones were defined as "observable developmental steps that describe progression from a beginning learner to the expected level of proficiency at the completion of training."[5] In July 2013 the ACGME began phasing in its "Next Accreditation System" (NAS), which required programs to demonstrate the educational outcomes for their trainees by documenting the progression of their residents through the various milestones.[6]

The outcomes approach carried many theoretical advantages. It was consistent with the Dreyfus model of the progression of learners through various stages from novice to master.[7] It required progression through a training program to be based on achieving educational milestones rather than on time served, thereby creating the possibility that some trainees could finish residency and fellowship programs more quickly.[8] The outcomes movement was aligned with cultural trends demanding increasing accountability from graduate medical education, for the intention was to evaluate residents on the basis of what they could actually do rather than on knowledge alone. The ACGME even promised that the NAS would reduce the heavy burden of documentation and paperwork for program directors, which over the preceding 20 years had led to significant unhappiness, burnout, and turnover.[9] The chief worry about the outcomes movement was that it was too reductionist. That is, some thought that by breaking medical training into small, discrete, measurable tasks, the graduate medical education community might have overemphasized the question of assessment and overlooked the formation of professional identity. Stated another way, the competencies focused on doing the work of a physician, not on the broader, integrative, holistic goal of *being* a physician.[10]

A second issue beset graduate medical education in the 2010s: the danger that there would be an insufficient number of residency positions to accommodate all US medical school graduates. As noted before, the Balanced Budget Act of 1997 capped the number of residency positions eligible for federal support at 1997 levels—around 100,000. Subsequently, the number of residency positions grew very slowly—primarily in the clinical subspecialties, supported by hospital revenues. Such an approach made sense in the 1990s, when common wisdom held that the nation already had a physician surplus. Several highly publicized studies in the 1980s and 1990s had advanced that notion, and, during testimony over the Balanced Budget Act, six prominent medical organizations, including the Association of American Medical Colleges and the American Medical Association, endorsed the limitation on residency slots.[11] In 2001, the chair of the Council on Graduate Medical Education (COGME), a public body that makes recommendations on workforce issues to the federal government, declared that the number of physicians being trained in the country was "about right."[12]

Workforce projections of the 1990s assumed the country's health system would fall under the control of group or staff model managed care plans, such as Kaiser Permanente. Such plans used far fewer physicians to care for their enrolled populations than did fee-for-service plans. Beginning in 2004, as managed care retreated, and as the country continued to grow, age, and economically prosper, the same authorities that in the 1990s declared a physician surplus now claimed there was an impending physician shortage. The work of Richard Cooper, the former dean of the Medical College of Wisconsin, was particularly important in precipitating a reexamination of the question. The nation's medical education community responded. In 2002, there were 125 US medical schools. By 2013, there were 141 schools, and others were in the planning stage. Many existing schools increased their class size. It was estimated that by the 2016–17 academic year, there will have been a 30 percent increase in medical school enrollments from 15 years before. However, the number of residency positions had scarcely budged, creating the specter that some US-trained medical and osteopathic students would be unable to obtain positions. The large cohort of international medical school graduates seeking US residency positions found itself in even greater jeopardy.[13]

Many medical educators worried, believing that the residency system had the responsibility to provide positions for US medical and osteopathic graduates. In the mid-2010s it was not clear how this would be done. The Association of American Medical Colleges and allies had tried to persuade Congress to increase its GME funding as part of the Affordable Care Act. This effort was unsuccessful, and although further efforts will undoubtedly be made, the problems of the burgeoning budget deficit made it unlikely that Congress would respond favorably, at least in the near future.[14] Some called for the states to fund more residency positions, given the growing workforce needs of many states. It had long been known that the primary determinant in where physicians decided to locate was where they did their residency and clinical fellowship, not where they went to medical school.[15] Others argued that hospitals should fund more positions from clinical revenues or that residents should accept lower stipends and benefits. Yet not all medical educators and commentators were sympathetic. Some pointed out that law school graduates were not guaranteed a position practicing law; a few suggested that residents and clinical fellows pay tuition, particularly in the high-earning specialties and subspecialties. As this book was completed, the issue had not been resolved.

In the 2010s a third development was transforming graduate medical education: information technology. Hospitals had used computers since the 1950s, largely at first for accounting purposes. In the 1970s many hospitals began providing computer printouts of laboratory results. In the 1990s, computerized ordering and electronic medical records came into use. At the same time, the development of the Internet made the search for medical information much easier than before, and web-based learning tools came into use.[16] By the 2000s, telemedicine was spreading, and the appearance of handheld personal digital assistants (PDAs) and smartphones freed house officers and physicians from being bound to a computer terminal to obtain information. House officers and physicians, particularly the younger ones, also partook actively in the use of social media. One article referred to house officers of the 2010s as "cyborgs."[17]

The potential of information technology to transform medical education and practice was unquestioned. The 2010s witnessed vigorous debate over both its potential benefits and inadvertent consequences. From an educational perspective, however, a different question arose: Had growing up in the digital age made medical students and house officers of the 2010s different from those of earlier generations? Certainly, childhood in America had changed. From 2001 to 2011, the average amount of time that US children spent online each day tripled.[18] A study in 2010 found that students 8 to 18 years of age spent more than 7.5 hours a day engaged with computers, cell phones, television, music, or video games.[19] For medical educators, the pertinent question was how the digital age affected the minds and hearts of learners.

Here, there was clearly a need for heightened awareness and understanding. A number of studies had suggested that regular use of the Internet contributed to a shortened attention span and difficulty concentrating or reading long texts. The Internet allowed for boundless information to be quickly obtained, but it did not promote the deep, thoughtful reflection needed for understanding and intellectual growth. Some authorities maintained that in young people who were constantly online, neurons developed differently, resulting in a fragmenting effect on the cohesiveness of mental processes.[20] In addition, there was evidence that since 2000 empathy had declined among college students. The major reason for this was thought to be that as young people spent more time with social media, they spent less time in direct face-to-face interactions with real people. Accordingly, their ability to read social cues, understand people, and develop appropriate social skills diminished.[21] In the 2010s, the effects of growing up in a digital environment were still only dimly perceived. However, the consequences for medical education were potentially profound, given the importance of producing doctors who can reflect and empathize.

Although new issues continued to confront residency training, the greatest challenge in the 2010s remained the traditional one: creating and maintaining a rich learning environment that allowed the intellectual, technical, emotional, and moral growth of house officers to be maximized. A number of opportunities were available to do so. The first, and one that was completely within the control of the educational community, was for the ACGME to revise its current (2011) duty-hour regulations. As seen throughout this book, there had long been a moral imperative to address the onerous work schedule of house officers, and the ACGME finally did so. However, as discussed in the last chapter, the rigidity of the rules requiring house officers to end shifts at precise, predetermined times created serious inadvertent consequences. The simple step of eliminating the "+4" required departure on days after call could do much to improve education, provide better continuity of care, and restore meaning to house officers' work. Such a step could easily be taken without jeopardizing the more important goals of an 80-hour work-week limit or the requirement of at least 10 hours off between shifts. Not surprisingly, leading thinkers in graduate medical education such as Vineet Arora and Kevin Volpp were calling for the ACGME to do so,[22] and the great majority of faculty and house officers were hoping for such a change.

House staff hours represented a thorny issue because competing goods needed to be kept in balance: continuity of care versus the need for rest and recuperation. This, as discussed before, represented one of the perpetual dilemmas of graduate medical education. The key for the residency system to flourish was to permit flexibility in its work rules because responsibilities for continuous patient care could not be automatically discharged at specific predictable times. As David Hellmann pointed out, few would argue that parenting should involve staying up with a child night and day, yet good parenting occasionally required a mother or father to be up at night with a sick child.[23] The same kind of commonsense reasoning needed to be applied to graduate medical education. House officers themselves protested the inflexibility of the system. One surgical resident explained, "You might expect that, as residents, we'd stand up and rejoice that these regulations have been passed. But I'll tell you, if you're the chief resident on the GI service and a case comes along that you may have one or two opportunities during your entire residency to do... well, many of us have to be dragged kicking and screaming out of the hospital."[24] What was needed was a system that inspired house officers to do their best rather than one that congratulated them for leaving and scolded them for staying late to tend to their patients' needs.

Despite the enormous controversy, work hours represented only one part of the learning environment. In an era of high patient throughput and work compression, medical educators had a second major opportunity to improve the learning environment: by ensuring that house officers not be assigned more patients than they could reasonably manage. Such an approach required wisdom and flexibility, for a "reasonable" patient load was subject to many factors, including the severity of illness and complexity of care, the maturity and capability of individual house officers, and the availability of support services. Nevertheless, it was clear in the 2010s that house officers were regularly assigned more patients than they could safely care for. Correction of this problem—for instance, by assigning some patients to nonteaching services, hospitalists, nurse practitioners, physician assistants, or faculty—was vital to allowing house officers more time for reflection and learning as well as for being careful and attentive to detail in patient management. Such a step was also essential for allowing house officers to become more engaged with their work. Environments with high patient volumes and low resident-to-patient ratios fostered attitudes among house officers that their job was to "get rid of patients." Better staffing ratios provided more time for house officers to experience the joy of the one-on-one caring that ideally was at the heart of medical care.[25] It was curious that the nursing profession had already recognized that care was unsafe when individual nurses were assigned too many patients at one time, and some states had even enacted legislation regulating the ratio of nurses to patients.[26] The medical profession had yet to acknowledge the problem of overload.

A third opportunity was to take steps to lessen the traditional economic exploitation of house officers for institutional service. Reducing the large patient loads for house officers would represent one such step. Another would be by providing larger numbers of ward clerks, secretaries, transporters, and other important assistants to help with many of the nonphysician duties of patient care. So enabled, house officers could spend more time on learning and on delivering good care, and the primacy of education over institutional service could at last be established.

A fourth opportunity was to improve the process of supervision. Better supervision was an important element to improving safety. It was also an important, underutilized educational tool. David Sklar, the editor of *Academic Medicine*, demonstrated how real-time faculty supervision could improve the diagnostic and therapeutic acumen of house officers while allowing the independence and self-esteem of residents to be preserved.[27] For residents, the opportunity to observe experienced, caring physicians modeling professional behavior at the bedside was also invaluable for internalizing many of the humanistic aspects of medical care.

Surprisingly little was known about effective supervision. Current supervisory practices had little empirical or theoretical basis, and the educational literature did not even contain a standard definition of "supervision."[28] It was clear that there were different levels of supervision, ranging from direct involvement with care to retrospective review of a resident's actions.[29] It was also clear that there were significant differences among physicians as to what constituted appropriate supervision. For instance, studies of anesthesiology faculty members found notable differences among them on when they allowed residents autonomy and on how much to allow.[30] There was also considerable disciplinary variation in the perceived effectiveness of supervision. In one study, 45 percent of residents in ophthalmology, 46 percent in neurology, and 44 percent in neurosurgery stated that they had experienced inadequate supervision at least once a week throughout the year, compared with 1.5 percent of residents in pathology and 3 percent in dermatology.[31] Without question, a research agenda stood before medical educators.

However, the need for research did not preclude deliberation and action. Too much was at stake, both for resident education and patient safety. Part of the solution involved providing faculty the time to become more involved with the work of their house officers—actually supervising residents instead of tending to their own direct patient care and providing supervision only as time allowed.[32] Another part of the solution required bringing about a cultural change in residency—creating a climate in which house officers felt they were truly free to call for help without being perceived as "weak."[33] As always, supervision needed to be undertaken carefully and judiciously. Supervision had to be balanced with the competing goal of allowing house officers progressive responsibility, lest residents emerge from training ill prepared to practice independently.

A fifth opportunity was for medical schools to restore teaching to a central place in the institutional value system. This required a second cultural change at medical schools: the willingness to take good teaching more fully into account when awarding faculty promotions, tenure, and salary increases.[34] Encouraging good teaching could certainly aid the efforts to improve supervision. It could also help restore house officers to a central place in the faculty's gaze. Residents in every specialty had always been the happiest when they felt they were important to their teachers, up to and including the department chair. A stronger faculty presence, particularly from the senior faculty, offered the opportunity to stimulate relationships, provide real mentoring, restore a sense of community to the residency experience, and invigorate specialty training on a personal, not just an intellectual, level.[35]

What might good teachers accomplish with house officers? Intellectually, they could emphasize cognitive processes—biological principles, critical analysis, problem solving, managing uncertainty, and the important distinctions between information and knowledge and knowledge and wisdom. Outstanding teachers could also discuss what was unknown as well as what was known, how unanswered questions might be solved, and how tomorrow's medicine might differ from that of today's. Doctors needed to be able to accommodate to the changes in diseases, medical knowledge, diagnostics, and therapeutics that would inevitably occur over the course of their professional lifetimes; these represented the skills necessary to do so. Such an approach required skills beyond knowing the latest antibiotic dosage by heart or how to shorten their patients' length of hospital stay by a few hours.[36] Ideally, some faculty would help residents acquire skills in important new areas such as clinical epidemiology and biomedical ethics, develop an understanding of health care disparities and the socioeconomic determinants of health and disease, acquire "cultural competence" (the ability to understand individuals from different ethnic, racial, religious, and socioeconomic backgrounds), and learn interdisciplinary team-based approaches to medical and surgical practice.

Outstanding teachers were also needed for transmitting the spirit and values, not just the content, of medicine. They could help residents understand the primacy of the patient, the value of caring, the management of complexity, the personal and ethical dimensions of care, the importance of life-long learning, and how to deal effectively with the human condition and quasi-religious aspects of medical care. They could instill many residents with the desire to leave medicine better than when they started through research, teaching, or working to develop safer and more effective systems of care in their future offices, hospitals, or health care systems. Arguably the most important idea an instructor provided a learner was a conception of how to be a physician. For this, training programs needed to develop and recruit outstanding individuals to the teaching faculty and reward those individuals for the time and work necessary to do that job well.

A sixth opportunity was to promote more vigorously an agenda of safety and quality in patient care. Certainly the steps enumerated above—more effective teaching, better supervision, greater flexibility in work hours, and manageable workloads—would aid that agenda. So would greater attention in the residency curriculum to learning the principles of systems-based practice improvement. In this regard, the ACGME took a major step in 2012 with the implementation of its Clinical Learning Environment Review (CLER) project. Here, the ACGME began working with hospitals sponsoring residency programs to involve residents in the recognition and reporting of errors and in the creation and implementation of specific strategies for improving safety and quality. "Graduate medical education must include training and active participation in quality and safety initiatives by every resident physician," CLER leaders declared.[37]

However, safety and quality also depended on graduate medical education performing its traditional task well: producing doctors who could think, solve problems, decipher unknowns, manage complexity, and care about their patients. What was often overlooked in discussions of safety and quality was that effective clinical systems still required highly competent clinicians.[38] Producing such doctors was the responsibility of residency training.

As one manifestation of the importance of individuals in patient safety, correct treatment depended on having the correct diagnosis. Yet, ironically, quality criteria in the 2010s did not include diagnostic accuracy. A physician achieved high quality scores in the treatment of "congestive heart failure," for example, if that was the diagnosis in the chart and the appropriate treatments for that condition were given—even if the diagnosis was incorrect, the cause of the patient's fluid retention was something other than congestive heart failure, and the treatment was in fact wrong for the patient's problem. In the early 2000s diagnostic errors were surprisingly common. Studies revealed a 20 to 25 percent incidence of incorrect diagnoses, despite the widespread use of imaging studies and other sophisticated laboratory technologies.[39] It was estimated that 74 percent of all diagnostic errors had a cognitive basis.[40] That was why the safety experts Mark L. Graber, Robert M. Wachter, and Christine K. Cassel wrote, "Diagnostic errors seem intensely personal: the 'system' appears to be the physician."[41]

Stated another way, despite the substantial and appropriate attention in the 2010s to creating better clinical systems, individuals still mattered. The pioneering safety expert Lucian L. Leape acknowledged this point. He told the American Board of Medical Specialties that "'systems' theory is truly a transforming concept that is already changing the way hospitals deal with accidental injury." He also pointed out, however, that "some errors *are* the result of misconduct or incompetence. In these cases it is the individual, not the systems that needs to be dealt with."[42] The issue facing medical educators was not to argue the relative importance of individuals and systems in improving safety and quality. Both were important. Rather, their task was to recognize that in an era of systems thinking, skilled clinicians were still indispensable for the safest and best practice of medicine. Hence, the traditional task of residency training, producing outstanding doctors, remained essential—and always would.

A seventh opportunity was to expand the teaching of residents to sites outside the inpatient wards of teaching hospitals. A fundamental tenet of graduate medical education had always been to locate specialty teaching in sites where patient care was delivered. This was essential if residents were to learn by doing and receive graded responsibility. For generations the teaching hospital had provided a marvelous educational laboratory. However, in the latter twentieth century, more and more clinical practice moved to nonhospital settings. By 2013, inpatient days per capita were only one-half of what they had been a generation previously.[43] Medical educators had the opportunity to adjust to this tectonic shift by taking greater advantage of ambulatory and community settings, private doctors' offices, same-day surgery facilities, and other nontraditional teaching sites. Such locations provided excellent opportunities to make initial diagnoses, manage chronic illnesses, perform a variety of technical and surgical procedures that had moved to outpatient settings, and learn about many of the emotional, sociological, economic, and ethical dimensions of medical care. Great care had to be exercised in doing so to make certain that high educational standards were maintained. If done properly, however, this single step could go far toward helping produce the types of doctors the country was thought to need in the twenty-first century.

Who would lead these changes? Many have said that the residency system needed a twenty-first-century Abraham Flexner, who would focus attention this time on graduate medical education rather than on medical schools. These sentiments, however, reflected a misunderstanding of the history of US medical education. Both the university medical school and the residency system were created by the pioneering faculty of the Johns Hopkins School of Medicine. Flexner popularized the Hopkins medical school model to the public at large, and he was spectacularly successful in doing so. However, the ideas were not his—a fact he openly acknowledged.[44] It is more accurate to say that graduate medical education needed another Johns Hopkins, not another Abraham Flexner.

In subsequent generations, the university contributed far less to graduate medical education—or any part of medical education—than at the beginning. Private medical insurance, the National Institutes of Health, Medicare and Medicaid, the managed care movement, and now, most likely, the Affordable Care Act all drive residency training much more than educational ideas generated by academic leaders. The same is true of cultural forces such as the civil rights movement, feminism, consumerism, changing attitudes toward poverty, and new attitudes about balancing work and personal life. Since the residency system was created, the university serves more as the guarantor of the status quo than as the fountainhead of new educational ideas. Accordingly, residency training, as the rest of medical education, became relatively fossilized—much grander in size and scope, but far less innovative, both in terms of protecting the integrity of the learning environment and in developing new educational models to address the emerging health care needs of the twenty-first century.

However, it was difficult to imagine who would lead the redesign of residency training if not university-based medical educators. Perhaps a single institution—most likely, though not necessarily, a high-prestige institution—would forge an enriching learning environment for residency training that could become the model for the twenty-first century, much as Johns Hopkins did for the twentieth. Leaders are needed from within the profession—individuals with vision, values, courage, conviction, optimism, and determination. Such individuals should recognize that good medical practice is a noble pursuit, and they would approach the task of educational change with gratitude for the privilege of being a physician, not with a preoccupation for income and power.

In this transformation, the ACGME possessed the opportunity to play an important and constructive role. As an accrediting agency, it could apply leverage to the system: Nonaccredited programs were ineligible to receive GME funding from Medicare. The ACGME had the authority to provide flexibility in the work-hour regulations it imposed. It also had the power to hold programs accountable to more exacting standards in regard to patient loads, unreasonable amounts of "scut work," supervision, and the provision of intellectually invigorating teaching. ACGME standards, in fact, had long contained explicit and expansive language on these points. As was the case with work hours prior to its 2003 regulations, however, these requirements had rarely been enforced. Many medical educators and house officers believed that the ACGME could contribute enormously to graduate medical education by turning its attention from the strict enforcement of rigid work hours to the more vigorous upholding of standards pertaining to these broader educational matters.

Much of what the ACGME would do depended on its new chief executive officer, Thomas J. Nasca, who succeeded David Leach in 2007. A noted internist and nephrologist, Nasca had served as dean of the Jefferson Medical College prior to joining the ACGME. Nasca, like Leach, had a deeply philosophical temperament. He wrote and spoke widely on the subject of professionalism, influenced in his view by the pioneering medical ethicist Edmund Pellegrino.[45] Nasca had a deep sense of humility and a strong desire to serve others. He attributed much of this to an encounter he had as an intern at the Mercy Hospital of Pittsburgh with the hospital president, Sister Ferdinand Clarke. On his way to see a sick patient at 4 a.m., Nasca passed Sister Clarke on her knees scrubbing floors by hand. He asked if he could help, whereupon she responded peacefully, "You take care of the patients and I'll take care of this." Through that exchange, her humility and sense of service were imprinted on him.[46] Nasca also had a sophisticated understanding of educational issues, a recognition of the complexity of balancing competing goods, and an understanding of the challenges to a self-regulating profession of being responsive to the society that supports it while still upholding and defending important professional principles. In the early 2010s, the newly independent ACGME's role was still unfolding, but there was reason to believe it would promote the betterment of graduate medical education.

Ultimately, for graduate medical education to implement the needed changes, it required a steady and sufficient supply of funds. Improvements large and small—the reduction of "scut work," better use of technology, improved call-room comfort, more time for attending physicians to spend with house officers, additional personnel to care for some of the patients previously managed by residents, the extension of residency training to ambulatory settings—all required additional financial resources. The opportunity costs of medical education were also enormous. Time that faculty members spent teaching detracted from the time they had available to generate clinical revenue. This was not an expense for third-party payers, but it represented considerable lost income for teaching hospitals and medical schools.[47] These and other costs of good graduate medical education explained why residency training had from the beginning been so resistant to fundamental change: Any successful effort to improve its quality depended on money, faculty time, or both, and these typically were in short supply.

Where would the money come from? For many years, academic leaders had advocated creating an "all-payer" system for financing graduate medical education. In such a system, all third-party payers, private and federal alike, would contribute proportionately to the funding of resident education on the grounds that everyone benefited from having well-trained doctors.[48] In the mid-2010s, however, the idea of creating an all-payer system had not developed traction. The insurance industry fiercely opposed it, and with federal budgets soaring, neither Democrats nor Republicans had made it a political priority. Indeed, the whole subject of GME financing had become controversial and confusing, largely because it had become entangled with the debate over how active a role the federal government should play in shaping the physician workforce.[49]

In the mid-2010s, the prospects for the future funding of graduate medical education were uncertain. In 2013 an IOM committee was preparing a report on the issue. Many academic leaders feared that the committee would actually recommend a decrease in federal GME payments. The likelihood of Medicare GME funding disappearing was remote, but the possibility of a reduction was real. Such an action would place more of the financial burden on hospitals and trainees. If that occurred, educational debt would undoubtedly continue to rise, the rush to the high-paying specialties and subspecialties would likely continue, and the medical profession would probably become even less accessible to young men and women from nonaffluent families. The Affordable Care Act contained a provision to provide $230 million in new funding for residency programs in primary care sponsored by community health centers. However, this funding was scheduled to run out in 2015, and further support depended on the uncertain process of obtaining additional congressional appropriations.[50]

Despite the angst and confusion, the medical profession had much more control over the ultimate outcome than it might have appeared. The argument for public funding had always been that graduate medical education was a public good. To the degree that the medical profession in the years ahead behaved as a guild, zealously protecting its own economic interests, the prospect of receiving generous outside help with GME financing was lessened. To the degree that doctors collectively behaved as a profession, subordinating their direct economic interests to the needs of patients and the public, the outlook for robust and secure GME funding was greatly improved. Physicians had more influence in the process than many imagined.

ALIGNING EDUCATION AND PATIENT CARE

Fortunately—for medical education and the nation at large—models could be found in the 2010s of residency programs successfully coping with many of the pressures working against good graduate medical education. A notable example was the experiment in internal medicine training conducted by faculty of the Brigham and Women's Hospital at the Faulkner Hospital in Boston (now called the Brigham and Women's Faulkner Hospital), a community teaching hospital closely affiliated with the Brigham that was staffed by Brigham internal medicine house officers. At Faulkner, as elsewhere, house officers in internal medicine struggled with the problems of high inpatient volume, rapid throughput of patients, and diminished availability of senior attending physicians. To combat these challenges, the Brigham faculty—led by Graham T. McMahon, an endocrinologist and medical educator; Joel Katz, the internal medicine residency program director; and Joseph Loscalzo, the chair of internal medicine at Women and Brigham's Hospital—created an experimental model at Faulkner called the

Integrated Teaching Unit (ITU). Compared with control teams, ITU teams were designed to be educationally driven, not service driven. A house officer on an ITU team received fewer patients and had a reduced workload. The average census per intern on the ITU teams was 3.5 patients, compared with 6.6 patients on the control teams. In addition, each ITU team worked with two designated attending physicians, carefully chosen for teaching skill, compared with control teams, which worked with multiple supervising attending physicians. The patient mixes managed by ITU and control teams appeared comparable.

By every measure the experiment proved a success. House officers on ITU teams spent twice as much time in direct learning and four times as much time in teaching activities as control-team trainees, and they felt they learned more. They also spent more time at the bedside with patients, enjoyed more time for reflection, and were more likely than control-team house officers to agree that the rotation was closer to their ideal of what a residency experience should be. McMahon and colleagues were particularly impressed with the much higher degree of satisfaction demonstrated by ITU house officers, who were more engaged with their work and derived more fulfillment from their training than did the control-team house officers. Faculty on the ITU teams also found that the experience provided them with a much more satisfying teaching experience than they derived from a conventional inpatient service. The experiment thus illustrated the importance of time for reflection and the active participation of superior faculty to the learning environment. The Faulkner experience reminded medical educators that what mattered most in residency training was not merely the hours of work but what residents did during those hours. As McMahon put it, "Relationships [of residents] matter," both with their patients and their teachers.[51]

A more ambitious project was undertaken at the Johns Hopkins Bayview Medical Center (the former Baltimore City Hospital), a major affiliate of the Johns Hopkins School of Medicine. Institutional leaders David B. Hellmann and Roy C. Ziegelstein listened to the concerns of Bayview house officers, who repeatedly pointed out that intense time pressures and high patient workloads did not adequately allow them to learn or heal. Accordingly, in 2007 Hellmann and Ziegelstein created a new program for internal medical house officers at Bayview, the Aliki Initiative, that aimed to develop "caring doctors who have a genuine and deep appreciation of the importance of knowing each patient's unique personal circumstances and who make patient care recommendations that apply the best evidence to the individual patient." The explicit goal of the program's founders was to enable physicians-in-training not only to master the mechanics of delivering medical care but to learn the art of healing.[52]

To accomplish this, Hellmann and Ziegelstein reduced the number of patients assigned to each resident on the Aliki team by one-half. Traditional internal medicine teams at Bayview admitted ten patients every fourth night on "long call" and four patients during an intervening "short call." The Aliki team admitted five patients on long call and two on short call. In addition, the Aliki house officers visited their patients after discharge at home or in institutional facilities, thereby receiving the opportunity to spend more time with patients both during and after hospitalization. With the reduced census, the Aliki team members had more time to read, reflect, participate in teaching sessions, make home visits, and engage in mentored experiences designed to improve their skills at history taking, counseling, and developing individualized treatment plans. The thrust of the Aliki experience was to help house officers develop an understanding of each patient as a unique person within his or her own home and community.

The Aliki rotation, which was required of all Bayview internal medicine house officers, quickly became the program's most popular feature. Initially house officers worried that fewer patients would mean less learning. They quickly discovered that the Aliki service provided sufficient clinical experience and that the additional time for reading, reflection, bedside teaching, conferences, home visits, and clinical discussions resulted in more learning than would be received on the standard rotations. Equally important, house officers on the Aliki service felt more fulfilled in their work. One intern remarked, "It's given me time to be the kind of doctor I've always wanted to be and do the things I should be doing for all my patients."[53] A senior resident at the end of her residency even said that "the Aliki rotation made her love medicine again and reminded her of why she once dreamed of becoming a physician."[54]

The key to the Aliki Initiative's success was the reduced patient load. This provided house officers, in the words of the program's leaders, with "the gift of time."[55] With this time, house officers were more attentive to detail, more reflective, and more engaged with their patients and teachers. They also had more time and energy for reading and teaching students. One Aliki house officer described how he detected one problem after another with his patients because of the opportunity to do a more thorough job while on that rotation. "Had I been managing twice the number of patients that month, none of this would have been possible."[56] This house officer also described how the gift of time helped him and his fellow residents find meaning in their work:

> When I think about how I train in a hospital with limited resources and a patient load that I can barely handle, I realize how lucky I am that the Aliki service even exists. I am thankful that my residency program has made it a priority for

> residents to experience the gratification of really doing the best job that we can for our patients and not just repeating the usual mistakes produced by a volume-driven system. I understand now why the Aliki rotation resurrected that senior resident's love for medicine. The Aliki service provided . . . us with a rare oasis in our training where we could practice the best medicine that we possibly could, rekindle the passion that brought us to our careers in the first place, and discover new passions.[57]

Neither the Faulkner nor the Aliki experiments developed new strategies for teaching residents. Rather, their contribution was in reaffirming the soundness of fundamental principles of medical education: the importance of time for reflection, a manageable patient census, and inspiring relationships with good teachers. Their applicability was especially strong to the medical fields, which did not have to ensure that trainees performed a sufficient number of procedures as the surgical disciplines did.

The Faulkner and Aliki experiments also illustrated a fundamental truth of graduate medical education: Good residency training is expensive. In the case of Faulkner Hospital, additional expenses were incurred to pay for the time of the extra faculty members on the ITU teams. This funding was provided by the hospital and the Department of Medicine of Brigham and Women's Hospital. In the Aliki Initiative, funding was needed to pay for hospitalists to care for the patients who otherwise would have been admitted to the Aliki team. This was provided by the philanthropist Aliki Perroti, for whom the program was named. To Johns Hopkins faculty, the interest and support of Mrs. Perroti raised new possibilities of what private philanthropy might contribute to graduate medical education in the twenty-first century.[58]

The problem in residency training in the 2010s was that the conditions at the Women and Brigham's Faulkner Hospital and the Johns Hopkins Bayview Medical Center were not commonly present. House officers learned and practiced medicine in the real world, where medical and surgical practice were so volume-driven and time-deprived that patient care, not just learning, sometimes suffered. Of course, as discussed earlier, many conditions could be treated quickly and effectively. Certainly, medical and surgical emergencies could not wait. The dilemma in medical practice, however, was that many patients required "slow medicine," and the American health care system was poorly organized to provide this type of care.

The need for "slow medicine" was apparent throughout the health care system. With many hospitalized patients, it was illustrated by unacceptably high rates of readmission for the same condition or a complication thereof soon after discharge.[59] For many outpatients, the lack of time with their physician was equally problematic. This was especially true in the primary care fields, where good medical practice required doctors to listen carefully, ask probing questions, pay attention to detail, address patient concerns, provide education and counseling, and elicit patient preferences on a variety of diagnostic and therapeutic matters. Doctors committed to good preventive care faced similar difficulties. The time required to thoroughly address preventive issues vastly exceeded the time of typical office visits.[60] In psychiatry, it became easier simply to provide patients with drugs than to engage in counseling and psychotherapy, even with patients who most readily stood to benefit from such treatment.[61] With many patients, especially elderly individuals, it was much quicker just to prescribe another drug than to explore what might be causing a patient's symptoms. (Of course, the more medications, the greater the chance of an adverse drug reaction or interaction, especially in older persons.) Neurologists, geriatricians, and pediatricians often encountered similar challenges, as did doctors in any field when caring for a patient of unusual complexity or difficulty.

In the early twenty-first century, there were widespread complaints about this situation from doctors and patients alike, none of whom liked dealing with complicated problems in brief office visits or overly short hospital stays.[62] As discussants at a conference at Harvard observed, "How medicine is practiced, and the inability to spend time with the patient, have created a real crisis in the perception [among doctors] of what medicine is all about."[63] Patients, too, frequently complained of assembly-line medicine—of receiving impersonal care from doctors who did not seem to know them or even to listen to them.[64] One frustrated patient wrote, "I can't find a doctor who's willing to listen to the most basic and relevant questions. They either don't listen, or cut me off short, or mumble something before they begin making an exit."[65] These changes in medical practice helped explain a variety of phenomena that developed in the 1990s and early 2000s: the widespread emergence of burnout among physicians (especially those in primary care),[66] the substitution of shared medical appointments for individual appointments,[67] the proliferation of popular literature instructing patients how to make certain they got their questions answered when their doctors were short on time,[68] and the development of "concierge" or "boutique" practice (a new form of practice in which doctors, for an annual retainer fee from each patient, limited the size of their practice so that they might provide patients prompt access, more time during appointments, and, in some cases, home visits).[69] At this time there was also a resurgence of interest in professionalism among physicians, a response attributed at least in part to a pushback among doctors to the time pressures of contemporary practice.[70]

Residents also learned medicine in a real-world health care system characterized by the excessive amount of care it provided (at least, to those with access to medical care). Overutilization ran contrary to the principles of good medical practice, which required patient-appropriate care, not all the tests and treatments that could be imagined. Health care analysts had long recognized that more medical care did not equate to better care or a healthier public, and for decades they had been concerned about the problem of provider-induced demand for potentially unnecessary services. However, this perspective had yet to permeate the practice of many physicians. Accordingly, it was estimated that as much as one-third of all health care delivered was unnecessary or inappropriate.[71] Diagnostic imaging studies were particularly prone to unnecessary use. It was estimated that as many as 50 percent of all "high-tech" imaging studies provided no useful information and might be unnecessary.[72] This culture of excess came with a price: substantial unnecessary costs and the burden of complications and adverse reactions, including deaths, from procedures or treatments that had little justification in the first place. For example, depending on the part of the body studied, computed tomographic (CT) scanning exposed patients to 100 to 500 times the radiation dose of a standard chest radiograph, and it was clear that the cancer risks created by unnecessary CT scanning were significant and growing.[73] The unbridled use of CT scanning gave rise to another phenomenon: the "incidentaloma." This new term referred to an unsuspected abnormal finding, almost always harmless, detected in asymptomatic patients who had undergone CT scanning for some other reason, often flimsy. Once these findings were known, physicians typically felt obligated to work them up, often with a biopsy, which led to additional costs, patient worry and discomfort, and an occasional complication such as bleeding or infection.[74]

Ironically, these circumstances in health care existed at a time when more and more voices were calling for doctors and hospitals to deliver "patient-centered care." In response, many hospitals for the first time started designing their facilities for the comfort and benefit of patients. Among the changes widely introduced were private rooms, more liberal visiting hours, rollout beds for family members, more comfortable waiting areas, better food, improved décor and layout, wider hallways and doors, softer colors, warmer lighting, and more convenient parking. Some hospitals even offered patients who could afford a steep extra charge the ambience of a luxury hotel, with skylights, sumptuous rooms, designer furniture, private chefs, and concierge service. In introducing these changes, hospitals were influenced by the growing consumerism pervading health care as well as by the notion of the "healing hospital," the idea that physical surroundings can affect patient outcomes. Hospitals that improved their amenities and service were at an advantage in the fierce competition to attract paying patients.[75]

The new attention to patient amenities, however, as important and well intended as it was, fell short of the meaning of "patient-centered care" that the IOM had in mind when it popularized the term in a 2001 report.[76] The report used this term to describe a model of care focusing on understanding the needs of the individual patient and tailoring specific treatment to the patient at hand. This type of care required patient-appropriate tests or treatments, not the performance of anything that could be done. True "patient-centered care" also required concerted attention to good communication with patients and the conveyance of kindness, compassion, and caring. However, this required time, which was in short supply. Wendy Levinson and Philip A. Pizzo pointed out that most full-time and private physicians wanted to communicate carefully with their patients and develop strong personal relationships. However, "They are under intense pressure to be productive, measured in numbers of patients observed in units of time. Perverse [payment] incentives have contributed to physicians developing 'efficient styles' that squeeze out time to listen because it is perceived to take too much time."[77] For both these reasons—the culture of excess and the emphasis on high throughput—the concept of "patient-centered care" remained more an ideal than an actuality.

Indeed, in the money-driven, profit-oriented, highly commercialized health care system of the early twenty-first century, it was not always clear whom medicine served. Did doctors exist to serve patients, or did patients exist to serve doctors? This was precisely the question Rosemary Gibson, a former program officer at the Robert Wood Johnson Foundation, and Janardan Prasad Singh, an economist at the World Bank, asked in their book, *The Treatment Trap*. Gibson and Singh described the culture of excess in American medical practice and the health care system's market-driven behavior, where doctors and hospitals, like actors in any business, thrived on selling customers as much as they could, whether needed or not. They quoted a seasoned nurse: "Health insurance used to be about giving people access to health care. Now it's about giving providers access to patients."[78] The reason for this was simple, Gibson and Singh wrote: "One person's overuse is another person's payment for college tuition or a mortgage on a McMansion."[79]

Who was looking out for patients? It was not necessarily the providers, who often churned patients in and out of hospitals and offices and provided paying patients an abundance of care, necessary or unnecessary. It was no accident that the early twenty-first century gave rise to an antimedical consumer campaign aimed at educating patients on how to survive their hospitalization or medical care. Books appeared with titles such as *How to Survive Your Doctor's Care, Surviving Health Care, Protect Yourself in the Hospital*, and *Special Treatment: How to Get the Same High-Quality Health Care Your Doctor Gets*.[80] Consumer's Union produced a report, *When to Say "Whoa" to Doctors: A Guide to Common Tests and Treatments You Probably Don't Need*.[81] Articles in lay publications regularly appeared with titles like "How to Survive a Hospital Stay," "How to Get Treated Like a Doctor without Going to Medical School," "Does the Doctor Work for You?," "The Danger of Too Many Tests," "Knowing When to Say 'No' to Tests," and "How to Improve Your Care."[82] All suggested that patients were on their own, vulnerable to exploitation. Proponents of this view dismissed the traditional assumption that doctors and other health care workers were staunch patient advocates. Indeed, so the argument went, patients now needed to protect themselves from the providers of health care. As Regina E. Herzlinger, a professor at Harvard Business School, wrote, "Patients learn—sometimes the hard way—to bring along an assertive, intelligent loved one to protect them during a hospital stay."[83]

Herein lay the era's deepest and most troubling threat to patient safety: not medical errors per se, but the growing possibility that patients needed protection from the providers of care. Many patients experienced a growing distrust of the health care system and a palpable skepticism toward the system's desire and capacity to do right by them. In the extreme, this view represented a caricature, of course. It overlooked the wonderful contributions of modern medicine and the unflinching efforts of countless, fundamentally good people working in health care trying to help patients every day. Yet the very fact that responsible individuals could raise this question spoke volumes as to the existence of a fundamental shift in American health care. Traditionally, it had been considered a prima facie truth that doctors (and everyone in health care) made the welfare of patients their primary concern. Now, that traditional belief no longer seemed self-evident. Words espousing the primacy of the patient continued to be voiced throughout health care, and no one was about to deny that they were in favor of "patient-centered care." However, such words often seemed hollow, as they were not consistently accompanied by deeds or actions. More and more a skeptical public expressed its lack of trust in the commitment of the medical profession to place the needs of patients first.

Thus, at the most fundamental level, the problems of residency training and medical practice were the same: learning and practicing medicine in a commercialized health care environment that gave mainly lip service to "patient-centered care." The emphasis on maximizing patient throughput and the culture of excess in delivering services served the needs of neither learners nor patients. High-quality learning was impossible in the absence of high-quality patient care. Accordingly, the fate of residency training, as always, was ultimately interrelated with the fate of the health care delivery system.

For professional leaders, these challenges presented a great opportunity: to work to create a health care system where service and patient-oriented values remained strong. To do so, they needed to help create systems of care where quality and safety were maximized, sufficient time was available to address patients' problems, appropriate care was emphasized, curiosity and learning flourished, and genuine caring remained central to the practice of medicine. To some, medicine's greatest need was to retain its focus on caring. The medical anthropologist Arthur Kleinman wrote, "Modern medical practice's greatest challenge may be finding a way to keep caregiving central to health care."[84] To be at their best, both medical education and patient care required competent clinical systems that judged themselves (and were judged by others) by how well they benefited those under their care, not simply by financial criteria.

Physicians as well as patients stood to benefit from a more patient-centered health care environment. In the early twenty-first century there was growing concern about the quality of professional life in medicine. Studies showed that job-related burnout had become a significant problem for physicians in practice and that burnout was more common among doctors than among other workers. Primary care physicians were at greatest risk. A major reason for burnout, especially for those in primary care, was decreasing professional satisfaction from work.[85] A patient-oriented system with enough time for doctors to develop meaningful relationships with patients and to address their patients' problems could go far toward restoring the meaning of medical work.

Evidence existed that this indeed was the case. For instance, Eric B. Larson and Robert Reid described a prototype outpatient clinic developed by Group Health, a Seattle-based nonprofit health insurance and care delivery system. In this experiment, Group Health reduced physician panels from approximately 2,300 to 1,800 patients, expanded the standard visit time from 20 to 30 minutes, and increased the size of the support staff. They found that these changes improved the patient experience and quality of care and reduced clinician burnout. These effects were sustained through the first two years of the clinic's operation.[86] The success of the Group Health experiment was consistent with a growing body of research that suggested that "enhancing meaning in work increases physician satisfaction and reduces burnout."[87] The challenge before American medicine was to implement such changes systematically.

Architects of health care reform faced a daunting task. In such a large, complex system, it was imperative that simplistic solutions be avoided, competing goods be balanced, the law of inadvertent consequences be respected, and accountability and transparency be present. It was also important to avoid unrealistic expectations of medicine. Even the best care could not eliminate accidents, disease, suffering, and death, nor could it substitute for preventive care, personal responsibility, and improvements in the social and economic determinants of health. All medical and surgical care carried the risk of harm to patients; uncertainty was a constant presence in every aspect of medical practice.

Discussion of specific proposals would require another voice in another book. However, the key point here is the recognition that definitive solutions could not be obtained simply by throwing more money into the system or relying on technological fixes. Rather, at its root health care renewal involved thorny moral questions about what type of health care Americans wanted to receive. Which types of care did Americans value? Did people truly wish to have deeply personal care? Did they wish to have strong doctor-patient relationships? Was medical care essentially a business, or, as Arnold Relman has long argued, an essential human service best pursued when organizations involved in the financing or delivery of care are nonprofit?[88] Most provocatively, did patients exist to serve the health care system, or did the health care system exist to serve patients? The challenges in health care were the same as elsewhere in American politics, where, as Irving Kristol once argued, the great seduction "was to believe that problems that were essentially moral and civic could be solved by economic means."[89]

Physicians, especially, incurred the responsibility of looking inward and asking tough questions of themselves. In particular, they needed to ask why they chose medicine as a career and what type of profession they believed medicine should be. The historian David J. Rothman wrote, "It is necessary to examine the internal, not the external, factors that have weakened professionalism," and he pointed out that "professionalism may well require some financial sacrifice."[90] Indeed, doctors had more leeway to spend time with patients and lessen the frequency of unnecessary tests and procedures than they often admitted—if they were willing to lower their income expectations. It was hard not to argue that physicians merited high incomes, but few—especially doctors—asked, "How much is enough?" Should individuals entering medicine expect that medical practice would provide highly comfortable incomes and lifestyles—or the opportunity, as in finance and business, to become Masters of the Universe? The oncologist and medical humanist Jerome Groopman declared, "I bet there are a lot of physicians who would say 'I'd rather be fulfilled and not make a football player's salary, but really enjoy my profession and return some level of civility and art to it.'"[91] These and other difficult moral questions lie at the root of health care reform.

Thus, the opportunity was present for the medical profession to help design and lead health care reform and participate in creating high-performing delivery systems that improved the welfare of patients. Indeed, the Physician Charter of 2002 explicitly called on doctors to do just that as one manifestation of medical professionalism.[92] This was not a task for doctors alone, of course. The health care system was too large and complex, and it included too many widely diverse interest groups. Physicians, however, were in a unique position to provide leadership, particularly in defining effective and appropriate care and in ensuring that professional and social values were preserved. Medical leadership was essential to helping establish financial incentives that rewarded and did not penalize professional behavior.[93] Michael E. Porter, a well-known professor at Harvard Business School, argued that "improving the value of health care is something only medical teams can do."[94] The sociologist Eliot Freidson argued that professionalism was "the third logic," an essential counterweight to the market and to bureaucracy in organizing work and establishing policy.[95] Many leading physicians agreed, including Relman, who viewed doctors as "the key to health care reform," and Jordan J. Cohen, president of the Association of American Medical Colleges from 1994 to 2006, who argued that "doctors have the professional responsibility to lead medicine out of its current predicament."[96]

For the medical profession, such leadership required a reversal of recent behavior. Since the 1970s, the profession had lost considerable authority, influence, and public trust. This shift arose from the growing perception that doctors were more concerned about their personal economic well-being than the welfare of their patients and that physicians were politically apathetic except when it came to protecting their own financial interests. With so much money pouring into health care, some doctors grew exceedingly rich, but public confidence in physicians' altruism and professionalism declined precipitously. Mark Schlesinger, who carefully studied this trend, observed, "Over a 30-year period, American medicine went from being perhaps the most trusted to being one of the least trusted social institutions."[97]

However, the past was not necessarily prelude. The historians of medicine Daniel M. Fox and Howard Markel, though warning that "historians have too much respect for contingency to dare to predict the future," observed that "interest groups' perception of self-interest can change."[98] Rajat K. Gupta, a former managing director of McKinsey & Company, spoke of the importance of "enlightened self-interest" serving as a catalyst for constructive social change, based on the recognition that the success of a business or an activity depends on the well-being of those being served.[99] Rosemary Stevens, another distinguished historian of medicine, noted that doctors might gain support for a more active policy role if they were able to define an agenda for political action in health care that resonated with broader notions of the public good. Of course, effacing self-interest to the needs of patients and society had always represented the ideal of medicine. That was why Stevens pointed out, "Public interest and professional self-interest are not necessarily, or even usefully, antagonistic."[100] The message for the medical profession was clear: In any health care environment, including the uncertain climate of the 2010s, doctors had much less to fear about their position and influence in society if they did their job well and made clear that service to patients and the public came first.

Could academic medical centers provide institutional leadership in health care reform? Many doubted this. Academic medical centers had financially prospered too much from the status quo. They had increased their throughput of patients with alacrity and billed plentifully for physician, laboratory, and radiological services. Billion-dollar annual budgets were commonplace, construction cranes were ubiquitous, and the size of their "clinical enterprises" had grown gargantuan. From this perspective, they had little reason to wish for change. One government official told a leading medical educator, "Medical schools and teaching hospitals are the last people I would expect to change anything."[101] Michael E. Whitcomb, the former editor of *Academic Medicine*, believed that the kinds of changes needed to improve patient care and medical education "are unlikely to come about unless influential individuals outside the profession make it clear to leaders within the profession that this must happen."[102]

Yet, as with individual physicians, an alternative narrative was possible. Academic medical centers were highly adapted to prospective hospital payment and to the fee-for-service system, but they were not as well prepared for many features of the impending Affordable Care Act, such as "value-based purchasing," "bundling," and the emphasis on creating affordable "medical homes." In the words of Darrell G. Kirch, who became president of the Association of American Medical Colleges in 2006, academic medical centers were "maladjusted and financially unsustainable" for the 2010s.[103] Many believed that payment reform could become the catalyst that finally prompted academic medical centers to become better stewards of resources and more attentive guardians of patient welfare. Some even believed that the time had come for academic medical centers to assume such a role simply because it was the right thing to do and much more in keeping with their traditional values. Thus, Jordan S. Cohen warned that the quest for growth at academic medical centers has "begun to obscure our quest for meaning" and that "our 'drive for size'" was "displacing our deep-seated aspiration to contribute in meaningful ways to the improvement of the human condition."[104] The future, of course, was contingent on many factors, but academic medical centers had the potential to become the nation's chief protectors and champions of patient welfare. If they succeeded in reinvigorating their core values, their chances of receiving more consistent public funding for their indispensable social missions of education, research, and charity care were likely to improve.[105]

At the center of academic medicine's potential contribution to health care renewal stood graduate medical education. Residency training had the opportunity to take on directly the prevailing culture of excess by more effectively teaching decision-making strategies and the appropriate use of medical resources. Faculty had the responsibility to teach residents to obtain tests and procedures when they were indicated, not just because they were available. Residency programs had the opportunity to teach learners how better to manage uncertainty and become problem solvers, not simply to do everything and see what happened. As seen in this book, that had been the promise of the "scientific practitioner" from the very beginning of the residency system. However, as also discussed in this book, the failure to produce enough doctors who could more closely approximate that ideal had been the residency system's greatest failing. Over time, this deficiency grew more significant as the scope and expense of medical care increased. But the basic fault line—the failure to produce enough practitioners who exercised these vital reasoning skills—was present all along.

Of course, many factors, such as "defensive medicine" and the powerful financial incentives to do more created by the fee-for-service system, contributed to the culture of excess besides poor decision making. Nevertheless, there was still a huge amount of excess care that resulted from this reason.

This was something doctors often did not wish to admit. It was understandably much easier for doctors to fix the blame outside on external factors than to look inwardly at their own behavior. A poll in 2013 revealed that most doctors denied "major responsibility" for cutting costs.[106] Yet those denials flew in the face of the evidence. The fee-for-service system did not account for the high rate of unnecessary surgery on patients treated at Veterans Hospitals because the physicians who worked there were paid a salary and had no financial incentive to provide unnecessary treatment.[107] External factors did not explain the common tendencies to obtain multiple imaging studies of the same organ when one would have sufficed, to obtain blood tests of hospitalized patients far more often than necessary, or to overuse antibiotics and screening tests. External factors also did not account for excessive testing that resulted from bedside sloppiness—for instance, the five negative imaging studies on the patient with "abdominal pain" in the emergency room, only because his doctors failed to do a complete examination that would have revealed his epididymitis; or the multiple negative imaging tests of another emergency room patient's liver to investigate a mild elevation of liver enzymes, only because his physicians did not recognize florid congestive heart failure (which also explained the laboratory abnormalities).[108] Most medical expenditures were under the control of physicians; no one forced doctors to order or do anything. The fact that poor decision making was not the only cause of excessive care and soaring costs did not lessen its significance. It represented a large problem, and it was something doctors could address on their own without waiting for other aspects of health care reform.

Fortunately, in the 2010s there was evidence of an emerging cultural shift in medicine, as some influential physicians began speaking out against overutilization. Policy leaders Donald M. Berwick and Andrew D. Hackbarth wrote of the importance of "eliminating waste in US health care," arguing that the opportunity for meaningful cost savings was "immense."[109] There was more and more discussion of pursing "value" in health care—that is, outcomes relative to cost. Steven E. Weinberger, the executive vice president of the American College of Physicians, argued that promoting high-value, cost-conscious care should be "a critical seventh general competency for physicians," to be enforced by the ACGME and the American Board of Medical Specialties in conjunction with their existing six competences.[110] David B. Reuben and Christine K. Cassel urged "physician stewardship of health care in an era of finite resources"; Sean Palfrey dared doctors to rely on their clinical skills "to practice low-cost medicine in a high-tech era."[111] In 2012, the American Board of Internal Medicine Foundation, working with *Consumer Reports*, announced its Choosing

Wisely initiative. In the initial iteration, nine leading medical organizations identified five tests or treatments within their purview that they believed were highly overused, in the hope that practitioners would use them with greater discretion.[112]

Physicians' behaviors have always been notoriously difficult to modify.[113] Accordingly, many believed that the best opportunity to influence doctors' decision-making practices came when those practices were learned and internalized—that is, during residency training.[114] There was much residency programs could do in this regard. They could introduce economic issues into the curriculum, inform house officers of the costs of tests and procedures, and improve the way residents learned how to use diagnostic tests. They could discuss case studies of inappropriate care (including underuse and misuse as well as overuse), both in large- and small-group formats. All programs could foster skills in diagnostic reasoning and communication to patients of benefits and harm. Surgical programs could reemphasize the fundamental principle of not subjecting patients to unnecessary operations. Eventually, these skills could be incorporated into high-stakes examinations such as board certification testing. Academic medical centers could help with this work by engaging in faculty development, honoring faculty for good teaching, and creating a culture that celebrated restraint. Perhaps academic medical centers, with the aid of the media, could lead a massive, top-down effort to foster appropriate care in American medicine, much as the one that recently aided the movement to reduce hospital errors.[115]

Most important, residency programs needed to bring such teaching to the bedside. General discussions of lists of evidence-based tests only went so far. Coronary angiography was a good test; that did not mean its use was justified by the presence of a beating heart. Residents needed to be taught to ask themselves a few key questions before ordering tests, most particularly, "Will the test result change my management of the patient?" On attending rounds or at residents' report, house officers could describe the rationale for the tests or procedures they ordered—or the reasons why they did not order certain others. Faculty members needed to ask residents why they did something, not just why they did not. The goal, to paraphrase William Osler, was to teach residents to view medical practice as "a way of thinking," not just "a way of life." Ideally, clinicians in every field would learn to approach every patient in every setting in a judicious, parsimonious fashion, and cost savings would be the inevitable outgrowth of good care.

The example of the Aliki Initiative at the Johns Hopkins Bayview Medical Center demonstrated that residency programs could achieve these objectives. Earlier, the educational success of the Aliki experiment was noted, a success made possible by reducing the residents' patient census and enhancing the quality of faculty teaching. Here, it is noteworthy that the Aliki Initiative also resulted in the consumption of fewer resources and the provision of better care. For instance, the 30-day heart failure readmission rate (a proxy for quality and cost) was 4 percent on the Aliki team, compared with 14 percent on the three standard teaching teams.[116] House officers on the Aliki rotation engaged in considerable discussion with faculty members and each other about unnecessary testing, something they rarely did on the standard rotations because of too little time. A group of house officers was thereby motivated to develop cost-reduction strategies for the hospital, the first of which saved $1 million per year in charges by reducing unnecessary ordering of cardiac enzymes.[117]

Here, then, was the link between residency training and health care reform. Parsimonious medical practice represented both better and less expensive care. It produced less harm from treatment, consumed less money, and allowed doctors to serve as better stewards of society's resources with less strain on their one-on-one relationships with patients. The key to making such care widely available lay in the residency system and the commitment of academic medical centers. The fact that other factors also contributed—in some cases, substantially—to the culture of excess did not excuse professional leaders from addressing a major factor under their own control.

Ultimately, it was likely that the problem of health care costs would be definitively addressed. After all, the country could never spend 100 percent of its gross domestic product on medical care. The question was at what point a solution would finally be achieved, and in what way. Compromises between the two, of course, were possible, but at some point there would probably be either heavy-handed, bureaucratic approaches—perhaps even explicit rationing—or a patient-oriented approach, as suggested here, wherein doctors, by doing what was best for the patient at hand, would allow more to be left over for others. If the latter course was chosen, it would have to be undertaken carefully. The economist Victor R. Fuchs pointed out, "Every dollar of waste is income to some individual or organization."[118] With forethought, however, careful transition strategies could help mitigate the potential economic dislocations.

Could responsible health renewal—reform that would benefit both residency training and patients—be accomplished? Could graduate medical education contribute to that process? The early 2010s were an uncertain time for health care in America. The country was emerging from a severe recession, the implications of the Affordable Care Act were not fully understood, many members of Congress were still trying to repeal the law, and the health care system had become highly commercialized. Yet it was also a time of tremendous opportunity. The capacity of medicine to prevent and relieve suffering was unprecedented, the promise of medical science unsurpassed, and the need for good doctors greater than ever as the population grew and aged. A significant amount of civic-mindedness remained within the medical profession, and there was residual good will from the public.[119] Bright, idealistic young men and women continued to choose medicine as a career. A new Medical College Admissions Test (MCAT), scheduled for introduction in 2015, placed much greater emphasis on the social and behavioral sciences, thereby explicitly acknowledging the importance of doctors having humanistic qualities and the ability to understand people as well as science.[120]

These circumstances provided all doctors, academicians and private practitioners alike, an opportunity to ask fundamental questions: Who are we? Why did we go into medicine? What do we want medical care to be? What are our responsibilities and obligations, not just our rights and entitlements? These circumstances also provided professional leaders an opportunity to take the high ground of developing a consensus view of what, ideally, medical education and the health system should look like. Rapid change is often unnerving, but professional leaders could take comfort in remembering that change in medicine has always been not only acceptable but also mandatory—provided that the interests of patients and society are served.

The key to success lay in remembering that good medical education could contribute to health care reform. Parsimonious medical practice—doing what the patient needed, not everything that could be done—ultimately is a learned habit, though one admittedly influenced by other concerns. The great opportunity for residency education was to improve the thinking and reasoning habits of ordinary practicing physicians in all specialties. A more careful approach to patient care offered the opportunity to eliminate much of the excess in American health care and thereby significantly reduce costs. Such an approach also offered the opportunity to improve quality by reducing the inevitable complications of care. The public undoubtedly would be grateful, both for the financial savings and for having a medical profession that more clearly put the welfare of patients first. Doctors and hospitals might find their interests more closely aligned with those of third-party payers. In such circumstances, the public might become more inclined to provide the types of resources necessary to improve the learning and patient care environment, including the provision of enough time to provide "slow medicine" to patients in need of it. Using language I employed in an earlier work, the potential existed for the "social contract" between medicine and society to be restored.[121] Was this scenario a possibility or a dream? That depended on many factors, not the least of which was what the medical profession decided to do.

NOTES

PREFACE

1. Cheryl Ulmer, Dianne Miller Wolman, and Michael M. E. Johns, eds., *Resident Duty Hours: Enhancing Sleep, Supervision, and Safety* (Washington, D.C.: National Academies Press, 2009).
2. Kenneth M. Ludmerer, *Learning to Heal: The Development of American Medical Education* (New York: Basic Books, 1985).
3. Kenneth M. Ludmerer, *Time to Heal: American Medical Education from the Turn of the Century to the Era of Managed Care* (New York: Oxford University Press, 1999).

CHAPTER 1

1. Audrey W. Davis, *Dr. Kelly of Hopkins: Surgeon, Scientist, Christian* (Baltimore, Md.: Johns Hopkins University Press, 1959), p. 38.
2. Kenneth M. Ludmerer, *Learning to Heal: The Development of American Medical Education* (New York: Basic Books, 1985).
3. John Harley Warner, *Against the Spirit of System: The French Impulse in Nineteenth-Century American Medicine* (Princeton: Princeton University Press, 1998), p. 28.
4. Warner, *Against the Spirit of System*, pp. 17–31.
5. Ludmerer, *Learning to Heal.*
6. C. D. O'Malley, ed., *The History of Medical Education* (Berkeley: University of California Press, 1970).
7. Whitfeld J. Bell Jr., "John Redman, Medical Preceptor (1722–1808)," in Whitfeld J. Bell Jr., *The Colonial Physician and Other Essays* (New York: Science History Publications, 1975), pp. 27–39.
8. "Report of the Committee on Medical Education," *T Am Med Assoc*, 17 (1867): 364.
9. William F. Norwood, *Medical Education in the United States before the Civil War* (Philadelphia: University of Pennsylvania Press, 1944); William G. Rothstein, *American Physicians in the Nineteenth Century: From Sects to Science* (Baltimore, Md.: Johns Hopkins University Press, 1972), pp. 85–131.
10. N. S. Davis, *Contributions to the History of Medical Education and Medical Institutions in the United States of America, 1776–1876* (Washington, D.C.: Government Printing Office, 1877), p. 46.
11. Rosemary A. Stevens, "Graduate Medical Education: A Continuing History," *J Med Educ*, 53 (1978): 3.

12. On the extramural schools, see Dale C. Smith, "The Emergence of Organized Clinical Instruction in the Nineteenth Century American Cities of Boston, New York and Philadelphia" (PhD diss., University of Minnesota, 1979), pp. 112–48; and Steven J. Peitzman, "'Thoroughly Practical': America's Polyclinic Medical Schools," *B Hist Med*, 54 (1980): 166–87.
13. Boston City Hospital, *Annual Report* (1866), pp. 12–13.
14. J. A. Curran, "Internships and Residencies: Historical Backgrounds and Current Trends," *J Med Educ*, 34 (1959): 873–84; David M. Davis, "The History of the Resident System," *T Stud Coll Physicians Phila*, 27 (1959): 76–81.
15. J. M. Toner, "Statistics of Regular Medical Associations and Hospitals of the United States," *T Am Med Assoc*, 24 (1873): 314–15.
16. Curran, "Internships and Residencies," pp. 874–75.
17. Charles E. Rosenberg, *The Care of Strangers: The Rise of America's Hospital System* (New York: Basic Books, 1987), pp. 58–68, 190–200.
18. Frederic A. Washburn, *The Massachusetts General Hospital: Its Development, 1900–1935* (Boston: Houghton Mifflin, 1939), p. 163.
19. Edward C. Churchill, ed., *To Work in the Vineyard of Surgery: The Reminiscences of J. Collins Warren, 1842–1927* (Cambridge: Harvard University Press, 1958), p. 75. Excellent firsthand descriptions of house officers' experience are found in this source, pp. 72–85, and in Arthur Ames Bliss, *Blockley Days: Memories and Impressions of a Resident Physician, 1883–1884* (privately printed, 1916).
20. The maintenance of order in the nineteenth-century hospital is a major theme in Rosenberg, *The Care of Strangers*.
21. Lakeside Hospital, *Annual Report* (1898), p. 85.
22. Bliss, *Blockley Days*, p. 72.
23. See, for instance, Committee of the Hospital Staff, *A History of the Boston City Hospital, from Its Foundation until 1904* (Boston: Municipal Printing Office, 1906), p. 135; and meeting of May 25, 1887, Minutes of the Medical Board, The Presbyterian Hospital in the City of New York, Archives and Special Collections, A. C. Long Health Sciences Library, Columbia University Medical Center, New York, N.Y.
24. J. M. T. Finney, *A Surgeon's Life* (New York: G. P. Putnam's Sons, 1940), p. 69.
25. Bliss, *Blockley Days*, p. 47.
26. Churchill, *To Work in the Vineyard of Surgery*, p. 73.
27. Meetings of April 11, 1896, and June 13, 1894, Minutes of the Medical Board, The Presbyterian Hospital in the City of New York.
28. Churchill, *To Work in the Vineyard of Surgery*, p. 173.
29. Washburn, *The Massachusetts General Hospital*, p. 159.
30. Washburn, *The Massachusetts General Hospital*, pp. 150–51.
31. George Rosen, *The Specialization of Medicine with Particular Reference to Ophthalmology* (New York: Froben Press, 1944), is the classic historical study of the process of specialization. Two other studies are particularly important: Rosemary Stevens, *American Medicine and the Public Interest* (New Haven: Yale University Press, 1971); and George Weisz, *Divide and Conquer: A Comparative History of Medical Specialization* (New York: Oxford University Press, 2006). Many accounts of the development of individual specialties have been provided, but especially notable is W. Bruce Fye, *American Cardiology: The History of a Specialty and Its College* (Baltimore, Md.: Johns Hopkins University Press, 1996).
32. "Some of the Wonders of Modern Surgery," *Atl Mon*, March 1868, p. 373.

33. See, for instance, Clarence John Blake to Dear blessed Mater, February 8, 1869, Folder 12, Clarence John Blake Papers, HMS c 19.1, Rare Books and Special Collections, Francis A. Countway Library of Medicine, Harvard Medical School, Boston, Mass.
34. John S. Billings, *Medical Education. Extracts from Lectures Delivered before the Johns Hopkins University, Baltimore, 1877–8* (Baltimore, Md.: Wm. K. Boyle & Son, 1878), p. 30.
35. Stevens, *American Medicine and the Public Interest*, p. 46.
36. Warner, *Against the Spirit of System*; Russell M. Jones, ed., *The Parisian Education of an American Surgeon: Letters of Jonathan Mason Warren (1832–1835)* (Philadelphia: American Philosophical Society, 1978). Warner (pp. 292–94) points out that early in the century Americans had dual motives for studying in France: acquiring more general clinical experience and studying a medical specialty. However, by the 1840s the desire to study a specialty had become the overriding objective.
37. Warner, *Against the Spirit of System*, pp. 291–329.
38. On German scholarship in nonmedical areas, see Jurgen Herbst, *The German Historical School in American Scholarship: A Study in the Transfer of Culture* (Ithaca, N.Y.: Cornell University Press, 1965); Carl Diehl, *Americans and German Scholarship, 1770–1870* (New Haven: Yale University Press, 1978); and Fritz K. Ringer, *The Decline of the German Mandarins: The German Academic Community, 1890–1933* (Cambridge: Harvard University Press, 1969).
39. The best study of American physicians in Germany remains the classic work by Thomas N. Bonner, *American Doctors and German Universities: A Chapter in International Intellectual Relations, 1870–1914* (Lincoln: University of Nebraska Press, 1963).
40. Clarence John Blake to Dear Pater, January 21, 1866, Folder 3, Blake Papers.
41. Clarence John Blake to Dear Pater, June 8, 1869, Folder 15, Blake Papers.
42. Billings, *Medical Education*, p. 30.
43. Of course there were exceptions, such as William Beaumont's studies of the physiology of digestion, William Gerhard's distinction between typhoid and typhus, and Oliver Wendell Holmes's discovery of the mode of transmission of puerperal fever.
44. Richard Shryock, "American Indifference to Basic Science during the Nineteenth Century," in Richard Shryock, *Medicine in America: Historical Essays* (Baltimore, Md.: Johns Hopkins University Press, 1966), pp. 71–89; and Nathan Reingold, "American Indifference to Basic Research: A Reappraisal," in George H. Daniels, ed., *Nineteenth-Century American Science: A Reappraisal* (Evanston, Ill.: Northwestern University Press, 1972), pp. 38–62.
45. Bonner, *American Doctors and German Universities*; Ludmerer, *Learning to Heal*, pp. 29–38.
46. Clarence John Blake to Dear Pater and Mater, February 8, 1866, Folder 5, Blake Papers.
47. Clarence John Blake to Dear Pater, April 2, 1866, Folder 6, Blake Papers.
48. Harvey Cushing, *The Life of Sir William Osler* (New York: Oxford University Press, 1940), p. 216.
49. A. McGehee Harvey, *Science at the Bedside: Clinical Research in American Medicine, 1905–1945* (Baltimore, Md.: Johns Hopkins University Press, 1981), pp. 3–30.
50. Abraham Flexner, *I Remember: The Autobiography of Abraham Flexner* (New York: Simon and Schuster, 1940), p. 162.

51. Lewellys F. Barker, *Time and the Physician: The Autobiography of Lewellys F. Barker* (New York: G. P. Putnam's Sons, 1942), p. 130.
52. Harvey, *Science at the Bedside*, p. 183.
53. Samuel J. Meltzer, "The Science of Clinical Medicine: What It Ought to Be and the Men to Uphold It," *JAMA*, 53 (1909): 510.
54. Graham Lusk, "Medical Education: A Plea for the Development of Leaders," *JAMA*, 52 (1909): 1230.
55. Meltzer, "The Science of Clinical Medicine," p. 511.
56. Quoted in Cushing, *The Life of Sir William Osler*, p. 225.

CHAPTER 2

1. On the development of higher education in the United States, see Laurence R. Veysey, *The Emergence of the American University* (Chicago: University of Chicago Press, 1965); and Burton J. Bledstein, *The Culture of Professionalism: The Middle Class and the Development of Higher Education in America* (New York: Norton, 1976).
2. Valuable studies of the early Johns Hopkins include Alan M. Chesney, *The Johns Hopkins Hospital and the Johns Hopkins University School of Medicine: A Chronicle*, 3 vols. (Baltimore, Md.: Johns Hopkins University Press, 1943, 1958, 1963); Richard H. Shryock, *The Unique Influence of the Johns Hopkins University on American Medicine* (Copenhagen: Ejnar Munksgaard, 1953); and Hugh Hawkins, *Pioneer: A History of the Johns Hopkins University, 1874–1889* (Ithaca, N.Y.: Cornell University Press, 1960).
3. Gert H. Brieger, "The California Origins of the Johns Hopkins Medical School," *B Hist Med*, 51 (1977): 339–52.
4. On Billings, see Carleton B. Chapman, *Order Out of Chaos: John Shaw Billings and America's Coming of Age* (Boston: Science History Publications, 1994); James H. Cassedy, *John Shaw Billings: Science and Medicine in the Gilded Age* (Bethesda, Md.: Xlibris, 2009); and A. McGehee Harvey, "John Shaw Billings: Forgotten Hero of American Medicine," *Perspect Biol Med*, 21 (1977): 35–57. Billings wrote a series of essays that illustrated his admiration of German medical education. See, for instance, John Shaw Billings, "Hospital Construction and Organization," in *Hospital Plans: Five Essays Relating to the Construction, Organization and Management of Hospitals* (New York: William Wood, 1875), pp. 1–46; John Shaw Billings, *Johns Hopkins Hospital. Reports and Papers Relating to Construction and Organization*, no. 1 (Baltimore, Md.: n.p., 1876); and John Shaw Billings, "On the Plans for the Johns Hopkins Hospital at Baltimore," *Med Record*, 12 (1877): 129–33, 145–48.
5. Henry M. Hurd, "Historical Address, October 5, 1914," delivered at the Twenty-fifth Anniversary of the Johns Hopkins Hospital, in Folder 25, Box 15, Henry M. Hurd Papers, the Alan Mason Chesney Medical Archives of the Johns Hopkins Medical Institutions, Baltimore, Md.
6. John Shaw Billings to Daniel Coit Gilman, June 23, 1876, Folder 4, Box 57, William H. Welch Papers, the Alan Mason Chesney Medical Archives of the Johns Hopkins Medical Institutions, Baltimore, Md.
7. See, for instance, John Shaw Billings to Daniel Coit Gilman, December 9, 1884, Folder 12, Box 57, Welch Papers.
8. "A Report to the Trustees of the Johns Hopkins University by Daniel C. Gilman," December 2, 1878, Folder 18, Box 97, Welch Papers. In the manuscript, the word

"Billings" is written in pencil in the margin by this sentence, suggesting that Billings gave Gilman the idea.

9. Quoted in Rosemary Stevens, *American Medicine and the Public Interest* (New Haven: Yale University Press, 1971), p. 58.
10. Chesney, *The Johns Hopkins Hospital*, vol. 1, p. 162.
11. Henry Mills Hurd, "A History of the First Quarter-Century of The Johns Hopkins Hospital 1889–1910," unpublished manuscript, chapter VIII, p. 1, Folder 8, Box 12, Hurd Papers.
12. William H. Welch to My dear Mother, November 27, 1893, Folder 22, Box 68, Welch Papers.
13. Lakeside Hospital, *Annual Report* (1891), p. 11.
14. William Stewart Halsted, "The Training of the Surgeon," *B Johns Hopkins Hosp*, 15 (1904): 272.
15. See, for instance, Jim Eppinger to Henry A. Christian, 1936, Volume 10, Henry A. Christian Papers, Archives HMS B68, Rare Books and Special Collections, Francis A. Countway Library of Medicine, Harvard Medical School, Boston, Mass.
16. On Osler, see Michael Bliss, *William Osler: A Life in Medicine* (New York: Oxford University Press, 1999); and Harvey Cushing, *The Life of Sir William Osler* (New York: Oxford University Press, 1940).
17. William Osler, "Letters to My House Physicians," *NY State Med J*, LII (1890): 334.
18. Report of William Osler, January 30, 1890, with meeting of January 30, 1890, Minutes of the Medical Board, Johns Hopkins Hospital [Medical Board]; William Osler, "L'Envoi," *Aequanimitas with Other Addresses to Medical Students, Nurses and Practitioners of Medicine*, 3rd ed. (Philadelphia: Blakiston Company, 1948), p. 450 (quotation).
19. Osler, "L'Envoi," p. 450.
20. On Halsted, see Howard Markel, *An Anatomy of Addiction: Sigmund Freud, William Halsted, and the Miracle Drug Cocaine* (New York: Vintage, 2012); Gerald Imber, *Genius on the Edge: The Bizarre Double Life of Dr. William Stewart Halsted* (New York: Kaplan, 2010); and W. G. MacCallum, *William Stewart Halsted, Surgeon* (Baltimore, Md.: Johns Hopkins Press, 1930). The once flamboyant Halsted had unintentionally become addicted to cocaine in New York in the early 1880s while experimenting with its use as a local anesthetic. His addiction radically changed his personality, and he was never able to shake it. Osler and Welch knew of this problem but kept it a secret.
21. Halsted, "The Training of the Surgeon," p. 272.
22. On Kelly, see Audrey W. Davis, *Dr. Kelly of Hopkins: Surgeon Scientist Christian* (Baltimore, Md.: Johns Hopkins Press, 1959).
23. Howard A. Kelly, "Methods of Teaching Gynecology," *Phila Med J*, 6 (1900): 391–93.
24. John Shaw Billings, "The Plans and Purposes of The Johns Hopkins Hospital," address at the opening of the Johns Hopkins Hospital, May 7, 1889, p. 26, bound in the Johns Hopkins Hospital, *Superintendent's Report* (1889–90).
25. Meeting of February 25, 1897, Minutes of the Advisory Board of the Medical Faculty and Committees, the Johns Hopkins University School of Medicine, the Alan Mason Chesney Medical Archives of the Johns Hopkins Medical Institutions, Baltimore, Md.
26. William H. Welch to Alexander C. Abbott, April 20, 1898, Folder 8, Box 1, Welch Papers.

27. Meeting of March 13, 1890, Minutes of the Medical Board, the Johns Hopkins Hospital.
28. The Johns Hopkins Hospital, *Superintendent's Report* (1904), p. 17.
29. A listing of chief residents through 1918, with their terms of service, is found in the Johns Hopkins Hospital, *Superintendent's Report* (1918), pp. 99–100. The average length of service of a Johns Hopkins surgical house officer who rose through the system to chief residency was eight years—six as assistant resident, two as chief resident. See Halsted, "The Training of the Surgeon," p. 271.
30. The Johns Hopkins Hospital, *Superintendent's Report* (1904), p. 17.
31. Billings, *Medical Education*, p. 8.
32. Letter of William Osler, January 30, 1890, with meeting of January 30, 1890, Minutes of the Medical Board, the Johns Hopkins Hospital, the Alan Mason Chesney Medical Archives of the Johns Hopkins Medical Institutions, Baltimore, Md.
33. William Welch, "On Some of the Humane Aspects of Medical Science," in William Henry Welch, *Papers and Addresses*, vol. 3 (Baltimore, Md.: Johns Hopkins University Press, 1920), p. 5.
34. John Shaw Billings, "Valedictory Address" (unpublished lecture), n.d., Box 44, John Shaw Billings Papers, New York Public Library, New York, N.Y.
35. Kenneth M. Ludmerer, *Learning to Heal: The Development of American Medical Education* (New York: Basic Books, 1985), pp. 47–71.
36. Abraham Flexner, *Medical Education in the United States and Canada* (New York: Carnegie Foundation for the Advancement of Teaching, 1910), p. 68; Abraham Flexner, *Medical Education in Europe* (New York: Carnegie Institution for the Advancement of Teaching, 1912), pp. 168, 171.
37. Ludmerer, *Learning to Heal*, pp. 63–71.
38. Quoted in Davis, *Dr. Kelly of Hopkins*, p. 59.
39. William Thayer, "Teaching and Practice," in William Sydney Thayer, *Osler and Other Papers* (Baltimore, Md.: Johns Hopkins Press, 1931), p. 191.
40. Morton White, *Social Thought in America: The Revolt against Formalism* (Boston: Beacon Press, 1957).
41. John Dewey, "Science as Subject-Matter and as Method," *Science*, 31 (1910): 122.
42. Lewellys F. Barker, *Time and the Physician: The Autobiography of Lewellys F. Barker* (New York: G. P. Putnam's Sons, 1942), p. 158.
43. Thayer, "Teaching and Practice," p. 208.
44. Flexner, *Medical Education in the United States and Canada*, p. 92.
45. Flexner, *Medical Education in the United States and Canada*, p. 92.
46. J. M. T. Finney, *A Surgeon's Life: The Autobiography of J. M. T. Finney* (New York: G. P. Putnam's Sons, 1940), p. 332.
47. Hugh Young, *A Surgeon's Autobiography* (New York: Harcourt, Brace and Company, 1940), p. 76. Halsted's appointments of youthful division chiefs, though in the end successful, at the time caused no small amount of dismay among the older physicians who had been working at the hospital in those fields. For instance, dedicated local physicians had been working without compensation in the Ear, Nose, and Throat Clinic since the hospital's opening, without even having been granted inpatient privileges. Crowe recounted their "indignation and surprise" in 1912 when he, four years out of medical school and with no experience in the specialty, was appointed by Halsted to supersede them (Samuel James Crowe, *Halsted of Johns Hopkins: The Man and His Men* [Springfield, Ill.: Charles C. Thomas, 1957], p. 149).
48. Crowe, *Halsted of Johns Hopkins*, p. 57.

49. Letter of William Osler, January 30, 1890, with meeting of January 30, 1890, Minutes of the Medical Board, the Johns Hopkins Hospital.
50. W. T. Councilman, "Osler in the Early Days at the Johns Hopkins Hospital," *Boston Med Surg J*, 182 (1920): 345.
51. Crowe, *Halsted of Johns Hopkins*, p. 57.
52. Barker, *Time and the Physician*, p. 120.
53. The Johns Hopkins Hospital, *Superintendent's Reports* (1904), p. 22.
54. Davis, *Dr. Kelly of Hopkins*, p. 93; Councilman, "Osler in the Early Days," pp. 341–45; Crowe, *Halsted of Johns Hopkins*, pp. 37–59; Finney, *A Surgeon's Life*, pp. 283–99; MacCallum, *William Stewart Halsted*, pp. 121–38.
55. Barker, *Time and the Physician*, p. 41 ("Uncle Hank" and "the Hurdlets"); Finney, *A Surgeon's Life*, pp. 99–100.
56. Edith Gittings Reid, *The Great Physician: A Short Life of Sir William Osler* (New York: Oxford University Press, 1931), pp. 117–18.
57. Meeting of May 13, 1912, Minutes of the Medical Board, the Johns Hopkins Hospital.
58. Finney, *A Surgeon's Life*, p. 106.
59. Finney, *A Surgeon's Life*, pp. 110, 209; Imber, *Genius on the Edge*, pp. 207, 295.
60. Chesney, *The Johns Hopkins Hospital*, vol. 2, pp. 181–82.
61. William Osler, "Teacher and Student," in Osler, *Aequanimitas*, p. 36.
62. Quoted in Bliss, *William Osler*, pp. 260–61.
63. Joseph H. Pratt, *A Year with Osler, 1896–1897* (Baltimore, Md.: Johns Hopkins Press, 1949), p. xiii.
64. Imber, *Genius on the Edge*, p. 238.
65. See, for instance, the description of the Johns Hopkins Hospital in the 1890s provided by Barker, *Time and the Physician*, pp. 84–105; and by Finney, *A Surgeon's Life*, pp. 88–105.
66. Barker, *Time and the Physician*, p. 100.
67. Donald Fleming, *William Welch and the Rise of Modern Medicine* (Boston: Little, Brown, 1954), p. 114.
68. This portrayal is found in Thomas B. Turner, *Heritage of Excellence: The Johns Hopkins Medical Institutions, 1914–1947* (Baltimore, Md.: Johns Hopkins University Press, 1974).
69. Turner, *Heritage of Excellence*, p. 269.
70. Councilman, "Osler in the Early Days," p. 344.
71. Fleming, *William Welch*, pp. 115–16; quotation, p. 116.
72. Howard Gardner, Mihaly Csikszentmihalyi, and William Damon, *Good Work: When Excellence and Ethics Meet* (New York: Basic Books, 2001); quotations, p. 5.
73. Ludmerer, *Learning to Heal*, esp. pp. 29–38, 123–38, and 207–18.
74. The Johns Hopkins Hospital, *Superintendent's Report* (1915), p. 15.
75. B. Noland Carter, "The Fruition of Halsted's Concept of Surgical Training," *Surgery*, 32 (1952): 518–27.
76. Attachment A, "Dr. Allen O. Whipple," with meeting of May 21, 1963, Minutes of the Medical Board, the Presbyterian Hospital in the City of New York, Archives and Special Collections, A. C. Long Health Sciences Center, Columbia University Medical Center, New York, N.Y.
77. Young, *A Surgeon's Autobiography*, pp. 240–41; quotation, p. 240.
78. Young, *A Surgeon's Autobiography*, pp. 245–46; Crowe, *Halsted of Johns Hopkins*, pp. 124–25.

79. Edwards A. Parks, "John Howland Award Address," *Pediatrics*, 10 (1952): 82–108; L. Emmett Holt Jr., "John Howland: Turning Point of American Pediatrics," *J Pediatr*, 69 (1966): 865–75; quotation, Parks, "John Howland Award Address," p. 95.
80. MacCallum, *William Stewart Halsted*, p. x.

CHAPTER 3

1. Kenneth M. Ludmerer, *Learning to Heal: The Development of American Medical Education* (New York: Basic Books, 1985).
2. Abraham Flexner, *Medical Education in the United States and Canada* (New York: Carnegie Foundation for the Advancement of Teaching, 1910).
3. Columbia University College of Physicians and Surgeons, Report of the Dean (1916), p. 10.
4. A. McGehee Harvey, *Science at the Bedside: Clinical Research in American Medicine, 1905–1945* (Baltimore, Md.: Johns Hopkins University Press, 1981), pp. 64–67; A. McGehee Harvey, *Adventures in Medical Research: A Century of Discovery at Johns Hopkins* (Baltimore, Md.: Johns Hopkins University Press, 1976), pp. 124–27.
5. Elias P. Lyon, "The Relation of the Laboratory Courses to the Work of the Clinical Years," *JAMA*, 66 (1916): 630.
6. Lyon, "The Relation of the Laboratory Courses," p. 629.
7. Lyon, "The Relation of the Laboratory Courses," p. 630.
8. For instance, these concerns arose in the basic science departments of Harvard Medical School. See E. E. Southard to Henry A. Christian, March 18, 1913, Volume 1; and Henry A. Christian to Walter B. Cannon, December 3, 1919, Volume 3, Henry A. Christian Papers, Archives HMS B68, Rare Books and Special Collections, Francis A. Countway Library of Medicine, Harvard Medical School, Boston, Mass.
9. For instance, private practitioners on the voluntary teaching faculties of Johns Hopkins and Georgetown resented their subordinate roles in the governance of their respective medical schools. See meeting of October 28, 1921, and "Report on the Resolutions Concerning Representation of the Part-Time Teaching Staff Adopted at the General Faculty Meeting on June 5, 1922," with meeting of December 8, 1922, Minutes, Advisory Board of the Medical Faculty, the Johns Hopkins University School of Medicine, the Alan Mason Chesney Medical Archives of the Johns Hopkins Medical Institutions, Baltimore, Md.; and meeting of November 8, 1923, Faculty Minutes, Georgetown University School of Medicine, Georgetown University Archives, Georgetown University, Washington, D.C.
10. In this early period of clinical research, the line between a private practitioner and clinical scientist was not as sharp as it later came to be. Some private practitioners, particularly those who had studied abroad or completed a residency, acquired sufficient scientific expertise to perform important clinical research while in practice. Consider Thomas S. Cullen, the epitome of the academic private practitioner. After completing a residency in gynecology at Johns Hopkins under Howard Kelly, he entered private practice in Baltimore. While in practice, he conducted extensive research on the pathology of the female reproductive tract, which resulted in more than 100 papers and several books, including two that became classics. In 1932, he left private practice to become a professor of gynecology at Johns Hopkins, a position he held until his retirement in 1939 (Minute, Thomas S. Cullen, with meeting of March 31, 1953, Minutes,

the Johns Hopkins Hospital Medical Advisory Board, the Alan Mason Chesney Medical Archives of the Johns Hopkins Medical Institutions, Baltimore, Md.).

11. Columbia University College of Physicians and Surgeons, Report of the Dean (1911), p. 2.
12. Massachusetts General Hospital, *Annual Report* (1914), Section B, pp. 13–14.
13. Flexner, *Medical Education in the United States and Canada*, p. 108.
14. Harvey Cushing, "Suggestions for the Further Development of the Peter Bent Brigham Hospital," 1917, Volume 14, Christian Papers.
15. Detailed discussion of the rise of the teaching hospital is provided in Ludmerer, *Learning to Heal*, pp. 152–65, 219–33.
16. Meeting of February 20, 1914, Minutes, Advisory Board of the Medical Faculty, the Johns Hopkins University School of Medicine.
17. Meeting of March 17, 1913, Minutes of the Meetings of the Faculty, College of Physicians and Surgeons of Columbia University, Archives and Special Collections, A. C. Long Health Sciences Library, Columbia University Medical Center, New York, N.Y.
18. Mount Sinai Hospital, *Annual Report* (1893), p. 22; Cleveland City Hospital, *Annual Report* (1872), p. 2; Lakeside Hospital, *Annual Report* (1898), p. 9; Massachusetts General Hospital, *Annual Report* (1871), p. 54; and Massachusetts General Hospital, *Annual Report* (1902), pp. 10, 260. Cleveland City Hospital was renamed as Lakeside Hospital in 1889.
19. James B. Herrick, "The Educational Function of Hospitals and the Hospital Year," *Am Med Assoc B*, 6 (1911): 106.
20. Massachusetts General Hospital, *Annual Report* (1899), p. 7.
21. Charles E. Rosenberg, *The Care of Strangers: The Rise of America's Hospital System* (New York: Basic Books, 1987).
22. Herrick, "The Educational Function of Hospitals and the Hospital Year," p. 106.
23. Edward D. Churchill, ed., *To Work in the Vineyard of Surgery: The Reminiscences of J. Collins Warren 1842–1927* (Cambridge: Harvard University Press, 1958), p. 72.
24. J. A. Curran, "Internships and Residencies: Historical Backgrounds and Current Trends," *J Med Educ*, 34 (1959): 878.
25. Curran, "Internships and Residencies," p. 878.
26. For instance, in 1937 only 62 of 5,557 medical graduates did not take an internship (*Graduate Medical Education: Report of the Commission on Graduate Medical Education* [Chicago: University of Chicago Press, 1940], p. 88). Reasons included poor health, disability, or choosing a nonclinical career such as basic research or public health.
27. Appendix B, with meeting of June 18–20, 1948, Agenda and Minutes of the Business Meetings of the Council on Medical Education and Hospitals, American Medical Association Archives, Chicago, Ill.
28. Grace Whiting Myers, *History of the Massachusetts General Hospital: June, 1872, to December, 1900* (Boston: Griffith-Stillings Press, 1929), p. 154. Medical staff members of the hospital did have the privilege of removing materials from the library.
29. Meeting of December 1–6, 1945, Agenda and Minutes of the Business Meetings of the Council on Medical Education and Hospitals.
30. See, for instance, meeting of December 17, 1914, Medical Board Minutes, the Babies Hospital; and meeting of June 25, 1935, Minutes of the Medical Board of the Neurological Institute of New York, both Archives and Special Collections,

A. C. Long Health Sciences Library, Columbia University Medical Center, New York, N.Y.

31. *Graduate Medical Education*, p. 43.
32. Memorandum of C. M. Peterson, August 25, 1934, with meeting of February 18–19, 1935, Agenda and Minutes of the Business Meetings of the Council on Medical Education and Hospitals.
33. Evarts A. Graham to J. Burus Amberson, December 16, 1935, Folder 20, Box 4, Evarts Ambrose Graham Papers, Washington University School of Medicine Archives, St. Louis, Mo.
34. See, for instance, the exchange between Nathan P. Colwell, Secretary of the Council on Medical Education and Hospitals, and Henry A. Christian, Chief of Internal Medicine at the Peter Bent Brigham Hospital, in Henry A. Christian to N. P. Colwell, January 26, 1925, and Colwell to Christian, January 30, 1925, both Volume 3, Christian Papers.
35. Columbia University College of Physicians and Surgeons, Report of the Dean (1932), p. 4.
36. Columbia University College of Physicians and Surgeons, Report of the Dean (1932), p. 253.
37. Meeting of June 14, 1932, Minutes, Board of Trustees, Mount Sinai Hospital, Archives, Mount Sinai Medical Center, New York, N.Y; Mount Sinai Hospital, *Annual Report* (1926), p. 70.
38. Meeting of February 1, 1937, Minutes, Advisory Board of the Medical Faculty, the Johns Hopkins University School of Medicine; meetings of November 23, 1921, May 28, 1923, and January 6, 1925, Medical Board Minutes, the Babies Hospital; Henry A. Christian to S. S. Goldwater, October 10, 1917, Volume 3, Christian Papers. The most difficult positions to fill were the January and April positions. Medical graduates understandably did not want to wait six or nine months after graduation to start their internship, and most medical schools were reluctant to grant fourth-year students permission to leave school before graduation.
39. *Graduate Medical Education*, p. 83.
40. *Graduate Medical Education*, p. 12.
41. Meeting of October 9, 1919, Faculty Minutes, Georgetown University School of Medicine, Georgetown University Archives, Georgetown University, Washington, D.C.
42. The thirteen medical schools that delayed conferring the MD degree until after the completion of an internship were Stanford, Northwestern, Marquette, Loyola, Wayne, the College of Medical Evangelists, Duke, Louisiana State, and the Universities of Minnesota, California, Illinois, Cincinnati, and Southern California (*Graduate Medical Education*, p. 256).
43. Victor Johnson, *A History of the Council on Medical Education and Hospitals of the American Medical Association, 1901–1959* (Chicago: American Medical Association, 1959).
44. *Graduate Medical Education*, p. 83. The licensing boards were located in Alabama, Delaware, Idaho, Illinois, Iowa, Louisiana, Michigan, New Hampshire, New Jersey, North Dakota, Oklahoma, Oregon, Pennsylvania, Rhode Island, South Dakota, Utah, Vermont, Washington, West Virginia, Wisconsin, and Wyoming.
45. *Graduate Medical Education*.
46. *Final Report of the Commission on Medical Education* (New York: Office of the Director of the Study, 1932), p. 143.
47. Herrick, "The Educational Function of Hospitals and the Intern Year," p. 107.

48. Meeting of October 18, 1925, Agenda and Minutes of the Business Meetings of the Council on Medical Education and Hospitals.
49. Memorandum on Single Service Internships, August 25, 1934, with meeting of October 26–27, 1934, Agenda and Minutes of the Business Meetings of the Council on Medical Education and Hospitals. Scores of hospitals with seventy-five beds or fewer regularly applied for approval. Descriptions of the educational problems at specific small community hospitals are found in meeting of February 16–18, 1941, Agenda and Business Meetings of the Council on Medical Education and Hospitals; Maurice A. Schnitker to Henry A. Christian, February 15, 1939, Volume 10, Christian Papers; and Harry Buhrmeister to Henry A. Christian, December 5, 1940, Volume 11, Christian Papers.
50. N. P. Colwell, "Progress in Medical Education," in US Department of the Interior Bureau of Education, *Report of the Commissioner of Education* (Washington, D.C.: Government Printing Office, 1913), p. 44.
51. N. P. Colwell, "What the American Medical Association Expects of the Teaching Hospital," *The Diplomate [of the National Board of Medical Examiners]*, December 1929, pp. 9–10.
52. I am indebted to the late Donald Fleming of Harvard University for this interpretation of Ford and Edison.
53. William Welch, "Medical Education in the United States," in William Henry Welch, *Papers and Addresses*, vol. 3 (Baltimore, Md.: Johns Hopkins Press, 1920), p. 124.
54. George Rosen, *The Specialization of Medicine with Particular Reference to Ophthalmology* (New York: Froben Press, 1944).
55. Francis M. Rackemann, *The Inquisitive Physician: The Life and Times of George Richards Minot* (Cambridge: Harvard University Press, 1956), p. 94. For more on Edsall, see Joseph C. Aub and Ruth K. Hapgood, *Pioneer in Modern Medicine: David Linn Edsall of Harvard* (Boston: Harvard Medical Alumni Association, 1970).
56. Peabody was struck down in 1927 at the age of 46 by a leiomyosarcoma of the stomach, an unusual form of stomach cancer. Famous as a sensitive and caring physician, not just as an outstanding clinical investigator, he wrote from his deathbed one of the most compelling essays ever on the doctor-patient relationship, "The Care of the Patient." Even today, the article's last sentence resonates with compassionate healers: "One of the essential qualities of the clinician is interest in humanity, for the secret of the care of the patient is in caring for the patient" (Francis W. Peabody, "The Care of the Patient," *JAMA*, 88 [1927]: 877–82). For more on Peabody, see Oglesby Paul, *The Caring Physician: The Life of Dr. Francis W. Peabody* (Boston: Francis A. Countway Library of Medicine/Harvard Medical Alumni Association, 1991).
57. Peter Bent Brigham Hospital, *Annual Report* (1915), p. 47.
58. Untitled manuscript by Henry A. Christian, 1913, Volume 1, Christian Papers.
59. Meeting of June 10, 1929, Peter Bent Brigham Hospital Executive Committee Minutes, 1921–1958, Storage Code HC4NM, Peter Bent Brigham Hospital Records, Brigham and Women's Hospital Archives, Boston, Mass.
60. Henry A. Christian to Frederick S. Lee, March 19, 1913, Volume 1, Christian Papers.
61. Peter Bent Brigham Hospital, *Annual Report* (1919), p. 56.
62. Peter Bent Brigham Hospital, *Annual Report* (1929), p. 84.
63. Henry A. Christian, "Pioneer Features of Staff Organization," 1938, Volume 46, Christian Papers.

64. Peter Bent Brigham Hospital, *Annual Report* (1946), p. 89.
65. *Graduate Medical Education*, p. 101.
66. Report of the Staff Committee on Professional Services on Residency and Graduate Training, with meeting of October 15, 1952, the Johns Hopkins University School of Medicine, Minutes of the Medical Faculty and Committees, the Alan Mason Chesney Medical Archives of the Johns Hopkins Medical Institutions, Baltimore, Md.
67. A splendid account of the residency system at Vanderbilt is found in Timothy C. Jacobson, *Making Medical Doctors: Science and Medicine at Vanderbilt since Flexner* (Tuscaloosa: University of Alabama Press, 1987).
68. Christian originally called his visiting professors "Visiting Physician, Pro Tem." The first, in 1913, was William S. Thayer of Johns Hopkins (Henry A. Christian to Alexander Cochrane, February 28, 1914, Volume 5, Christian Papers).
69. *Graduate Medical Education*, p. 99.
70. See, for instance, Henry A. Christian to James B. Conant, April 17, 1936, Volume 4, Christian Papers.
71. Essentials in a Hospital Approved for Residencies in Specialties, with meeting of February 12, 1933, Agenda and Minutes of the Business Meetings of the Council on Medical Education and Hospitals.
72. *Graduate Medical Education*, p. 116.
73. Columbia University College of Physicians and Surgeons, Report of the Dean (1941), p. 5.
74. *Graduate Medical Education*, p. 117.
75. The Johns Hopkins Hospital, *Superintendent's Report* (1922), p. 25. Among those who accompanied Palmer were A. Raymond Dochez, Dana Atchley, William Ladd, and Robert Loeb, each of whom subsequently had notable academic careers.
76. Presbyterian Hospital in the City of New York, *Annual Report* (1934), p. 56. Some of the projects carried out by the ophthalmology residents included a study of the injection of fluid and air into the vitreous as a treatment for detached retina, an investigation of the intraocular administration of adrenal gland extracts in patients with glaucoma, a study of capillary fragility in retinal hemorrhage, and an investigation of the effect of sulfanilamide on experimental keratitis of the rabbit. See Presbyterian Hospital in the City of New York, *Annual Report* (1936), p. 54, and (1938), p. 56.
77. Columbia University College of Physicians and Surgeons, Report of the Dean (1940), p. 8.
78. Henry Schmitz to Henry A. Christian, January 22, 1929, and Roberto Escamilla to Henry A. Christian, June 12, 1935, both Volume 9, Christian Papers.
79. *Graduate Medical Education*, p. 100.
80. For instance, of 502 individuals who worked as an intern or resident at the Peter Bent Brigham Hospital during its first quarter-century, 233 had attended Harvard Medical School, while 272 had come from other schools. Ninety alumni ultimately remained in Boston, an additional 22 settled elsewhere in Massachusetts, 72 went to New York State, and the rest dispersed among 37 states and 13 foreign countries. Data from Register of Former Members of the Staff, Peter Bent Brigham Hospital, *Annual Report* (1937), pp. 157–234.
81. Prior to air travel, a trip from San Francisco to the East Coast involved a five-day train ride, with an annoying depot change and transfer of trains in Chicago. The trip typically cost $150 to $250, which equaled a month's salary for many junior faculty members. Lane Hospital, the Stanford teaching hospital, did not appoint

its first resident from a medical school other than Stanford until 1929. It required population growth and the emergence of air travel for West Coast teaching hospitals to become competitive with the more established hospitals. See N. C. Gilbert to Henry A. Christian, December 6, 1940, and Arthur L. Bloomfield to Henry A. Christian, November 15, 1940, both Volume 13, Christian Papers; and David A. Rytand, *Medicine and The Stanford University School of Medicine circa 1932: The Way It Was* (Palo Alto, Calif.: Stanford University School of Medicine Alumni Association, 1984), pp. 29, 51.

82. J. Arthur Myers, *Masters of Medicine: An Historical Sketch of the College of Medical Sciences University of Minnesota 1888–1966* (St. Louis, Mo.: Warren H. Green, 1968).
83. Charles W. Mayo, *Mayo: The Story of My Family and My Career* (Garden City, N.Y.: Doubleday, 1968), p. 23.
84. An account of life as a resident at the Rockefeller Institute is found in Paul, *The Caring Physician*, pp. 26–33.
85. Henry A. Christian to Reginald Fitz, January 30, 1912, Volume 3, Christian Papers.
86. Peter Bent Brigham Hospital, *Annual Report* (1923), p. 121.
87. James A. Gannon Jr. to Soma Weiss, n.d., Folder 128, Box 2, Soma Weiss Papers, MC 823, Rare Books and Special Collections, Francis A. Countway Library of Medicine, Harvard Medical School, Boston, Mass.
88. I am indebted to W. Bruce Fye for this information about the Mayo Clinic. See also W. Bruce Fye, "The Origins and Evolution of the Mayo Clinic from 1864 to 1939," *B Hist Med*, 84 (2010): 323–57.
89. Gordon B. Myers to Henry A. Christian, December 22, 1936, Volume 10, Christian Papers.
90. David M. Davis, "The History of the Resident System," *T Stud Coll Physicians Phila*, 27 (1959): 79.
91. Jacobson, *Making Medical Doctors*, pp. 174–75.
92. William P. Longmire Jr., *Alfred Blalock: His Life and Times* (privately printed, 1991), p. 36.
93. Harvey, *Adventures in Medical Research*, p. 26.
94. Harvey, *Adventures in Medical Research*, p. 229.
95. Henry A. Christian to Reginald Fitz, January 30, 1912, Volume 3, Christian Papers.
96. Peter Bent Brigham Hospital, *Annual Report* (1919), p. 60.
97. Henry A. Christian to Charles P. Curtis, June 23, 1926, Volume 5, Christian Papers.
98. Peter Bent Brigham Hospital, *Annual Report* (1938), p. 113. "Laggard" was a relative term, given that the same year house officers at the hospital published 23 papers (p. 84).
99. Data from Register of Former Members of the Staff, Peter Bent Brigham Hospital, *Annual Report* (1937), pp. 157–234.
100. George Weisz, *Divide and Conquer: A Comparative History of Medical Specialization* (New York: Oxford University Press, 2006); quotation, p. xix.
101. Peter Bent Brigham Hospital, *Annual Report* (1938), pp. 116–17.
102. Galen S. Wagner, Bess Cebe, Marvin P. Rozear, and E. A. Stead Jr., *What This Patient Needs Is a Doctor* (Durham, N.C.: Carolina Academic Press, 1978), p. 157.
103. Wagner, Cebe, Rozear, and Stead Jr., *What This Patient Needs Is a Doctor*, p. 157.
104. John Laszlo and Francis A. Neelon, *The Doctors' Doctor: A Biography of Eugene A. Stead Jr., MD* (Durham, N.C.: Carolina Academic Press, 2006), p. 262.

105. Ross Golden to Henry A. Christian, November 16, 1918, Volume 7, Christian Papers.
106. Aub and Hapgood, *Pioneer in Modern Medicine*, p. 312.
107. *Graduate Medical Education*, p. 142.
108. World War I, of course, created significant stresses for medical education. Many staff members were called overseas, leaving a greater burden for those at home. To increase the supply of physicians, many internship programs were reduced in length—from 24 months to 16, or from 16 months to 12—making training harder and more intense. However, during the war, residency programs grew in both size and number.
109. Lakeside Hospital, *Annual Report* (1914), p. 30, and (1915), p. 31.
110. Massachusetts General Hospital, *Annual Report* (1932), pp. 18–20.
111. Massachusetts General Hospital, *Annual Report* (1921), p. 8.
112. Lakeside Hospital, *Annual Report* (1925), p. 17.
113. Paul Beeson to Soma Weiss, November 26, 1940, Folder 48, Box 1, Weiss Papers.
114. R. L. Duffus and L. Emmett Holt Jr., *L. Emmett Holt: Pioneer of a Children's Century* (New York: D. Appleton-Century, 1940), p. 136. The most notable of these assistants was John Howland, the pioneering pediatrician at Johns Hopkins, who early in his training spent time with Holt.
115. Quoted in Robert K. Richards, *Continuing Medical Education: Perspectives, Problems, Prognosis* (New Haven: Yale University Press, 1978), p. 18.
116. Roswell T. Pettit to Henry A. Christian, December 7, 1928, Volume 10, Christian Papers.
117. William H. Brown to George H. Humphreys, October 6, 1944, Folder "Hosps Mt. Sinai 1944," Box 366, Office of the Executive VP for Health Sciences/Dean of the Faculty of Medicine, Central Files, Archives and Special Collections, A. C. Long Health Sciences Library, Columbia University Medical Center, New York, N.Y.
118. Detailed accounts of the New York Post-Graduate Medical School are provided in the annual reports of the Dean of the Columbia University College of Physicians and Surgeons.
119. George H. Humphreys to I. Snapper, October 12, 1944, Folder "Hosps Mt. Sinai 1944," Box 336, Office of the Executive VP for Health Sciences/Dean of the Faculty of Medicine, Central Files.
120. Columbia University College of Physicians and Surgeons, Report of the Dean (1931), p. 11.

CHAPTER 4

1. Peter Bent Brigham Hospital, *Annual Report* (1943), p. 26.
2. The Johns Hopkins Hospital, *Superintendent's Report* (1924), pp. 61–62.
3. Ernst P. Boas, *The Unseen Plague: Chronic Disease* (New York: J. J. Augustin, 1940).
4. Henry A. Christian to Mrs. Hooper, October 3, 1912, Volume 1, Henry A. Christian Papers, Archives HMS B68, Rare Books and Special Collections, Francis A. Countway Library of Medicine, Harvard Medical School, Boston, Mass.
5. "Report of the Staff Committee on Professional Services on Residency and Graduate Teaching," with meeting of October 15, 1952, Executive Committee Minutes, the Johns Hopkins Hospital, the Alan Mason Chesney Archives of the Johns Hopkins Medical Institutions, Baltimore, Md.

6. See, for instance, Peter Bent Brigham Hospital, *Annual Report* (1928), p. 135 (Christian's remarks); Peter Bent Brigham Hospital, *Annual Report* (1932), p. 62 (Cushing's remarks); and J. M. T. Finney, *A Surgeon's Life* (New York: G. P. Putnam's Sons, 1940), p. 62.
7. George Crile Jr., "Surgery, in the Days of Controversy," *JAMA*, 262 (1989): 256–258 (Cleveland Clinic); Homer W. Humiston to Henry A. Christian, January 29, 1927, Volume 8, Christian Papers (Mayo Clinic). According to Humiston, individuals in Mayo's three-year surgical residency received relatively little operative experience. However, after residency, many became a "first assistant" to a Mayo surgeon, a position that provided abundant operating experience.
8. In surgery, junior house officers were allowed to do minor procedures, with supervision. As they progressed up the pyramid surgical residents were given the opportunity to perform simple procedures without direct supervision and more complex operations with supervision from the chief resident or an attending surgeon. Surgical faculty were almost always present in the surgical suite or in the hospital, readily available to scrub in if a resident needed help. Chief residents had the authority to perform operations themselves or to delegate a case to a junior. Typically, they assigned simpler cases to the assistant residents and did the more challenging or interesting operations themselves. The chief of surgery or a faculty member assisted the chief resident (or even did the operation himself, with the chief resident assisting) if the chief resident was performing a procedure for the first time or taking on an especially difficult case.

   To many surgical residents, brimming with eagerness and impatience, the time they had to wait before receiving operative responsibility often seemed interminable. However, when that time came, they were customarily ready, and the transition from assistant to operator typically went seamlessly. One former surgical resident at Johns Hopkins described the experience of his cohort in doing their first appendectomy and cholecystectomy. "We had assisted The Resident and the visiting staff so many, many times at operation after operation, that by the time we undertook the procedures on our own, it hardly seemed as if, in fact, we were doing so for the first time" (Mark M. Ravitch, "The Surgical Residency: Then, Now, and Future," *Pharos*, Winter 1987, p. 13).
9. "Presentation of Certificates of Fellowship, June 23, 1923," in Folder "Education—Fellows, Residents," 3–PR20, Cleveland Clinic Archives, Cleveland, Ohio.
10. Edward D. Churchill to Philip B. Price, January 10, 1957, Folder 22, Box 3, Edward D. Churchill Papers, Rare Books and Special Collections, Francis A. Countway Library of Medicine, Harvard Medical School, Boston, Mass.
11. William Dock to Henry A. Christian, November 6, 1936, Volume 10, Christian Papers.
12. Quoted in Oglesby Paul, *The Caring Physician: The Life of Francis W. Peabody* (Francis A. Countway Library of Medicine/Harvard Medical Alumni Association, 1991), p. 116.
13. Peter Bent Brigham Hospital, *Annual Report* (1928), p. 131.
14. See, for instance, Peter Bent Brigham Hospital, *Annual Report* (1928), pp. 133–34.

15. Soma Weiss, Notes for Meeting of Interns and Resident Staff, n.d., Folder 48, Box 1, Soma Weiss Papers, MC 823, Rare Books and Special Collections, Francis A. Countway Library of Medicine, Harvard Medical School, Boston, Mass. The Hungarian-born Weiss succeeded Christian, serving as the Hersey Professor of the Theory and Practice of Physic at Harvard Medical School and Physician-in-Chief at the Peter Bent Brigham Hospital from 1939 to 1942, before tragically dying of a ruptured Berry aneurysm (dilated blood vessels in the brain) days after his 43rd birthday. A splendid clinical investigator, he described the changes in the pulmonary vessels caused by mitral stenosis, the role of left ventricular failure in the development of acute pulmonary edema, and, with Robert W. Wilkins, the relationship between heart failure and vitamin B_1 (thiamine) deficiency in beriberi. Dynamic and charismatic, he inspired many physicians who worked at "the Brigham" in the late 1930s and early 1940s, including Paul Beeson and Eugene Stead. Dr. Beeson frequently spoke to me of the enormous influence Weiss had on him and others.
16. Peter Bent Brigham Hospital Medical Service, Instructions for Clinical Clerks, Folder 39, Box 1, Weiss Papers.
17. In anticipation, perhaps, of Andy Warhol's famous comment that everyone has his "fifteen minutes of fame," medical educators understood the ephemeral nature of medical knowledge and the fact that few scientific investigations proved lasting. To encourage residents to evaluate work critically, medical teachers began reciting a now-familiar aphorism: "So often in medicine this week's pearl is next week's glass bead." To my knowledge the origin of this aphorism is unknown.
18. Entry of Coons, 1937, Massachusetts General Hospital, Medical Interns' Autobiographies, 1927–1940, Archives, Massachusetts General Hospital, Boston, Mass.
19. Peter Bent Brigham Hospital, *Annual Report* (1921), p. 118.
20. M. Kaufman to Henry A. Christian, April 27, 1944, Volume 51, Christian Papers.
21. Benson B. Roe to Edward Churchill, November 5, 1950, Folder 32, Box 5, Churchill Papers.
22. A. McGehee Harvey, *Adventures in Medical Research: A Century of Discovery at Johns Hopkins* (Baltimore, Md.: Johns Hopkins University Press, 1974), pp. xii–xiii.
23. Entry of Henry H. Brewster, 1938, Massachusetts General Hospital, Medical Interns' Autobiographies.
24. *Graduate Medical Education: Report of the Commission on Graduate Medical Education* (Chicago: University of Chicago Press, 1940), p. 135.
25. Charles W. Mayo, *Mayo: The Story of My Family and My Career* (Garden City, N.Y.: Doubleday, 1968), p. 339.
26. Quoted in Michael Bliss, *Harvey Cushing: A Life in Surgery* (New York: Oxford University Press, 2005), p. 426.
27. Mayo, *Mayo*, p. 91.
28. Mayo, *Mayo*, p. 103.
29. Finney, *A Surgeon's Life*, p. 340.
30. Peter Bent Brigham Hospital, *Annual Report* (1938), p. 112.
31. Henry A. Christian, "Hospital Mosaics," Address at Mortgage Redemption Dinner of Beth Israel Hospital, June 4, 1944, Volume 51, Christian Papers.
32. Mayo, *Mayo*, p. 82.
33. Peter Bent Brigham Hospital, *Annual Report* (1944), p. 57.

34. S. Burt Wolbach to Henry A. Christian, July 2, 1947, Volume 53, Christian Papers.
35. Lewellys F. Barker, *Time and the Physician: The Autobiography of Lewellys F. Barker* (New York: G. P. Putnam's Sons, 1942), p. 166.
36. Joseph C. Aub and Ruth K. Hapgood, *Pioneer in Modern Medicine: David Linn Edsall of Harvard* (Boston: Harvard Medical Alumni Association, 1979), p. 130.
37. See, for instance, C. W. McClure to Dr. Christian, July 25, 1918, Volume 7, Christian Papers; and Henry Buhrmeister to Henry A. Christian, August 10, 1935, Volume 10, Christian Papers.
38. Henry A. Christian to Frank Billings, November 2, 1914, Volume 1, Christian Papers; Peter Bent Brigham Hospital, *Annual Report* (1919), p. 58.
39. Minutes of the Hospital Committee, April 5, 1937, with meeting of April 7, 1937, Executive Faculty Minutes, Washington University School of Medicine, Washington University School of Medicine Archives, St. Louis, Mo.
40. See, for instance, meeting of October 9, 1930, Medical Board Minutes, the Babies Hospital, Archives and Special Collections, A. C. Long Health Sciences Library, Columbia University Medical Center, New York, N.Y.; meeting of April 18, 1922, Peter Bent Brigham Hospital Executive Committee Minutes, 1921–1958, Storage Code HC4NM, Peter Bent Brigham Hospital Records, Brigham and Women's Hospital Archives, Boston, Mass.
41. Henry A. Christian to Joseph B. Howland, November 13, 1920, Volume 6, Christian Papers.
42. Kenneth M. Ludmerer, *Learning to Heal: The Development of American Medical Education* (New York: Basic Books, 1985), pp. 152–65, 219–33.
43. For an important sociological study of the management of error, see Charles L. Bosk, *Forgive and Remember: Managing Medical Failure* (Chicago: University of Chicago Press, 1979).
44. *Regulations for Residents and House Officers*, Massachusetts General Hospital, 1931, p. 13, located in Folder 2, Box 12, Edward D. Churchill Papers, Rare Books and Special Collections, Francis A. Countway Library of Medicine, Harvard Medical School, Boston, Mass.
45. Meeting of November 24, 1930, Minutes of the Medical Board, the Presbyterian Hospital in the City of New York, Archives and Special Collections, A. C. Long Health Sciences Library, Columbia University Medical Center, New York, N.Y. Ideally, the physicians caring for the patient were present at the time the autopsy was performed, though in practice this often proved impractical.
46. W. G. MacCallum, *William Halsted: Surgeon* (Baltimore, Md.: Johns Hopkins Press, 1930), p. 132.
47. See, for instance, the letters from Henry A. Christian to J. B. Howland of November 26, 1926, March 18, 1921, and April 21, 1921, all Volume 6, Christian Papers.
48. Charles E. Rosenberg, *The Care of Strangers: The Rise of America's Hospital System* (New York: Basic Books, 1987).
49. Massachusetts General Hospital, *Annual Report* (1928), p. 5.
50. For instance, see Harry Buhrmeister to Henry A. Christian, December 5, 1940, Volume 11, Christian Papers, for a description of the deficiencies of the residency program at a small community hospital, this one in Lafayette, Indiana. Of course, exceptions occurred, such as the excellent training programs at Newark Beth Israel Hospital, which are described inAlan M. Kraut and Deborah A. Kraut, *Covenant of Care: Newark Beth Israel and the Jewish Hospital in America* (New Brunswick, N.J.: Rutgers University Press, 2007).

51. For more on American teaching hospitals of the period, see Kenneth M. Ludmerer, *Time to Heal: American Medical Education from the Turn of the, Century to the Era of Managed Care* (New York: Oxford University Press, 1999), pp. 102–124.
52. John Nunemaker to Henry A. Christian, September 19, 1940, Volume 11, Christian Papers.
53. Massachusetts General Hospital, *Annual Report* (1936), pp. 26–32; quotation, p. 32.
54. Tinsley R. Harrison to Henry A. Christian, February 24, 1941, Volume 12, Christian Papers.
55. Ludmerer, *Time to Heal*, p. xxii.
56. William P. Longmire Jr., *Alfred Blalock: His Life and Times* (privately printed, 1991), p. 215.
57. Evarts A. Graham to Nathaniel Allison, February 18, 1928, Folder 18, Box 3, Evarts Ambrose Graham Papers, Washington University School of Medicine Archives, St. Louis, Mo. For more on Graham, see C. Barber Mueller, *Evarts A. Graham: The Life, Lives, and Times of the Surgical Spirit of St. Louis* (Hamilton, Ont.: BC Decker, 2002).
58. See, for instance, Peter Bent Brigham Hospital, *Annual Report* (1938), p. 117.
59. The University of Southern California School of Medicine provides a typical example. See Paul S. McKibben to N. P. Colwell, August 21, 1931, Folder "Re 3rd Year Add. (1931)," Dean's Office Files, University of Southern California School of Medicine, Norris Medical Library, University of Southern California, Los Angeles, Calif.
60. *Graduate Medical Education*, p. 255.
61. Peter Bent Brigham Hospital, *Annual Report* (1925), p. 123 ("not too large"); newspaper clipping, "Standards Listed for Ideal Hospital," February 12, 1937, Volume 44, Christian Papers ("hurried in his work").
62. The Johns Hopkins Hospital, *Superintendent's Report* (1925), pp. 24–25; The Johns Hopkins Hospital, *Superintendent's Report* (1940), pp. 4–5. It may be helpful to note why the hospital length of stay was so long at this time. In part this resulted from the custom of admitting patients on a Thursday or Friday for diagnostic studies or elective surgery scheduled for the following Monday. Even more, it was a consequence of the prevailing practice of imposing prolonged bed rest following a heart attack, a surgical procedure, giving birth, and in many other conditions. The lack of chronic care facilities in the community led to extremely long stays for some patients, especially those convalescing from a neurological problem or orthopedic surgery. As an extreme example, in 1944 the orthopedic service of the Peter Bent Brigham Hospital had a patient occupying a hospital room for nearly a year and another for a year and a half (Meeting of April 19, 1944, Peter Bent Brigham Hospital Executive Committee Minutes).
63. Peter Bent Brigham Hospital, *Annual Report* (1913–14), p. 40.
64. Peter Bent Brigham Hospital, *Annual Report* (1928), p. 145.
65. Peter Bent Brigham Hospital, *Annual Report* (1925), p. 79.
66. Massachusetts General Hospital, *Annual Report* (1923), p. 129.
67. John E. Deitrick and Robert C. Berson, *Medical Schools in the United States at Mid-Century* (New York: McGraw-Hill, 1953), pp. 61–62.
68. Report on the Semi-Private Situation at the Presbyterian Hospital, with meeting of June 15, 1937, Minutes of the Medical Board, the Presbyterian Hospital in the City of New York.

69. "Resolutions Passed by the Board of Trustees at its Meeting on June 11, 1945," Folder 10, Dean's Office Files (Byron L. Robinson, 1941–46), I.D. Number 20DB009, Special Collections Division, University of Arkansas for Medical Sciences Library, Little Rock, Ark. For more on relations between "town" and "gown," including the inevitable tensions that were present, see Ludmerer, *Time to Heal*, pp. 115–18.
70. Peter Bent Brigham Hospital, *Annual Report* (1925), p. 144.
71. David Strayhorn to Henry A. Christian, November 25, 1936, Volume 10, Christian Papers.
72. Paul B. Magnuson, *Ring the Night Bell: The Autobiography of a Surgeon* (New York: Little, Brown, 1960), p. 37.
73. Magnuson, *Ring the Night Bell*, p. 37 ("why"); Thomas B. Turner, *Heritage of Excellence: The Johns Hopkins Medical Institutions, 1914–1947* (Baltimore, Md.: Johns Hopkins University Press, 1974), p. 269 ("new knowledge").
74. Medical Board, Recommendations of the Committee on Diets, November 1930, Folder 11, Box 54, Society of the New York Hospital, Secretary/Treasurer Papers (1811–1933), Archives, the New York Hospital-Cornell Medical Center, New York, N.Y.
75. Ludmerer, *Time to Heal*, pp. 41–51, 102–24, 249–59.
76. Stephen A. Hoffmann, *Under the Ether Dome: A Physician's Apprenticeship at Massachusetts General Hospital* (New York: Charles Scribner's Sons, 1986), p. 286.
77. James Wynn to Henry A. Christian, November 11, 1921, Volume 8, Christian Papers.
78. Susan E. Lederer, *Subjected to Science: Human Experimentation in America before the Second World War* (Baltimore, Md.: Johns Hopkins University Press, 1997).
79. Emily K. Abel, "'In the Last Stages of Irremediable Disease': American Hospitals and Dying Patients before World War II," *B Hist Med*, 85 (2011): 29–56.
80. Hospital Committee Meeting, January 2, 1923, with meeting of January 3, 1923, Executive Faculty Minutes, Washington University School of Medicine.
81. Meeting of October 1, 1940, Minutes of the Executive Committee of the Board of Governors, the Society of the New York Hospital, Archives, the New York Hospital-Cornell Medical Center, New York, N.Y.
82. A Communication from the Senior Class of Woman's Medical College of Pennsylvania, with meeting of June 22, 1917, Minutes of Faculty Meetings, Woman's Medical College of Pennsylvania, Legacy Center (Archives and Special Collections), Drexel University College of Medicine, Philadelphia, Pa. A faculty committee assigned to investigate the matter found that the charges were substantiated.
83. Mayo, *Mayo*, p. 104. For more on conditions at municipal hospitals, see Harry F. Dowling, *City Hospitals: The Undercare of the Underprivileged* (Boston: Harvard University Press, 1982).
84. See, for instance, meeting of February 16, 1937, Transactions of the Medical Board of the New York Hospital, Archives, the New York Hospital-Cornell Medical Center, New York, N.Y.
85. Maxwell Finland to Harry F. Dowling, April 7, 1981, Folder 9, Box 2, Maxwell Finland Papers, Rare Books and Special Collections, Francis A. Countway Library of Medicine, Harvard Medical School, Boston, Mass. Eugene Stead ended this practice when he became chair of internal medicine at Emory.

86. Memorandum of December 10, 1931, on medical activities of internes, Folder 326–7, Box "Hospital Records 1894–1937," Hospital Records, Georgetown University Archives, Georgetown University, Washington, D.C.
87. Ludmerer, *Time to Heal*, pp. 63, 94.
88. Rosenberg, *The Care of Strangers*, pp. 286–309.
89. So rigid were class distinctions at that time that authorities at some teaching hospitals considered the separation of private from semiprivate patients to be even more important than not allowing either group of paying patients to mix with ward patients. See, for instance, Report on the Semi-Private Situation at the Presbyterian Hospital, with meeting of June 15, 1937, Minutes of the Medical Board, the Presbyterian Hospital in the City of New York.
90. Quoted in William H. Welch, "On Some of the Humane Aspects of Medical Science," *Johns Hopkins University Circulars*, June 1886, p. 103.
91. Finney, *A Surgeon's Life*, pp. 126–27. For more on the repugnance of American physicians with the calloused treatment of patients they observed in Germany, see Thomas Neville Bonner, *American Doctors and German Universities: A Chapter in International Intellectual Relations 1870–1914* (Lincoln: University of Nebraska Press, 1963), pp. 104–5. Curiously, Abraham Flexner defended the treatment of patients in Germany, though he stood virtually alone in this. See Abraham Flexner, *Medical Education in Europe* (New York: Carnegie Foundation for the Advancement of Teaching, 1912), p. 166.
92. William Osler, "The Master-Word in Medicine," in William Osler, *Aequanimitas with Other Addresses to Medical Students, Nurses and Practitioners of Medicine*, 3rd ed. (Philadelphia: Blakiston Company, 1932), pp. 349–71.
93. Allen Kennedy to Henry A. Christian, January 5, 1941, Volume 12, Christian Papers.
94. Kristin Celello, *Making Marriage Work: A History of Marriage and Divorce in the Twentieth-Century United States* (Chapel Hill: University of North Carolina Press, 2009); Martha R. Fowlkes, *Behind Every Successful Man: Wives of Medicine and Academe* (New York: Columbia University Press, 1980).
95. Osler, "The Student Life," in Osler, *Aequanimitas*, p. 415.
96. Osler, "Internal Medicine as a Vocation," in Osler, *Aequanimitas*, p. 136.
97. Finney, *A Surgeon's Life*, pp. 384–85.
98. Mayo, *Mayo*, pp. 253 ("rarely saw"), 347 ("friendly strangers"), 347 ("price a father"), 193 ("Mother's loneliness"), 193 ("cried like a child"), 84 ("I'd never advise").
99. Quoted in Richard H. Shryock, *The Unique Influence of The Johns Hopkins University on American Medicine* (Copenhagen: Ejnar Munksgaard, 1953), p. 36.
100. Lisabeth Cohen, *A Consumers' Republic: The Politics of Mass Consumption in Postwar America* (New York: Alfred A. Knopf, 2003); Nancy Tomes, "Merchants of Health: Medicine and Consumer Culture in the United States, 1900–1940," *J Am Hist*, September 2001, pp. 519–547; Nancy Tomes, "The 'Information Rx,'" in David J. Rothman and David Blumenthal, eds., *Medical Professionalism in the New Information Age* (New Brunswick, N.J.: Rutgers University Press, 2010), pp. 40–65; and Nancy Tomes, "An Undesired Necessity: The Commodification of Medical Service in the Interwar United States," in Susan Strasser, ed., *Commodifying Everything: Relationships of the Market* (New York: Routledge, 2003), pp. 97–118.
101. Allen Whipple and Albert Lamb to Medical Board of the Presbyterian Hospital, February 28, 1921, with meeting of April 4, 1921, Minutes of the Medical Board, the Presbyterian Hospital in the City of New York.

102. *Regulations for Residents and House Officers*, Massachusetts General Hospital, p. 11.
103. Warren T. Vaughan to Henry A. Christian, December 1918, Volume 7, Christian Papers.

CHAPTER 5

1. Entries of Thomas Sterling Claiborne ("especially interested"), 1932, and Morton Morris Pinckney ("candy shop"), 1930, Massachusetts General Hospital, Medical Interns' Autobiographies, 1927–1940, Massachusetts General Hospital Archives, Boston, Mass. See also entry of John W. Norcross, 1935.
2. See, for instance, entries of James A. Halsted, 1930, and William H. Beckman, 1935, Massachusetts General Hospital, Medical Interns' Autobiographies.
3. Entry of Richard B. Capps, 1931, Massachusetts General Hospital, Medical Interns' Autobiographies.
4. Entry of Burness E. Moore, 1940, Massachusetts General Hospital, Medical Interns' Autobiographies.
5. See, for instance, entries of E. F. Bland, 1927, and Morton Morris Pinckney, 1930, Massachusetts General Hospital, Medical Interns' Autobiographies. This should not be a surprise, given the smaller differences in income between specialists and general practitioners, and among specialists in different fields, at this time.
6. Entry of Conger Williams, 1938, Massachusetts General Hospital, Medical Interns' Autobiographies.
7. Rarely, physicians in general practice applied for residency positions, hoping at this later date to gain entry to a specialty. In general they were at a competitive disadvantage with fourth-year students or current interns who were seeking a residency.
8. Henry A. Christian, "How to Select an Interneship," *J Phi Rho Sigma*, November 1924, p. 1, in Volume 37, Henry A. Christian Papers, Archives HMS B68, Rare Books and Special Collections, Francis A. Countway Library of Medicine, Harvard Medical School, Boston, Mass.
9. Christian, "How to Select an Interneship," pp. 1, 4.
10. Wallace B. Hamby, "The Making of a Neurosurgeon and What Came of It: An Autobiography," unpublished manuscript, August 1974, 3-PR10 Hamby, Cleveland Clinic Archives, Cleveland, Ohio.
11. Meeting of February 12, 1933, Agenda and Minutes of the Business Meetings of the Council on Medical Education and Hospitals, American Medical Association Archives, Chicago, Ill.
12. Thayer Hobson to Edward D. Churchill, November 7, 1955, Folder 10, Box 4, Edward D. Churchill Papers, Rare Books and Special Collections, Francis A. Countway Library of Medicine, Harvard Medical School, Boston, Mass.
13. Donald C. Balfour to Evarts Graham, December 21, 1939, Folder 1, Box 1, Evarts A. Graham Papers, Washington University School of Medicine Archives, St. Louis, Mo.
14. Henry A. Christian, "The Teaching of Medicine at the Peter Bent Brigham Hospital," *B Harvard Med School Alumni Assoc*, January 1929, p. 6.
15. "Internship Examination Scheme," 1937, Folder 7, Box 5, Elliott Cutler Papers, Rare Books and Special Collections, Francis A. Countway Library of Medicine, Harvard Medical School, Boston, Mass.

16. Hospital Committee meeting, December 3, 1923, with meeting of December 5, 1923, Executive Faculty Minutes, Washington University School of Medicine, Washington University School of Medicine Archives, St. Louis, Mo.
17. Elliott C. Cutler to B. C. MacLean, May 24, 1937, Folder 7, Box 5, Cutler Papers.
18. Carl H. Lenhart to Elliott C. Cutler, May 19, 1937, Folder 7, Box 5, Cutler Papers.
19. Ralph M. Hueston to A. C. Furstenberg, December 6, 1938, Folder G-J 1938, Box 42, University of Michigan Medical School Records, Michigan Historical Collections, Bentley Historical Library, University of Michigan, Ann Arbor, Mich.
20. George Whipple to Lewis H. Weed, September 26, 1927, October 1, 1927, and October 13, 1927; Lewis H. Weed to George Whipple, September 28, 1927, and October 11, 1927; all Folder "G. Whipple Mar 1927–Dec 1927," Box 46, Correspondence Files, Office of the Dean of the Medical Faculty, the Johns Hopkins School of Medicine, Record Group 3, Series B, Archive of the Johns Hopkins University School of Medicine, the Alan Mason Chesney Medical Archives of the Johns Hopkins Medical Institutions, Baltimore, Md.
21. J. R. T. to Henry A. Christian, May 26, 1918, Volume 7, Christian Papers. For more on the problems encountered by African-Americans, women, and Jews when seeking hospital positions, see Kenneth M. Ludmerer, *Time to Heal: American Medical Education from the Turn of the Century to the Era of Managed Care* (New York: Oxford University Press, 1999), pp. 94–95.
22. Supplement 22, with meeting of November 8, 1942, Agenda and Minutes of the Business Meetings of the Council on Medical Education and Hospitals.
23. See, for instance, Winthrop Pennock to Worth Hale, November 27, 1929, Folder 1062, Dean's Subject File, Harvard Medical School, Harvard Medical School Archives, Rare Books and Special Collections, Francis A. Countway Library of Medicine, Harvard Medical School, Boston, Mass.; Willard C. Rappleye to Dear Dr., 1935, Folder 1946–1948, Residents and Interns: Correspondence, 1936–1989, Box 301, Office of the Executive Vice President for Health Sciences/Dean of the Faculty of Medicine, Central Files, Archives and Special Collections, A. C. Long Health Sciences Library, Columbia University Medicine Center, New York, N.Y.
24. Meeting of October 1, 1928, Minutes of the Medical Board, the Johns Hopkins Hospital, the Alan Mason Chesney Medical Archives of the Johns Hopkins Medical Institutions, Baltimore, Md.
25. Elliott C. Cutler to Herman L. Blumgart, May 11, 1937, Folder 7, Box 5, Cutler Papers.
26. Helen Eastman Martin, *The History of the Los Angeles County Hospital (1878–1968) and the Los Angeles County-University of Southern California Medical Center (1968–1979)* (Los Angeles: University of Southern California Press, 1979), p. 77. Conditions could also be extremely unpleasant for the few African-Americans who served as house officers in desegregated hospitals. For instance, sometimes they encountered racial epithets scrawled on lavatory walls or found themselves relegated to the most inconvenient and unkempt bathroom and sleeping facilities.
27. See, for instance, the list of grievances filed by interns at the Georgetown University Hospital in 1931. Intern Statement, September 15, 1931, Folder 326–7, Box "Hospital Records 1894–1931," Georgetown University Hospital Records, Georgetown University Archives, Georgetown University, Washington, D.C.
28. Soma Weiss to Harry A. Bray, December 22, 1931, Folder 92, Box 2, Soma Weiss Papers, MC 823, Rare Books and Special Collections, Francis A. Countway Library of Medicine, Harvard Medical School, Boston, Mass.

29. Meeting of March 12, 1923, Minutes of the Medical Board, the Johns Hopkins Hospital, the Alan Mason Chesney Medical Archives of the Johns Hopkins Medical Institutions, Baltimore, Md.
30. See, for instance, meeting of June 10, 1929, Executive Committee Minutes, 1921–1958, Peter Bent Brigham Hospital, Storage Code HC4NM, Peter Bent Brigham Hospital Records, Brigham and Women's Hospital Archives, Boston, Mass.; and meeting of April 1, 1947, Minutes of the Medical Board, the Johns Hopkins Hospital.
31. Patricia Scollard Painter, *Henry Ford Hospital: The First 75 Years* (Detroit, Mich.: Henry Ford Health System, 1997), p. 36.
32. Entry of John T. Edsall, 1929, Massachusetts General Hospital, Medical Interns' Autobiographies.
33. Samuel A. Levine to Henry A. Christian, August 8, 1939, Volume 11, Christian Papers.
34. Meetings of February 1, 1937, and October 3, 1938, Minutes of the Medical Board, the Johns Hopkins Hospital.
35. On seasonality, see letter of December 31, 1973, Chief Resident Letters, Massachusetts General Hospital, Massachusetts General Hospital Department of Medicine Archives, Boston, Mass.; Peter Bent Brigham Hospital, *Annual Report* (1926), p. 120.
36. Meeting of August 2, 1926, Executive Faculty Minutes, University of Colorado School of Medicine, Denison Memorial Library, University of Colorado Health Sciences Center, Denver, Colo.
37. Hamby, "The Making of a Neurosurgeon," p. 111 (Cleveland Clinic); meeting of February 4, 1929, Minutes of the Medical Board, the Johns Hopkins Hospital (Johns Hopkins); H. B. Howard to Henry A. Christian, March 27, 1918, and Henry A. Christian to H. B. Howard, March 27, 1918, both Volume 6, Christian Papers (Peter Bent Brigham Hospital).
38. Meeting of April 21, 1925, Minutes of the Medical Board, the Mount Sinai Hospital Archives, the Mount Sinai Medical Center, New York, N.Y.
39. The Georgetown University Hospital is one example. See Memorandum "Internes," Folder 326–7, Box "Hospital Records 1894–1931," Georgetown University Hospital Records.
40. H. J. Stander to Otto H. Schwarz, September 13, 1940, Folder 6, Box 6, Henricus J. Stander Papers, Archives, the New York Hospital-Cornell Medical Center, New York, N.Y.
41. Edward D. Churchill to Leo Eloesser, April 1, 1937, Folder 8, Box 3, Churchill Papers.
42. Charles P. Wilson to Henry A. Christian, December 16, 1937, Volume 10, Christian Papers.
43. Charles W. Mayo, *Mayo: The Story of My Family and My Career* (Garden City, N.Y.: Doubleday, 1968), p. 82. This same resident claimed he found holding retractors and hemostats during surgery to be "profoundly moving" (p. 79), a statement few surgical house officers would have made. He certainly had "the right stuff" for surgery, if he is to be believed.
44. D. W. Dunlop to Soma Weiss, February 18, 1941, Folder 96, Box 2, Weiss Papers.
45. Wang Kai-Hsi, "A Brief Report of Two Years of Postgraduate Surgical Training in America," 1947, Folder 1, Box 102, Jerome P. Webster Papers, Archives and Special Collections, A. C. Long Health Sciences Library, Columbia University Medical Center.

46. Francis M. Rackemann, *The Inquisitive Physician: The Life and Times of George Richards Minot* (Cambridge: Harvard University Press, 1956), p. 174.
47. Peter Bent Brigham Hospital, *Annual Report* (1924), pp. 122–23, quotation, p. 123.
48. J. M. T. Finney, *A Surgeon's Life: The Autobiography of J. M. T. Finney* (New York: G. P. Putnam's Sons, 1940), p. 108.
49. Presbyterian Hospital in the City of New York, *Annual Report* (1934), p. 47; Kai-Hsi, "A Brief Report."
50. Peter Bent Brigham Hospital, *Annual Report* (1923), p. 124. The discovery of insulin helped lead to the discovery of liver treatment for pernicious anemia. George Minot, who developed the liver treatment, fell ill with diabetes in October 1921. His life was saved in January 1923, when he became one of the first patients to receive insulin. This allowed him to regain his health and perform the work that later saved the lives of countless victims of pernicious anemia (Rackemann, *The Inquisitive Physician*, pp. 120–40).
51. Lewis Thomas, *The Youngest Science: Notes of a Medicine-Watcher* (New York: Bantam, 1984), p. 35.
52. See, for instance, the entries of Thomas Coolidge, 1927, J. H. Fay, 1927, and James Graeser, 1927, Massachusetts General Hospital, Medical Interns' Autobiographies.
53. Edwards A. Park, "John Howland Award Address," *Pediatrics*, 10 (1952): 104.
54. Laurent Feiner to Charles A. Elsberg, May 24, 1920, with meeting of June 4, 1920, Minutes of the Medical Board of the Neurological Institute of New York, Archives and Special Collections, A. C. Long Health Sciences Library, Columbia University Medical Center, New York, N.Y.
55. This definition of "burnout" is taken from Jodie Eckleberry-Hunt, Anne Van Dyke, David Lick, and Jennifer Tucciarone, "Changing the Conversation from Burnout to Wellness: Physician Well-being in Residency Training Programs," *J Grad Med Educ*, 1 (2009): 225–30. Rare does not mean nonexistent. For an example of an episode of burnout in a house officer at the Peter Bent Brigham Hospital, see meeting of December 18, 1939, Executive Committee Minutes, 1921–1958, Peter Bent Brigham Hospital.
56. Howard Gardner, Mihaly Csikszentmihalyi, and William Damon, *Good Work: When Excellence and Ethics Meet* (New York: Basic Books, 2001);Teresa Amabile and Steven Kramer, "Do Happier People Work Harder?," *NY Times*, September 4, 2011, p. SR 7.
57. Entry of Frank B. Sutts, 1932, Massachusetts General Hospital, Medical Interns' Autobiographies.
58. Paul B. Magnuson, *Ring the Night Bell: The Autobiography of a Surgeon* (Birmingham: University of Alabama School of Medicine, 1986), p. 55 (Pennsylvania); Thomas Bourne Turner, *Part of Medicine, Part of Me: Musings of a Johns Hopkins Dean* (Baltimore, Md.: Williams and Wilkins, 1981), p. 36 (Johns Hopkins).
59. Thomas, *The Youngest Science*, p. 36.
60. Peter Bent Brigham Hospital, *Annual Report* (1938), p. 114.
61. Roy Cohn to Edward Churchill, October 27, 1938, Folder 8, Box 3, Churchill Papers.
62. Hugh Young, *A Surgeon's Autobiography* (New York: Harcourt, Brace and Company, 1940), p. 244.
63. Jerome Lowenstein, *The Midnight Meal and Other Essays about Doctors, Patients, and Medicine* (Ann Arbor: University of Michigan Press, 2005).
64. Janet Farrar Worthington, "Home, Sweet Dome," *Hopkins Med*, Winter 2011, pp. 45–46.
65. Peter Bent Brigham Hospital, *Annual Report* (1938), pp. 115–16.

66. Peter Bent Brigham Hospital, *Annual Report* (1939), p. 79.
67. Philips D. Edson to Henry A. Christian, December 1927, Volume 8, Christian Papers.
68. Maurice A. Schnitker to Henry A. Christian, February 28, 1940, Volume 11, Christian Papers.
69. Reginald Fitz to Henry A. Christian, March 9, 1918, Volume 7, Christian Papers. Fitz, who was planning to marry in England, only wished that Christian "were going to be [there] to stamp the ceremony with [his] official seal" (Reginald Fitz to Henry A. Christian, June 21, 1918, Volume 7, Christian Papers).
70. Warren Vaughan to Henry A. Christian, 1931, Volume 9, Christian Papers.
71. Eugene A. Stead Jr. to Henry A. Christian, August 17, 1941, Volume 12, Christian Papers.
72. Peter Bent Brigham Hospital, *Annual Report* (1949), p. 40.
73. J. A. Curran, "Internships and Residencies: Historical Backgrounds and Current Trends," *J Med Educ*, 34 (1959): 882.
74. Peter Bent Brigham Hospital, *Annual Report* (1927), p. 72.
75. Charles P. Wilson to Henry A. Christian, February 7, 1927, Volume 7, Christian Papers.
76. See, for instance, *Regulations for Residents and House Officers*, Massachusetts General Hospital, p. 21, located in Folder 2, Box 12, Edward D. Churchill Papers, Rare Books and Special Collections, Francis A. Countway Library of Medicine, Harvard Medical School, Boston, Mass.
77. *Graduate Medical Education: Report of the Commission on Graduate Medical Education* (Chicago: University of Chicago Press, 1940), p. 90.
78. *Graduate Medical Education*, p. 162.
79. Meeting with House Staff and New Interns, Folder 48, Box 1, Weiss Papers.
80. See, for instance, Peter Bent Brigham Hospital, *Annual Report* (1922), p. 122.
81. This highly effective treatment, an exceptional example of clinical investigation leading to rational therapy, became widely used for a short time, before being superseded by sulfa drugs. See Scott H. Podolsky's excellent book, *Pneumonia before Antibiotics: Therapeutic Evolution and Evaluation in Twentieth-Century America* (Baltimore, Md.: Johns Hopkins University Press, 2006).
82. One surgical chair felt compelled to defend his house staff. "We have reached the point where the necessary daily work may be more than our staff can perform without undue physical strain. The 'old timers' may think that the newer generations are unwilling or unable to work as hard as they did. That is not true" (Peter Bent Brigham Hospital, *Annual Report* [1940], p. 74).
83. Robert M. Heyssel, "The House Officer: Student or Employee?," unpublished address, n.d., in Box 1, House Staff Training Programs, General Administration Information, the Johns Hopkins Hospital, No. 507745, the Alan Mason Chesney Medical Archives of the Johns Hopkins Medical Institutions, Baltimore, Md.
84. Massachusetts General Hospital, *Annual Report* (1934), p. 29.

CHAPTER 6

1. Presbyterian Hospital in the City of New York, *Annual Report* (1939), p. 52.
2. See, for instance, Report of the Surgical Service, Barnes Hospital, *Annual Report*, 1928–29.
3. *Graduate Medical Education: Report of the Commission on Graduate Medical Education* (Chicago: University of Chicago Press, 1940), p. 101.
4. "A Review of the Program of the Medical Center," with meeting of July 7, 1937, Minutes of the Medical Board, the Presbyterian Hospital in the City of New York,

Archives and Special Collections, A. C. Long Health Sciences Library, Columbia University Medical Center, New York, N.Y.; Report of the Committee on Medical Specialties, Massachusetts General Hospital, December 19, 1935, Folder 8, Box 1, Evarts Ambrose Graham Papers, Washington University School of Medicine Archives, St. Louis, Mo.

5. Table 6.1 is taken from *Graduate Medical Education*, p. 257.
6. Rosemary Stevens, *American Medicine and the Public Interest* (New Haven: Yale University Press, 1971), pp. 158–59.
7. Meeting of January 5, 1937, Transactions of the Medical Board of the New York Hospital, Archives, the New York Hospital-Cornell Medical Center, New York, N.Y.
8. Meeting of June 23, 1930, Agenda and Minutes of the Business Meetings of the Council on Medical Education and Hospitals, American Medical Association Archives, Chicago, Ill.
9. Paul B. Magnuson, *Ring the Night Bell: The Autobiography of a Surgeon* (New York: Little, Brown, 1960), pp. 209–10.
10. Among the scholarship that has identified features of "progressive" reform continuing through the administration of Franklin D. Roosevelt, see Barry D. Karl, *The Uneasy State: The United States from 1915 to 1945* (Chicago: University of Chicago Press, 1983); William A. Link, *American Epoch: A History of the United States since 1900* (New York: McGraw-Hill, 1993); and Alice Kessler-Harris, *In Pursuit of Equity: Women, Men and the Quest for Economic Citizenship in 20th-Century America* (New York: Oxford University Press, 2003).
11. Loyal Davis, *Fellowship of Surgeons: A History of the American College of Surgeons* (Springfield, Ill.: Charles C. Thomas, 1960), pp. 133–34.
12. Davis, *Fellowship of Surgeons*, esp. pp. 173, 204–5, and 386–89. In 2007 the organization was renamed the Joint Commission.
13. Table 6.2 is derived from Council on Medical Education and Hospitals, "Background and Development of Residency Review and Conference Committees," *JAMA*, 165 (1957): 62.
14. *Graduate Medical Education*, pp. 102–3.
15. *Graduate Medical Education*, p. 113.
16. *Graduate Medical Education*, p. 114.
17. See, for instance, John Alexander to R. C. Buerki, September 18, 1936, Folder 8, Box 1, Graham Papers.
18. *Graduate Medical Education*, pp. 137–39.
19. "Background and Development of Residency Review and Conference Committees," pp. 60–64.
20. Paul E. Spangler to Edward D. Churchill, June 23, 1947, Folder 42, Box 1, Edward D. Churchill Papers, Rare Books and Special Collections, Francis A. Countway Library of Medicine, Harvard Medical School, Boston, Mass.
21. For instance, the American Board of Surgery received 1,507 applicants to its "Founders Group" (physicians in practice granted board certification without taking the board examination), of whom 938 were accepted. In internal medicine, 1,800 internists were certified without examination. "Report of the Board of Certification in Surgery, Meeting, May, 1939," Folder 56, Box 8, Elliott Cutler Papers, Rare Books and Special Collections, Francis A. Countway Library of Medicine, Harvard Medical School, Boston, Mass.; William Gerry Morgan, *The American College of Physicians: Its First Quarter Century* (Philadelphia: American College of Physicians, 1940), p. 99.

22. Edward D. Churchill to Henry J. Stanford, February 7, 1947, Folder 41, Box 1, Churchill Papers.
23. *Graduate Medical Education*, p. 133.
24. Francis G. Blake to Soma Weiss, June 12, 1936, Folder 21, Box 1, Soma Weiss Papers, MC 823, Rare Books and Special Collections, Francis A. Countway Library of Medicine, Harvard Medical School, Boston, Mass.
25. A. McGehee Harvey, "The Influence of William Stewart Halsted's Concepts of Surgical Training," *Johns Hopkins Med J*, 148 (1981): 215–36, esp. pp. 220–23.
26. Robert J. Bartz, "Generalists First: The Movement to Refashion General Practice in Post–World War II America" (PhD dissertation, University of California, San Francisco, 2005), pp. 23–24.
27. Evarts A. Graham to Edward D. Churchill, August 27, 1948, Folder 43, Box 1, Churchill Papers.
28. *Graduate Medical Education*, p. 10.
29. Edward C. Rosenow, *History of the American College of Physicians: Executive Perspectives, 1959–1977* (Philadelphia: American College of Physicians, 1984); Davis, *Fellowship of Surgeons*; Kenneth M. Ludmerer, *Time to Heal: American Medical Education from the Turn of the Century to the Era of Managed Care* (New York: Oxford University Press, 1999), pp. 88–90.
30. Meeting of January 4, 1940, Harvard University Medical Faculty, Administrative Board Records, Harvard Medical Archives, Rare Books and Special Collections, Francis A. Countway Library of Medicine, Harvard Medical School, Boston, Mass.
31. Edward L. Munson, "The Needs of Medical Education as Revealed by the War," *AMA B*, 13 (1919): 204–13.
32. Ludmerer, *Time to Heal*, pp. 131–34.
33. See, for instance, Russell Wood to Henry A. Christian, November 13, 1922, and George C. Turnbull to Henry A. Christian, December 22, 1927, both Volume 8, Henry A. Christian Papers, HMS B68, Rare Books and Special Collections, Francis A. Countway Library of Medicine, Harvard Medical School, Boston, Mass.
34. Douglas Donald to Henry A. Christian, October 12, 1921, Volume 8, Christian Papers.
35. Much material pertaining to the creation of the American Federation for Clinical Research is found in the Christian Papers, Volume 13.
36. A. C. Furstenberg, "Graduate Medical Education with Special Reference to Plans for Post-War Requirements," Folder "G-K, 1944," Box 47, University of Michigan Medical School Records, Michigan Historical Collections, Bentley Historical Library, University of Michigan, Ann Arbor, Mich.
37. A splendid example of this process is cardiology. See the notable study by W. Bruce Fye, *American Cardiology: The History of a Specialty and Its College* (Baltimore, Md.: Johns Hopkins University Press, 1996). Similarly, thoracic surgery was begun by general surgeons who took a particular interest in surgery of the chest. However, as the field rapidly developed in the 1930s and 1940s, their experience came to be considered inadequate as a model for the future training of thoracic surgeons. Accordingly, formal training programs, a subspecialty board, and a certifying examination were created. John Alexander to Carl Eggers, January 24, 1946, and Carl Eggers to Edward D. Churchill, February 19, 1946, both Folder 24, Box 1, Edward D. Churchill Papers, Rare Books and Special Collections, Francis A. Countway Library of Medicine, Harvard Medical

School, Boston, Mass. Much material on the emergence of thoracic surgery as a subspecialty of surgery is found in Box 1 of the Churchill Papers.
38. The Peter Bent Brigham Hospital, *Annual Report* (1925), p. 80.
39. Rosemary Stevens, *American Medicine and the Public Interest* (New Haven: Yale University Press, 1971), pp. 218–43.
40. *Surgery, Obstetrics & Gynecology*, which began in 1905, was published by the American College of Surgeons. In 1995 its name was changed to the *Journal of the American College of Surgeons*.
41. The tangled history of gynecology is well illustrated at Johns Hopkins, where a combined department of obstetrics and gynecology was created only in the late 1950s as a condition to lure Allan C. Barnes to accept the chairmanship. Meeting of April 27, 1959, Advisory Board of the Medical Faculty and Committees, the Johns Hopkins University School of Medicine, the Alan Mason Chesney Medical Archives of the Johns Hopkins Medical Institutions, Baltimore, Md. For more on gynecology at Johns Hopkins, seeJohn A. Rock, Timothy R. B. Johnson, and J. Donald Woodruff, eds., *Department of Gynecology and Obstetrics, the Johns Hopkins Hospital University School of Medicine, the Johns Hopkins Hospital: The First 100 Years* (Baltimore, Md.: Williams & Wilkins, 1991).
42. *Graduate Medical Education*, p. 139.
43. For internal medicine, these trends are illustrated in Fye, *American Cardiology*, and Russell C. Maulitz and Diana E. Long, eds., *Grand Rounds: One Hundred Years of Internal Medicine* (Philadelphia: University of Pennsylvania Press, 1988). An excellent account of the tension between generalism and specialization between 1920 and 1950 is Christopher Lawrence and George Weisz, eds., *Greater Than the Parts: Holism in Biomedicine 1920–1950* (New York: Oxford University Press, 1988).
44. Stevens, *American Medicine and the Public Interest*, pp. 161, 256.
45. *Graduate Medical Education*, p. 105.
46. Edward Churchill, "Outline for Address at Suffolk County Medical Society Dinner Meeting," February 26, 1947, Folder 11, Box 6, Churchill Papers.
47. *Graduate Medical Education*, p. 39.
48. Churchill, "Outline for Address at Suffolk County Medical Society Dinner Meeting."
49. *Final Report of the Commission on Medical Education* (New York: Office of the Director of the Study, 1932), p. 328.
50. Lewis Mayers and Leonard V. Harrison, *The Distribution of Physicians in the United States* (New York: General Education Board, 1924).
51. See, for instance, meeting of February 8, 1926, Minutes of the Medical Board, the Johns Hopkins Hospital, the Alan Mason Chesney Medical Archives of the Johns Hopkins Medical Institutions, Baltimore, Md. To house officers, the imperative to repeat laboratory studies was even greater when they received patients transferred from another hospital, for they usually deemed anyone's clinical laboratories other than their own to be unreliable.
52. Meeting of November 13, 1930, Medical Board Minutes, the Babies Hospital, Archives and Special Collections, A. C. Long Health Sciences Library, Columbia University Medical Center, New York, N.Y.
53. Hospital Communication of July 18, 1940, with meeting of September 26, 1940, Minutes of the Executive Committee of the Staff, Hospital of the Woman's Medical College of Pennsylvania, Legacy Center (Archives and Special Collections), Drexel University College of Medicine, Philadelphia, Pa.

54. Winford Smith to Members of the Medical Board, October 21, 1931, Folder "Johns Hopkins Hospital—Dr. W. Smith Correspondence 1929–1931," Box 4XY, Correspondence Files, Office of the Dean of the Medical Faculty, the Johns Hopkins School of Medicine, Record Group 3, Series B, Archives of the Johns Hopkins University School of Medicine, the Alan Mason Chesney Medical Archives of the Johns Hopkins Medical Institutions, Baltimore, Md.
55. Winford Smith to Members of the Medical Board, October 21, 1931 (note #54).
56. Meeting of November 24, 1931, Minutes of the Medical Board of the Neurological Institute of New York, Archives and Special Collections, A. C. Long Health Sciences Library, Columbia University Medical Center, New York, N.Y.
57. Winford Smith to Members of the Medical Board, October 21, 1931 (note #54).
58. Lewellys F. Barker, *Time and the Physician* (New York: G. P. Putnam's Sons, 1942), p. 237.

CHAPTER 7

1. The theme of World War II as a watershed in American history has been developed in William H. Chafe, *The Unfinished Journey: America since World War II*, 2nd ed. (New York: Oxford University Press, 1991), and other notable works.
2. Clark Kerr, *The Uses of the University*, 3rd ed. (Cambridge: Harvard University Press, 1982).
3. Harvard Medical School, *Dean's Report* (1965–66), p. 1.
4. Alexander T. Bunts to J. R. Forsythe, February 23, 1943, Folder 3, Box 1, Alexander T. Bunts, MD, Correspondence/War Correspondence from Fellows, ll-F82, Cleveland Clinic Archives, Cleveland, Ohio.
5. Meeting of March 10, 1944, Peter Bent Brigham Hospital Executive Committee Minutes, 1921–1958, HC4NM, Peter Bent Brigham Hospital Records, Brigham and Women's Hospital Archives, Rare Books and Special Collections, Francis A. Countway Library of Medicine, Harvard Medical School, Boston, Mass. The entire medical profession performed heroically during World War II. It is difficult to know who contributed more—those who cared for the sick and wounded in the theaters of war, or the depleted staffs tending to the civilian population at home. For more on medical education during World War II, see Kenneth M. Ludmerer, *Time to Heal: American Medical Education from the Turn of the Century to the Era of Managed Care* (New York: Oxford University Press, 1999), pp. 125–35.
6. For instance, the University of Maryland. See meeting of February 14, 1946, Faculty Minutes, University of Maryland School of Medicine, Historical and Special Collections, Health Sciences Library, University of Maryland at Baltimore, Baltimore, Md.
7. For instance, the Cleveland Clinic, University of Maryland, University of Michigan, Massachusetts General Hospital, and Mount Sinai Hospital (New York). See Alexander T. Bunts to C. C. McClure, March 26, 1943, Folder 3, Box 1, Bunts Correspondence; meeting of October 23, 1945, Faculty Minutes, University of Maryland School of Medicine; A. C. Furstenberg to Stacy P. Mettier, Folder "1944 C," Box 47, University of Michigan Medical

School Records, Michigan Historical Collections, Bentley Historical Library, University of Michigan, Ann Arbor, Mich.; Massachusetts General Hospital, *Annual Report* (1946), pp. 41–42; Mount Sinai Hospital, *Annual Report* (1945), pp. 25–26.

8. Supplement 4, with meeting of November 8, 1942 ("opportunities"), and meeting of November 19, 1944 ("temporarily"), Agenda and Minutes of the Business Meetings of the Council on Medical Education and Hospitals, American Medical Association Archives, Chicago, Ill.
9. Postwar Medical Education, March 10, 1945, Folder "Bulletins, Association of American Medical Colleges, 1945–48," Dean's Office Files, University of Southern California School of Medicine, Norris Medical Library, University of Southern California, Los Angeles, Calif.
10. Meeting of December 1–6, 1945, Agenda and Minutes of the Business Meetings of the Council on Medical Education and Hospitals.
11. "The American Board of Surgery," December 3, 1946, Folder 40, Box 1, Edward D. Churchill Papers, Rare Books and Special Collections, Francis A. Countway Library of Medicine, Harvard Medical School, Boston, Mass.
12. John E. Deitrick and Robert C. Berson, *Medical Schools in the United States at Mid-Century* (New York: McGraw-Hill, 1953), p. 276.
13. Charles F. Wilkinson Jr. to A. C. Furstenberg, January 7, 1947, Folder "1947 W-Z," Box 50, University of Michigan Medical School Records, Michigan Historical Collections, Bentley Historical Library, University of Michigan, Ann Arbor, Mich.
14. Francis D. Moore and Nathan P. Couch, eds., "Careers in Surgery: A Surgical Alumni Seminar, Peter Bent Brigham Hospital Fiftieth Anniversary Celebration," May 28, 1963, p. 142, Rare Books and Special Collections, Francis A. Countway Library of Medicine, Harvard Medical School, Boston, Mass.
15. For more on the factors promoting specialization, seePatricia L. Kendall, "Medical Specialization: Trends and Contributing Factors," in Robert H. Coombs and Clark E. Vincent, eds., *Psychosocial Aspects of Medical Training* (Springfield, Ill.: Charles C. Thomas, 1971), pp. 449–97.
16. Vernon W. Lippard, *A Half-Century of American Medical Education: 1920–1970* (New York: Josiah Macy Jr. Foundation, 1974), p. 96.
17. The prominence of the state of New York in graduate medical education has continued through the present.
18. The exception was general surgery, where most programs continued to maintain a pyramid system until the late twentieth century.
19. Citizens Commission on Graduate Medical Education, *The Graduate Education of Physicians* (Chicago: American Medical Association, 1966), p. 15.
20. Meeting of August 5, 1952, Minutes of the Medical Board, the Presbyterian Hospital in the City of New York, Archives and Special Collections, A. C. Long Health Sciences Library, Columbia University Medical Center, New York, N.Y.; meeting of April 3, 1956, Minutes of the Board of Governors, the Society of the New York Hospital, Archives, the New York Hospital-Cornell Medical Center, New York, N.Y.
21. Massachusetts General Hospital, *Annual Report* (1979), p. 10.
22. David M. Davis, "The History of the Resident System," *T Stud Coll Physicians Phila*, 27 (1959): 78.

23. Alan M. Kraut and Deborah A. Kraut, *Covenant of Care: Newark Beth Israel and the Jewish Hospital in America* (New Brunswick, N.J.: Rutgers University Press, 2007).
24. Moore and Couch, "Careers in Surgery," p. 30.
25. National Center for Health Services Research, *Financing and Reimbursement of Graduate Medical Education* (Ann Arbor: University of Michigan Library, 1977).
26. Report of Joint Residency Committee, with meeting of February 25, 1975, Minutes of the Medical Board, the Presbyterian Hospital in the City of New York; Massachusetts General Hospital, *Annual Report* (1979), p. 10.
27. Council on Medical Education and Hospitals, *The Student and the Matching Program* (Chicago: American Medical Association, 1955), p. 9. This pamphlet is found in Papers of the General Directors Office, Massachusetts General Hospital, AC 41, Carton 3, Folder "Internships—Matching Plans [1952–1956, 1963]," Massachusetts General Hospital Archives, Boston, Mass.
28. The Match was co-sponsored by the American Medical Association, the Association of American Medical Colleges, the American Hospital Association, the American Catholic Hospital Association, and the American Protestant Hospital Association. For the first year the program was officially named "the National Interassociation Committee on Internships" before permanently changing its name to the "National Intern Matching Program." Students who did not "match" entered the "scramble," feverishly seeking to find the best unfilled internship opportunity in the days that followed the announcement of that year's Match results. The only time the Match was challenged was in 2002, when Paul Jung, a fellow at Johns Hopkins, led a class-action lawsuit against it on antitrust grounds. The suit was dismissed. For more information, see F. J. Mullin, "Internship Appointments," *JAMA*, 145 (1951): 1339–41; F. J. Mullin and John M. Stalnaker, "Hospitals and Interns Benefit from Intern Matching Plan," *Hospitals*, 26 (1952): 81–86, 147–48; John M. Stalnaker, "The Matching Plan Pays Off," *Hospitals*, 27 (1953): 62–66; F. J. Mullin and John M. Stalnaker, "The Matching Plan for Internship Placement: A Report of the First Year's Experience," *J Med Educ*, 27 (1952): 193–200; Alvin E. Roth, "The Origins, History, and Design of the Resident Match," *JAMA*, 289 (2003): 909–12; "Appellate Court Affirms Jung Lawsuit Dismissal," AAMC Press Release, June 5, 2006. Although the Match represented a distinct improvement to the previous system, programs still had the opportunity to apply untoward pressures on students. "We would like you to stay," the distinguished chair of a prominent clinical department said to a high-ranking medical student from his own institution. "To do so, you must agree to rank us first on your list in the Match, and you must tell me now if you will do that. If you cannot commit to us at this time, I shall rank you low enough that you will have no chance of matching with us." Though fictional here, such episodes in fact commonly occurred at some of the most prestigious teaching hospitals. This problem is discussed in meeting of April 11, 1973, Minutes, Faculty Executive Committee, University of Southern California School of Medicine, Dean's Office, University of Southern California School of Medicine, Los Angeles, Calif.; meeting of October 18, 1974, College Committee Minutes, Board of Trustees, Thomas Jefferson University Archives and Special Collections, Thomas Jefferson University, Philadelphia, Pa.; and meeting of March 11, 1976, Executive Committee, Folder "Ex Com March–April 1976," Box 13, University

of Michigan Medical School Records, Michigan Historical Collections, Bentley Historical Library, University of Michigan, Ann Arbor, Mich.

29. Ludmerer, *Time to Heal*, pp. 260–67.
30. Meeting of September 30, 1971, Committee on Internship, Folder "Hospital Medical Board 1971," Dean's Office Files (Winston K. Shorey, 1961–1974), ID Number 20DB016, Special Collections Division, University of Arkansas for Health Sciences Library, Little Rock, Ark.
31. Moore and Couch, "Careers in Surgery," p. 142.
32. "Report of the Advisory Committee on Internships to the Council on Medical Education and Hospitals of the American Medical Association," *JAMA*, 151 (1953): 500.
33. Annual Report of Medical Services (1959), Massachusetts General Hospital, Folder 82, Box 8, John H. Knowles Papers, Rockefeller Archive Center, North Tarrytown, N.Y.
34. Council on Medical Education and Hospitals, *The Student and the Matching Program*, p. 4. The complete results of the first Match, indicating the number of interns sought and the number matched for each hospital participating in the program, are found in Massachusetts General Hospital, General Director's Office, AC 41, Carton 3, Folder "Internships—Matching Plans [1951–1955]," Massachusetts General Hospital Archives, Boston, Mass.
35. Mullin and Stalnaker, "The Matching Plan for Internship Placement," p. 193.
36. Lippard, *A Half-Century of American Medical Education*, p. 96. A valuable account of this subject is found in Rosemary Stevens, Louis Wolf Goodman, and Stephen S. Mick, *Alien Doctors: Foreign Medical Doctors in American Hospitals* (New York: John Wiley and Sons, 1978).
37. I used this term in *Time to Heal*, pp. 181–87.
38. Kenneth M. Ludmerer, "The Origins of Mount Sinai School of Medicine," *J Hist Med All Sci*, 45 (1990): 469–89.
39. Ludmerer, *Time to Heal*, pp. 256–59.
40. Ludmerer, *Time to Heal*, pp. 249–56.
41. Deitrick and Berson, *Medical Schools in the United States at Mid-Century*, pp. 278–80.
42. Citizens Commission on Graduate Medical Education, *The Graduate Education of Physicians*; Lowell T. Coggeshall, *Planning for Medical Progress through Education* (Evanston, Ill.: Association of American Medical Colleges, 1966).
43. August G. Swanson, "Graduate Education: Once for the Exceptional, Now Essential for All," *J Med Educ*, 48 (1973): 183.
44. See, for instance, the observations of Eugene Stead, the iconic chairman of internal medicine at Duke from 1947 to 1967, in Barton F. Haynes, ed., *A Way of Thinking: A Primer on the Art of Being a Doctor. Essays by Eugene A. Stead, Jr., M.D.* (Durham, N.C.: Carolina Academic Press, 1995), p. 70.
45. Massachusetts General Hospital, *Annual Report* (1953), p. 52.
46. Peter Bent Brigham Hospital Surgical Service, *Principles and Procedures* (Boston: Harvard Medical School, 1953), p. 21, located in Peter Bent Brigham Hospital Records, Brigham and Women's Hospital Archives, Rare Books and Special Collections, Francis A. Countway Library of Medicine, Harvard Medical School, Boston, Mass.
47. Francis D. Moore, ed., *Three Surgical Decades: Brigham Surgery and the Residency Program* (Boston: privately printed, 1980), p. 123.

48. Peter Bent Brigham Hospital Service, *Principles and Procedures*, p. 21.
49. W. Bruce Fye, *American Cardiology: The History of a Specialty and Its College* (Baltimore, Md.: Johns Hopkins University Press, 1996).
50. Leo Eloesser to Edward D. Churchill, November 27, 1936, Folder 12, Box 1, Churchill Papers. Much information about the development of thoracic surgery is found in the Churchill Papers.
51. Edward D. Churchill to Lyman A. Brewer III, November 1, 1954, Folder 29, Box 1, Churchill Papers.
52. "Year 64–65," Folder 77, Box 7, Knowles Papers.
53. Columbia-Presbyterian Medical Center, *Annual Report* (1962), pp. 85–86.
54. "Fellowship Training Program in Cardiology" and "Fellowship Training Program in Gastroenterology," both excerpted from meeting of April 8, 1981, of the Joint Committee on House Staff and Postdoctoral Programs, the Johns Hopkins Hospital, House Staff Training Programs, General Administration Information, the Alan Mason Chesney Medical Archives of the Johns Hopkins Medical Institutions, Baltimore, Md.
55. Meeting of May 9, 1978, Minutes, Medical Service Staff Meetings, Columbia-Presbyterian Medical Center, Office of the Chairman, Department of Medicine, College of Physicians and Surgeons of Columbia University, New York, N.Y.
56. For instance, see "The Undesirably Long Curriculum," with meeting of May 21, 1956, and meeting of December 18, 1961, both Minutes of the Advisory Board of the Medical Faculty and Committees, the Johns Hopkins University School of Medicine, the Alan Mason Chesney Medical Archives of the Johns Hopkins Medical Institutions, Baltimore, Md.
57. Joseph F. Kelley to William Michener, November 12, 1973, with meeting of December 6, 1973, Faculty Board Committee Minutes, 11–TA, Cleveland Clinic Archives, Cleveland, Ohio.
58. See, for instance, meeting of December 18, 1961, Minutes of the Advisory Board of the Medical Faculty and Committees, the Johns Hopkins University School of Medicine.
59. Peter Bent Brigham Hospital, *Annual Report* (1961), p. 16.
60. I was present at that conference.
61. Meeting of March 17, 1967, College Committee Minutes, Board of Trustees, Thomas Jefferson University, Thomas Jefferson University Archives and Special Collections, Thomas Jefferson University, Philadelphia, Pa. See also Mary D. Overpeck, "Physicians in Family Practice 1931–67," *Public Health Rep*, 85 (1970): 485–94.
62. Patricia L. Kendall and Hanan C. Selvin, "Tendencies toward Specialization in Medical Training," in Robert K. Merton, George G. Reader, and Patricia L. Kendall, eds., *The Student-Physician: Introductory Studies in the Sociology of Medical Education* (Cambridge: Harvard University Press, 1957), pp. 153–74.
63. Committee on Medical Care Teaching of the Association of Teachers of Preventive Medicine, eds., *Readings in Medical Care* (Chapel Hill: University of North Carolina Press, 1958).
64. Committee on Medical Care Teaching, *Readings in Medical Care*, p. 210.
65. Kendall and Selvin, "Tendencies toward Specialization in Medical Training," pp. 155, 166–67, 174.
66. A thoughtful account of general practice in the 1940s, 1950s, and 1960s is provided in Robert J. Bartz, "Generalists First: The Movement to Refashion

General Practice in Post–World War II America" (PhD dissertation, University of California, San Francisco, 2005), p. 123. Bartz points out (p. 123) that in the 1950s and 1960s general practitioners came to be defined "not by what they were but by what they were not."

67. John O. Boyd Jr. to Evarts A. Graham, November 8, 1951, Folder 20, Box 4, Evarts Ambrose Graham Papers, Washington University School of Medicine Archives, St. Louis, Mo.
68. Committee on Medical Care Teaching, *Readings in Medical Care*, p. 190.
69. Meeting of September 3, 1959, Transactions of the Medical Board of the New York Hospital, Archives, the New York Hospital-Cornell Medical Center, New York, N.Y.
70. Graph showing percentages of Cornell graduates by types of internship, with meeting of September 18, 1973, Transactions of the Executive Faculty, Cornell University College of Medicine, Archives, the New York Hospital-Cornell Medical Center, New York, N.Y. See also Robert E. Coker Jr., Norman Miller, and Alice Levine, "Study of Choice of Specialties in Medicine," Folder 811, Box 66, Knowles Papers.
71. Information on the AMA's support of the rotating internship is found widely in medical school and teaching hospital archives. See, for instance, the letters in Folder "Internships 1910–1957," the Johns Hopkins Hospital, House Staff Training Programs, General Administration Information, the Alan Mason Chesney Medical Archives of the Johns Hopkins Medical Institutions, Baltimore, Md. See also Lippard, *A Half-Century of American Medicine*, pp. 104–5.
72. Citizens Commission on Graduate Medical Education, *The Graduate Education of Physicians*.
73. Max Michael Jr., "Phasing Out the Freestanding Internship," *JAMA*, 218 (1971): 1690–91; Bartz, "Generalists First."
74. Bartz, "Generalists First," pp. 144–45.
75. "Missions, Goals, Objectives of the University of Arkansas College of Medicine," with meeting of March 20, 1975, Executive Committee, Folder "Committees—Executive Com. June '75–Jan 1976," Dean's Office Files (Thomas A. Bruce, 1974–1975), ID Number 20DB017, Special Collections Division, University of Arkansas for Health Sciences Library, Little Rock, Ark.
76. Rosemary Stevens, *American Medicine and the Public Interest* (New Haven: Yale University Press, 1971), p. 301; Carol Black, "Role of Public Policy—UK," manuscript of presentation at ABIM Foundation Summer Forum, 2010.
77. Eliot Freidson, *Professionalism: The Third Logic* (Chicago: University of Chicago Press, 2001).
78. See, for instance, E. W. Fonkalsrud, "Reassessment of Surgical Subspecialty Training in the United States," *Arch Surg*, 104 (1972): 759–60.
79. Stanley J. Reiser, *Medicine and the Reign of Technology* (New York: Cambridge University Press, 1978).
80. Winford Smith to Members of the Medical Board, October 21, 1931, Folder "Johns Hopkins Hospital—Dr. W. Smith Correspondence 1929–1931," Box 4XY, Correspondence Files, Office of the Dean of the Medical Faculty, the Johns Hopkins School of Medicine, Record Group 3, Series B, Archive of the Johns Hopkins University School of Medicine, the Alan Mason Chesney Medical Archives of the Johns Hopkins Medical Institutions, Baltimore, Md.; meeting of December 6, 1973, Transactions of the Medical Board of the

New York Hospital; meeting of February 21, 1961, Minutes of the Medical Board, the Mount Sinai Hospital, Archives, the Mount Sinai Medical Center, New York, N.Y.

81. Meeting of August 4, 1959, Corporate Board of Trustees Minutes, Thomas Jefferson University, Thomas Jefferson University Archives and Special Collections, Thomas Jefferson University, Philadelphia, Pa.
82. Meeting of November 1, 1972, Minutes of the Medical Board, the Presbyterian Hospital in the City of New York.
83. University Hospitals of Cleveland, *Director's Report* (1955), p. 20. See also University Hospitals of Cleveland, *Director's Report* (1959), p. 18.
84. Table 7.1 was compiled from information in Attachment C, with meeting of May 21, 1968, Minutes of the Medical Board, the Presbyterian Hospital in the City of New York.
85. "Report on a Laboratory Facility at the Columbia-Presbyterian Medical Center," with meeting of May 21, 1968, Minutes of the Medical Board, the Presbyterian Hospital in the City of New York.
86. I was one of the students.
87. Massachusetts General Hospital, *Annual Report* (1964), p. 59.
88. Mark E. Silverman and W. Bruce Fye, eds., *J. Willis Hurst: His Life and Teachings* (Mahwah, N.J.: Foundation for Advances in Medicine and Science, 2007), p. 109.
89. Silverman and Fye, *J. Willis Hurst*, p. 98.
90. J. Willis Hurst, *The Quest for Excellence: The History of the Department of Medicine at Emory University School of Medicine* (Atlanta: Scholars Press, 1997), p. 239.
91. Ludmerer, *Time to Heal*, p. 101.
92. Meeting of April 10, 1985, Minutes of the Medical Board, the Presbyterian Hospital in the City of New York.
93. Massachusetts General Hospital, *Annual Report* (1976), p. 85.

CHAPTER 8

1. George Crile Jr., *The Way It Was: Sex, Surgery, Treasure, and Travel* (Kent, Ohio: Kent State University Press, 1992), p. 162.
2. Robert H. Ebert, "The Dilemma of Medical Teaching in an Affluent Society," in John H. Knowles, ed., *The Teaching Hospital: Evolution and Contemporary Issues* (Cambridge: Harvard University Press, 1962), pp. 66–83.
3. Kenneth M. Ludmerer, *Time to Heal: American Medical Education from the Turn of the Century to the Era of Managed Care* (New York: Oxford University Press, 1999), pp. 162–79.
4. Report on Financing of Hospital and Clinic Operations, April 15, 1952, Folder 7, Box 252, Series 359, Chancellor's Office Administrative Files 1936–1959, Record Series 359, University Archives, Department of Special Collections, the University Library, University of California, Los Angeles, Los Angeles, Calif.
5. Table 8.1 is adapted from John H. Knowles, "Medical School, Teaching Hospital, and Social Responsibility: Medicine's Clarion Call," in Knowles, *The Teaching Hospital*, p. 107.
6. Employer-based private medical insurance became wildly popular in the late 1940s and early 1950s, owing to new federal tax deductions granted employers for providing medical insurance benefits. With the costs of hospitalization soaring, medical insurance became a highly sought-after benefit, and, because of favorable tax treatment, it was less costly to businesses than increasing wages.

7. The Peter Bent Brigham Hospital, *Annual Report* (1953), pp. 57–64; meeting of March 8, 1944, Peter Bent Brigham Hospital Executive Committee Minutes, 1921–1958, Storage Code HC4NM, Peter Bent Brigham Hospital Records, Brigham and Women's Hospital Archives, Rare Books and Special Collections, Francis A. Countway Library of Medicine, Harvard Medical School, Boston, Mass.
8. Data on the conversion of ward to semiprivate beds at many important teaching hospitals are found in Attachment F, with meeting of May 15, 1959, Minutes of the Medical Board, the Presbyterian Hospital in the City of New York, Archives and Special Collections, A. C. Long Health Sciences Library, Columbia University Medical Center, New York, N.Y.
9. John S. O'Shea, "Individual and Social Concerns in American Surgical Education: Paying Patients, Prepaid Health Insurance, Medicare and Medicaid," *Acad Med*, 85 (2010): 854–62.
10. Meeting of May 6, 1954, Transactions of the Medical Board of the New York Hospital, Archives, the New York Hospital-Cornell Medical Center, New York, N.Y; meeting of November 7, 1962, Ad Hoc Committee on Medicine at the Massachusetts General Hospital, Folder 45, Box 4, John H. Knowles Papers, Rockefeller Archive Center, North Tarrytown, N.Y.
11. Report of the Committee on the Residency Program, with meeting of March 7, 1956, Minutes of the Medical Board, the Presbyterian Hospital in the City of New York.
12. Attachment F, with meeting of May 15, 1959, Minutes of the Medical Board, the Presbyterian Hospital in the City of New York.
13. Report of the Staff Committee on Professional Services on Residency and Graduate Training, with meeting of October 15, 1952, Minutes, Advisory Board of the Medical Faculty, the Johns Hopkins University School of Medicine, the Alan Mason Chesney Medical Archives of the Johns Hopkins Medical Institutions, Baltimore, Md.
14. Meeting of November 28, 1962, Ad Hoc Committee on Medicine at the Massachusetts General Hospital, Folder 45, Box 4, Knowles Papers.
15. Paul S. Russell, "Surgery in a Time of Change," in Knowles, *The Teaching Hospital*, p. 58.
16. Provision of Medical Service for Paying Patients by Residents, with agenda items for meeting of May 15–16, 1961, Executive Council Meetings and Agendas, Association of American Medical Colleges, Association of American Medical Colleges Archives, Washington, D.C.
17. The 50 percent figure was the experience of many teaching hospitals. See, for instance, the New York Hospital, Chief Residents' Luncheon, December 8, 1964, Folder 3, Box 5, Associate Director of Professional Services Papers, Society of the New York Hospital (Kady, Carver, Baldridge), Archives, the New York Hospital-Cornell Medical Center, New York, N.Y.
18. Ludmerer, *Time to Heal*, pp. 221–36.
19. Steven Shea and Mindy Thompson Fullilove, "Entry of Black and Other Minority Students into U.S. Medical Schools," *N Engl J Med*, 313 (1985): 934–35. These requirements applied to nursing homes as well as to hospitals.
20. Allan L. Friedlich to Edward D. Churchill, August 30, 1961, Folder 115, Box 10, Knowles Papers.
21. Massachusetts General Hospital, *Annual Report* (1966), p. 10.
22. Robert H. Ebert, "The Dilemma of Medical Teaching in an Affluent Society," in Knowles, *The Teaching Hospital*, p. 80.

23. Stephen P. Strickland, *Politics, Science, and Dread Disease: A Short History of United States Medical Research Policy* (Cambridge: Harvard University Press, 1972), p. 249.
24. Meeting of June 13, 1972, Executive Faculty, Folder "Feb-June 1972," Box 132, University of Michigan Medical School Records, Michigan Historical Collections, Bentley Historical Library, University of Michigan, Ann Arbor, Mich.
25. Martin Bergmann, I. Jerome Flance, and Herman T. Blumenthal, "Thesaurosis Following Inhalation of Hair Spray: A Clinical and Experimental Study," *N Engl J Med*, 258 (1958): 471–76.
26. See, for instance, Russell, "Surgery in a Time of Change," p. 58; and John E. Deitrick and Robert C. Berson, *Medical Schools in the United States at Mid-Century* (New York: McGraw-Hill, 1953), p. 139.
27. Attachment D, with meeting of February 3, 1960, Minutes of the Medical Board, the Presbyterian Hospital in the City of New York.
28. John Laszlo and Francis A. Neelon, *The Doctors' Doctor: A Biography of Eugene A. Stead Jr., MD* (Durham, N.C.: Carolina Academic Press, 2006), pp. 105 (quotation), 115, 198–99.
29. Lowell T. Coggeshall, *Planning for Medical Progress through Education* (Evanston, Ill.: Association of American Medical Colleges, 1965), p. 23. Hospitalizations far longer than 10 days were frequent. It was standard practice, for instance, for a patient to remain in the hospital for 21 days following an uncomplicated myocardial infarction (heart attack). Blue Cross and other private insurers regularly paid for hospitalizations even longer than 21 days, as long as there was a medical justification.
30. See, for instance, the statement of a distinguished group of surgical educators, "Report to American Surgical Association of the Committee on Graduate Surgical Education," April 1, 1953, Folder 34, Box 2, Edward D. Churchill Papers, Rare Books and Special Collections, the Francis A. Countway Library of Medicine, Harvard Medical School, Boston, Mass.
31. Doctor X, *Intern* (New York: Harper & Row, 1965), p. 362.
32. Statement on Underlying Educational Policy, p. 16, with meeting of May 21, 1956, Minutes, Advisory Board of the Medical Faculty, the Johns Hopkins University School of Medicine.
33. Francis D. Moore, ed., *Three Surgical Decades: Brigham Surgery and the Residency Program* (Boston: privately printed, 1980), p. 81.
34. Moore, *Three Surgical Decades*, p. 81.
35. Presbyterian Hospital in the City of New York, *Annual Report* (1958), p. 64. Writing these words was Robert F. Loeb, director of the Medical Service, coeditor of a major textbook of medicine, and author of a famous aphorism delineating the three "rules" of internal medicine: "If something works, keep doing it. If what you are doing is not working, do something else. Never send the patient to the surgeon."
36. Stead's leadership transformed Duke into one of the nation's preeminent training programs in internal medicine and one of the country's finest medical schools. Helpful sources on Stead include Laszlo and Neelon, *The Doctors' Doctor*; Galen S. Wagner, Bess Cebe, and Marvin P. Rozear, eds., *E. A. Stead, Jr.: What This Patient Needs Is a Doctor* (Durham, N.C.: Carolina Academic Press, 1978); Barton F. Haynes, ed., *A Way of Thinking: A Primer on the Art of Being a Doctor. Essays by Eugene A. Stead, Jr.* (Durham, N.C.: Carolina Academic Press, 1995); and Barton F. Haynes, ed., *A Way of Working: Essays on the Practice of Medicine. Essays by Eugene A. Stead, Jr.* (Durham, N.C.: Carolina Academic Press, 2001).

37. These articles are reprinted in Haynes, *A Way of Working*, pp. 59–63 ("Training Is No Substitute") and pp. 97–106 ("The Role of the University").
38. Haynes, *A Way of Thinking*, p. 23.
39. Wagner, Cebe, and Rozear, *E. A. Stead, Jr.*, p. 36.
40. Wagner, Cebe, and Rozear, *E. A. Stead, Jr.*, p. 37.
41. Haynes, *A Way of Thinking*, p. 129 (italics in original).
42. Moore, *Three Surgical Decades*, p. 120.
43. Peter Bent Brigham Hospital Surgical Service, *Principles and Procedures* (Boston: Harvard Medical School, 1953), p. 12.
44. Peter Bent Brigham Hospital Surgical Service, *Principles and Procedures*, p. 10.
45. Moore's views of how a surgical training program should be conducted are described in detail in Moore, *Three Surgical Decades*, pp. 1–36.
46. Table, "Performance on American Board of Internal Medicine Examinations of Candidates Taking First Written Examination 1962–1968, by Type of Hospital," with meeting of January 22, 1970, Faculty Board Committee Minutes, 11–TA, Cleveland Clinic Archives, Cleveland, Ohio. The statistics cited referred to the written examination in internal medicine. At this time, the American Board of Internal Medicine also required an oral examination. Results were comparable to those on the written examination.
47. Peter Bent Brigham Hospital Surgical Service, *Principles and Procedures*, p. 11.
48. Richard H. Saunders, "The University Hospital Internship in 1960: A Study of the Programs of 27 Major Teaching Hospitals," *J Med Educ*, 36 (1961): 561–76.
49. Philip A. Tumulty, *The Effective Clinician: His Methods and Approach to Diagnosis and Care* (Philadelphia: W. B. Saunders, 1973), p. 7.
50. Tumulty, *The Effective Clinician*, p. 4.
51. Tumulty, *The Effective Clinician*, p. 6.
52. Tumulty, *The Effective Clinician*, p. 14.
53. Tumulty, *The Effective Clinician*. For more on Tumulty see T. E. Van Metre, "Philip A. Tumulty," *Trans Am Clin Climatol Assoc*, 101 (1990): liv–lvii.
54. I was in that group of medical students. Baughman became the head of the division of cardiology at Johns Hopkins and then the director of the Advanced Heart Disease Program at Brigham and Women's Hospital (the new name of the Peter Bent Brigham Hospital, the Peter Breck Brigham Hospital, and the Boston Hospital for Women after their merger in 1980) until his untimely death in 2009 when struck by a car while jogging.
55. Peter Bent Brigham Hospital Surgical Service, *Principles and Procedures*, p. 6.
56. Peter Bent Brigham Hospital, *Annual Report* (1949), p. 42.
57. Peter Bent Brigham Hospital Surgical Service, *Principles and Procedures*, p. 9.
58. Peter Bent Brigham Hospital Surgical Service, *Principles and Procedures*, p. 9.
59. Peter Bent Brigham Hospital Surgical Service, *Principles and Procedures*, p. 12.
60. Lester A. Steinberg to John Knowles, March 25, 1965, Folder 226, Box 19, Knowles Papers.
61. Ludmerer, *Time to Heal*, pp. 151–61. A notable champion of this viewpoint was Max Finland, a prominent clinical scientist at Boston City Hospital and Harvard Medical School. Diminutive in stature, gargantuan in intellect and kindness, and one of the most important specialists in infectious diseases of his generation, Finland "taught that there is an almost inverse relationship between continuing professional development and economic reward." A. Martin Lerner, "Some Personal Thoughts Concerning the Detroit Medical Center," *Mich Med*, 69 (1970): 577.

62. See, for instance, a statement of John Knowles, in response to a letter of April 18, 1961, Folder 115, Box 10, Knowles Papers.
63. Massachusetts General Hospital, *Annual Report* (1954), p. 35.
64. Georgetown University Medical Center, Purposes and Objectives, with agenda items for meeting of February 28, 1972, Administrative Council Meetings, Georgetown University Medical Center, Office of the Dean, Georgetown University School of Medicine, Washington, D.C.
65. Daniel M. Fox, *Health Policies, Health Politics: The British and American Experience, 1911–1965* (Princeton: Princeton University Press, 1986).
66. Meeting of December 1, 1955, Transactions of the Medical Board of the New York Hospital.
67. Deitrick and Berson, *Medical Schools in the United States at Mid-Century*, pp. 61–62.
68. Milton S. Grossman to John H. Knowles, June 6, 1967, Folder 302, Box 26, Knowles Papers.
69. Meeting of October 15, 1969, Minutes of the Private Patients Committee, Medical Board of the New York Hospital, Archives, the New York Hospital-Cornell Medical Center, New York, N.Y.
70. David G. Rothman, *Strangers at the Bedside: A History of How Law and Bioethics Transformed Medical Decision-Making* (New York: Basic Books, 1991); Susan E. Lederer, *Subjected to Science: Human Experimentation in America before the Second World War* (Baltimore, Md.: Johns Hopkins University Press, 1997).
71. This practice carried no harmful intent. It was meant to help socialize medical students into their new role as physicians. In the 1970s and 1980s, however, as the patient rights and consumer movements grew stronger, medical educators realized that this practice did not meet emerging standards of transparency, and the custom was dropped. After that, a medical student said to a patient something like "Hello. I'm Jane Smith, a third-year medical student."

CHAPTER 9

1. A splendid review of the sociological literature on graduate medical education is found in Renée C. Fox, *The Sociology of Medicine: A Participant Observer's View* (Englewood Cliffs, N.J.: Prentice-Hall, 1989), pp. 108–41. Helpful sociological studies of internship during this period include Emily Mumford, *Interns: From Students to Physicians* (Cambridge: Harvard University Press, 1970); and Stephen J. Miller, *Prescription for Leadership: Training for the Medical Elite* (Chicago: Aldine, 1970). The major studies of residency are Charles L. Bosk's analysis of surgical residency, *Forgive and Remember: Managing Medical Failure* (Chicago: University of Chicago Press, 1979); and Donald Light's study of psychiatry training, *Becoming Psychiatrists: The Professional Transformation of Self* (New York: W. W. Norton, 1980).
2. Evarts A. Graham to Charles R. Reynolds, January 21, 1947, Folder 50, Box 7, Evarts Ambrose Graham Papers, Washington University School of Medicine Archives, St. Louis, Mo.
3. Harry E. Dowling, *City Hospitals: The Undercare of the Underprivileged* (Cambridge: Harvard University Press, 1982).
4. Attachment F, with meeting of May 15, 1959, Minutes of the Medical Board, the Presbyterian Hospital in the City of New York, Archives and Special Collections, A. C. Long Health Sciences Library, Columbia University Medical Center, New York, N.Y.

5. "Faculty Board Residency Review, Department of Pediatrics," with meeting of July 6, 1971, Faculty Board Committee Minutes, Cleveland Clinic, 11–TA, Cleveland Clinic Archives, Cleveland, Ohio.
6. The institution was the New York Hospital. See meeting of October 1, 1959, Transactions of the Medical Board of the New York Hospital, Archives, the New York Hospital-Cornell Medical Center, New York, N.Y.
7. These cultural shifts have been discussed by many writers, including George E. Mowry and Blaine A. Brownell, *The Urban Nation: 1920–1980*, rev. ed. (New York: Hill and Wang, 1981); Richard Wightman Fox and T. J. Jackson Lears, eds., *The Culture of Consumption: Critical Essays in American History 1880–1980* (New York: Pantheon, 1983); and John Kenneth Galbraith, *The Affluent Society* (Boston: Houghton Mifflin, 1958).
8. Meeting of April 5, 1958, Minutes of the Medical Board, the Mount Sinai Hospital, Archives, the Mount Sinai Medical Center, New York, N.Y.; Meeting of April 12, 1977, Minutes of the Medical Service Staff Meetings, Columbia-Presbyterian Medical Center, Office of the Chairman, Department of Medicine, College of Physicians and Surgeons of Columbia University, New York, N.Y.
9. Letter of January 11, 1965, Chief Resident Letters, Massachusetts General Hospital Department of Medicine, Massachusetts General Hospital Department of Medicine Archives, Boston, Mass.
10. House officers tended to reserve their worst behavior for private doctors not affiliated with the hospital, or "LMDs" (local medical doctors). When LMDs referred patients to the hospital, residents were notoriously slow to keep them informed or send them discharge summaries. Frequently house officers disparaged the clinical skill of LMDs to their faces. The faculty at Johns Hopkins observed this behavior in its own house staff: "Consider, then, the reaction of the rural practitioner, his patient and the patient's family to the house officer who says: 'Send him sixty miles by ambulance if you want to, but I'll have to see him in the Accident Room before I can decide whether or not he'll be admitted.' The practitioner must be both thick-skinned and desperate to brave such response a second time" (Report of the Sub-Committee on Professional Relations of the Staff Conference Committee 1959–1960, with meeting of April 26, 1960, Minutes of the Medical Board, the Johns Hopkins Hospital, the Alan Mason Chesney Medical Archives of the Johns Hopkins Medical Institutions, Baltimore, Md.).
11. Massachusetts General Hospital, *Annual Report* (1951), p. 34; Massachusetts General Hospital, *Annual Report* (1967), p. 50.
12. See, for instance, Existing Fringe Benefits of the House Staff of Cleveland Clinic Foundation—1970, with meeting of April 26, 1971, Cleveland Clinic Faculty Board Committee Minutes.
13. Table 9.1 is taken from Dennis K. Wentz and Charles V. Ford, "A Brief History of the Internship," *JAMA*, 252 (1984): 3392. Table 9.2 is taken from meeting of January 19, 1961, Minutes of the Executive Committee of the Board of Governors, the Society of the New York Hospital, Archives, the New York Hospital-Cornell Medical Center, New York, N.Y. Table 9.3 is taken from Attachment H, with meeting of June 24, 1975, Minutes of the Joint Administrative Board, New York Hospital-Cornell Medical Center, Archives, the New York Hospital-Cornell Medical Center, New York, N.Y. In my archival research, I repeatedly found one hospital after another raising its salary scale to remain competitive with other hospitals in its area. I found no evidence of collusion among hospitals to set salaries at a particular level.

14. Minutes of the meeting of the Educational Policy and Curriculum Committee, December 16, 1982, with meeting of December 22, 1982, Minutes, Advisory Board of the Medical Faculty, the Johns Hopkins University School of Medicine, the Alan Mason Chesney Medical Archives of the Johns Hopkins Medical Institutions, Baltimore, Md. See also Robert E. Dedmon, "The Resident and the Medical Student," *JAMA*, 169 (1959): 329–33.
15. See, for instance, the discussion of this point in Presbyterian Hospital in the City of New York, *Annual Report* (1952), pp. 103–8.
16. Dr. X., *Intern* (New York: Harper and Row, 1965), p. 9.
17. A. McGehee Harvey to Russell A. Nelson, September 11, 1958, Folder "Medicine 1958," the Johns Hopkins Hospital, House Staff Training Programs, the Alan Mason Chesney Medical Archives of the Johns Hopkins Medical Institutions, Baltimore, Md.
18. Meeting of May 23, 1968, Graduate Staff Training Program Committee, Medical Board of the New York Hospital, Minutes (May 1968–November 1968), Archives, the New York Hospital-Cornell Medical Center, New York, N.Y.
19. For instance, in 1950 the Massachusetts General Hospital established such a fund, which permitted house officers to borrow up to $1,000 in any 12-month period, with no interest charged until residency had been completed. Between 1952 and 1955, 79 house officers borrowed $67,780 from the fund. See Massachusetts General Hospital, *Annual Report* (1950), p. 39, and (1955), p. 51.
20. Joel H. Goldberg, "House Officers Are Getting Living Wage at Last," *Hosp Physician*, March 1970, p. 67.
21. Differences between teaching and community hospitals of this era are explored extensively in Mumford, *Interns*. As Mumford points out (pp. 214–17), the role of community hospitals should not be disparaged. The challenge for medical students in selecting an internship was to find a program tailored to that person's desires and needs. For students planning to enter general practice, community hospitals were usually better choices than most university teaching hospitals, which seldom offered rotating internships and often disparaged general practice as a career. Many community hospitals, particularly the large ones, had excellent teachers on their medical staffs and close affiliations with medical schools. Later, some of these hospitals evolved into major teaching hospitals of their own right.
22. Cecelia M. Roberts, *Doctor and Patient in the Teaching Hospital: A Tale of Two Life-Worlds* (Lexington, Mass.: D.C. Heath, 1977), pp. 60–64.
23. Dr. X, *Intern*, p. 306.
24. Richard H. Saunders Jr., "The University Hospital Internship in 1960: A Study of the Programs of 27 Major Teaching Hospitals," *J Med Educ*, 36 (1961): 561–676.
25. Dr. X, *Intern*, p. 173.
26. Dr. X, *Intern*, p. 74.
27. Emergency rooms were more challenging places to work after World War II than before. Changing demographic and economic conditions transformed emergency rooms into sites that served large numbers of individuals with minor complaints who had nowhere else to go for medical care, not just the acutely ill or injured. This resulted in much larger numbers of patient visits, much more work for the medical and nursing staffs, and greater challenges in quickly recognizing someone who was seriously ill. See Beatrix Hoffman, "Emergency Rooms: The Reluctant Safety Net," in Rosemary A. Stevens, Charles E. Rosenberg, and

Lawton R. Burns, eds., *History and Health Policy in the United States: Putting the Past Back In* (New Brunswick, N.J.: Rutgers University Press, 2006), pp. 250–72.

28. Supervision was no easy task. Interns needed latitude and freedom. If a resident took over too quickly, the intern's confidence could easily be damaged. Good residents knew when and how to lend a hand, either with an overwhelming workload or a particularly difficult clinical problem. An excellent account of the learning trajectory of interns and residents is found in Molly Cooke, David M. Irby, and Bridget C. O'Brien, *Educating Physicians: A Call for Reform of Medical School and Residency* (San Francisco: Jossey-Bass, 2010), pp. 115–16.
29. Letter of December 23, 1965, Chief Resident Letters, Massachusetts General Hospital Department of Medicine.
30. For house officers, few chores were as irksome as dictating discharge summaries. The patients had already gone home, and residents' attention had moved to other patients. House officers often created work for themselves by making the summaries longer than necessary, and once behind, it was difficult to catch up. Yet few problems frustrated hospital administrators more than delinquent charts, for hospital accreditation could be lost if too many charts were not up-to-date. Various incentives and penalties, including the threat of withholding pay, were regularly discussed, but the problem remained at hospitals everywhere.
31. Committee on Teaching and Education, meeting of June 18, 1962, Folder 61, Box 6, John H. Knowles Papers, Rockefeller Archive Center, North Tarrytown, N.Y.
32. Peter Bent Brigham Hospital Surgical Service, *Principles and Procedures* (Boston: Harvard Medical School, 1953), p. 35.
33. William Hollingsworth, *Taking Care: The Legacy of Soma Weiss, Eugene Stead, and Paul Beeson* (Chapel Hill, N.C.: Professional Press, 1994), p. 111.
34. Letter of December 29, 1958, Chief Resident Letters, Massachusetts General Hospital Department of Medicine.
35. Galen S. Wagner, Bess Cebe, and Marvin P. Rozear, eds., *E. A. Stead, Jr.: What This Patient Needs Is a Doctor* (Durham, N.C.: Carolina Academic Press, 1978), p. 141.
36. As a medical intern at Barnes Hospital, I cared for an elderly woman in terminal condition whose family had instructed us to do everything possible for her. One night while on "long call" I successfully addressed serious problems she had developed at 7 p.m., 10 p.m., and 1 a.m. Just as I was getting ready to go to bed at 4 a.m., the nurses summoned me to see her. I remember thinking to myself, "Why doesn't this woman just die so that I can get some sleep?" The patient responded to my early-morning ministrations, but a day later, after some sleep, I was mortified for having entertained those thoughts. The memory of this incident still troubles me today.
37. Meeting of November 2, 1961, Transactions of the Medical Board of the New York Hospital.
38. As a clinical clerk at the Johns Hopkins Hospital, I witnessed this episode.
39. Richard C. Friedman, J. Thomas Bigger, and Donald S. Kornfeld, "The Intern and Sleep Loss," *N Engl J Med*, 285 (1971): 201–3.
40. Barton F. Haynes, ed., *At the Heart of Medicine: Essays on the Practice of Surgery and Surgical Education by David C. Sabiston, Jr., M.D.* (Durham, N.C.: Carolina Academic Press, 2006), p. 12.
41. Haynes, *At the Heart of Medicine*, p. 6.
42. Letter of January 3, 1968, Chief Resident Letters, Massachusetts General Hospital Department of Medicine.

43. Letter of December 29, 1978, Chief Resident Letters, Massachusetts General Hospital Department of Medicine.
44. Maxwell Finland and William B. Castle, eds., *The Harvard Medical Unit at Boston City Hospital* (Boston: Harvard Medical School, 1983), vol. II, p. 1237.
45. Mumford, *Interns*, pp. 81–86.
46. University Hospitals of Cleveland, *Director's Report* (1958), p. 5.
47. Haynes, *At the Heart of Medicine*, p. 70.
48. Hollingsworth, *Taking Care*, p. 212.
49. Hollingsworth, *Taking Care*, p. 205. On Beeson, see also Richard Rapport, *Physician: The Life of Paul Beeson* (Fort Lee, N.Y.: Barricade, 2001).
50. Laszlo and Neelon, *The Doctors' Doctor*, p. 79.
51. Conversation with David M. Kipnis, August 9, 2010. This opportunity launched Kipnis's interest in energy metabolism and diabetes, and he proceeded to have an unusually distinguished academic career.
52. Wagner, Cebe, and Rozear, *E. A. Stead, Jr.*, p. 220.
53. Hollingsworth, *Taking Care*, p. 99.
54. Hollingsworth, *Taking Care*, p. 109.
55. Wagner, Cebe, and Rozear, *E. A. Stead, Jr.*, p. 196.
56. Hollingsworth, *Taking Care*, p. 208.
57. Dr. X, *Intern*, p. 50.
58. Dr. X, *Intern*, p. 54.
59. Terry Mizrahi, *Getting Rid of Patients: Contradictions in the Socialization of Physicians* (New Brunswick, N.J.: Rutgers University Press, 1986).
60. Massachusetts General Hospital, *Annual Report* (1966), p. 9.
61. Policy Memorandum 2, January 30, 1946, University of Colorado Medical Center Reports, Veterans Administration Hospital Background and Development, Denison Medical Library, University of Colorado Health Sciences Center, Denver, Colo. See also Benjamin J. Lewis, *VA Medical Program in Relation to Medical Schools* (Washington, D.C.: US Government Printing Office, 1970); David M. Worthen, "The Affiliation Partnership between U.S. Medical Schools and the Veterans Administration," *Alabama J Med Sci*, 24 (1987): 83–89; and John A. Gronvall, "The VA's Affiliation with Academic Medicine: An Emergency Post-War Strategy Becomes a Permanent Partnership," *Acad Med*, 64 (1989): 61–66.
62. Meeting with Dr. Jarrett, January 27, 1965, in Folder "Training Program Reviews—1964," the Johns Hopkins Hospital, House Staff Training Programs—Reviews, the Alan Mason Chesney Medical Archives of the Johns Hopkins Medical Institutions, Baltimore, Md.
63. Meeting of September 9, 1971, Transactions of the Medical Board of the New York Hospital.
64. See, for instance, Peter Bent Brigham Hospital, *Annual Report* (1948), p. 58; and Presbyterian Hospital in the City of New York, *Annual Report* (1949), p. 38.
65. Attachment F, with meeting of May 15, 1959, Minutes of the Medical Board, the Presbyterian Hospital in the City of New York.
66. Philip J. Snodgrass, *A Life in Academic Medicine* (New York: iUniverse, 2007), pp. 39–40; quotation, p. 40.
67. J. Willis Hurst, *The Quest for Excellence: The History of the Department of Medicine at Emory University School of Medicine* (Atlanta: Scholars Press, 1997), p. 312.
68. Wagner, Cebe, and Rozear, *E. A. Stead, Jr.*, p. 47.
69. Francis A. Moore, ed., *Three Surgical Decades: Brigham Surgery and the Residency Program* (Boston: privately printed, 1980), p. 122.

70. Meeting of June 4, 1970, Transactions of the Medical Board of the New York Hospital.
71. Albert W. Wu, "Medical Error: The Second Victim," *Brit Med J*, 320 (2000): 726–27.
72. Bosk, *Forgive and Remember*.
73. See, for instance, Albert W. Wu, Susan Folkman, Stephen J. McPhee, and Bernard Lo, "Do House Officers Learn from Their Mistakes?," *JAMA*, 265 (1991): 2089–94.
74. Meeting of July 10–11, 1984, Minutes of Meeting, American Board of Medical Specialties Executive Committee, American Board of Medical Specialties Archives, Chicago, Ill.
75. Meeting of March 14, 1974, Faculty Board Committee Minutes, Cleveland Clinic.
76. Meeting of July 13, 1972, Faculty Board Committee Minutes, Cleveland Clinic.
77. Meeting of May 13, 1981, Faculty Board Committee Minutes, Cleveland Clinic.
78. Roberts, *Doctor and Patient in the Teaching Hospital*, p. 115.
79. Meeting of January 3, 1966, Minutes of the Meetings of the Executive Committee of the Medical Staff, Howard University Hospital, Office of the Medical Director, Howard University Hospital, Washington, D.C.
80. Thomas Duffy, "The House of God *Redux*," in Martin Kohn and Carol Donley, eds., *Return to The House of God: Medical Resident Education 1978–2008* (Kent, Ohio: Kent State University Press, 2008), p. 191.
81. Duffy, "The House of God *Redux*," p. 191.
82. Duffy, "The House of God *Redux*," p. 191.
83. Meetings of March 2, 1977, March 16, 1977, and March 30, 1977, Minutes of the Medical Board, the Presbyterian Hospital in the City of New York; John H. Knowles to Donald Martin, December 29, 1958, Chief Resident Letters, Massachusetts General Hospital Department of Medicine; John Salvaggio, *New Orleans' Charity Hospital: A Story of Physicians, Politics, and Poverty* (Baton Rouge: Louisiana State University Press, 1992), p. 168; and Report of House Staff Policy Review Committee, September 1971, Folder "Residency Training 1952–1971," the Johns Hopkins Hospital, House Staff Training Programs, General Administration Information, the Alan Mason Chesney Medical Archives of the Johns Hopkins Medical Institutions, Baltimore, Md.
84. For instance, see the discussion of this problem at the Columbia Presbyterian Medical Center, meeting of April 20, 1977, Minutes of the Medical Board, the Presbyterian Hospital in the City of New York.
85. Report of House Staff Policy Review Committee [Johns Hopkins], September 1971 (quotations); "Report of the Committee Appointed by the Medical Board to Study Present Methods for Periodic Review of Clinical Experience of the Departments and Divisions of the Hospital and to Make Appropriate Recommendations," with meeting of May 26, 1959, Minutes of the Medical Board, the Johns Hopkins Hospital, the Alan Mason Chesney Medical Archives of the Johns Hopkins Medical Institutions, Baltimore, Md.
86. George Crile Jr., *The Way It Was: Sex, Surgery, Treasure, and Travel, 1907–1987* (Kent, Ohio: Kent State University Press, 1992), p. 162.
87. I was that intern. I discovered my poor evaluation years later while a chief resident of the medical service at Barnes Hospital. At "pizza rounds" one Friday afternoon, the program director said to me, "You're a terrific chief resident. But we were really worried about you when you started. You've improved enormously, and we sure are proud of you now." I was stunned by the comment because

I thought I had always performed well relative to my level of experience (and, indeed, had received awards for my clinical work). Armed with a master key to the department of medicine's offices, I waited until 9 p.m. that night, went into the office of the department chair, David M. Kipnis, in search of my personnel folder, praying that Dr. Kipnis would not suddenly appear to find me rifling through his office. There in the folder I found the chief resident's evaluation of my first month as an intern, citing me for having asked him for help. Also in the folder were evaluations from later in the year that spoke of my "enormous improvement," "newly found confidence," and having outgrown my "early insecurity."

88. Massachusetts General Hospital, *Annual Report* (1958), pp. 60–61; Robert S. Palmer to Daniel Ellis, January 26, 1970, Folder 295, Box 25, Knowles Papers; Walter T. St. Goar to M.G.H. Staff Members, February 9, 1970, Folder 295, Box 25, Knowles Papers; Edward B. Benedict to John V. Lawrence, June 30, 1969, Folder 296, Box 25, Knowles Papers.
89. Salvaggio, *New Orleans' Charity Hospital*, p. 146.
90. Thomas Bourne Turner, *Part of Medicine, Part of Me: Musings of a Johns Hopkins Dean* (Baltimore, Md.: Williams and Wilkins, 1981), p. 37.
91. Peter Bent Brigham Hospital, *Annual Report* (1949), p. 40.
92. *Graduate Medical Education: Report of the Commission on Graduate Medical Education* (Chicago: University of Chicago Press, 1940).
93. [Johns Hopkins] House Staff Policy Review Committee, Subcommittee on Guidelines for Controlling Size and Duration of Training, 1971, Folder "Size," the Johns Hopkins Hospital, House Staff Training Programs, General Administration Information.
94. Saunders, "The University Hospital Internship in 1960."
95. Johns Hopkins House Staff Policy Review Committee, Subcommittee on Guidelines for Controlling Size and Duration of Training.
96. Saunders, "The University Hospital Internship in 1960."
97. Meeting of October 23, 1979, Minutes of the Medical Board, the Presbyterian Hospital in the City of New York.
98. Saunders, "The University Hospital Internship in 1960," esp. p. 645.
99. Saunders, "The University Hospital Internship in 1960," pp. 650–51; quotation, p. 650.
100. *The Graduate Education of Physicians: The Report of the Citizens Commission on Graduate Medical Education* (Chicago: American Medical Association, 1966), p. 59.
101. [Johns Hopkins] House Staff Policy Review Committee, Subcommittee on Guidelines for Controlling Size and Duration of Training.
102. John E. Deitrick and Robert C. Berson, *Medical Schools in the United States at Mid-Century* (New York: McGraw-Hill, 1953), p. 287.
103. *The Graduate Education of Physicians*, p. 58.
104. Meeting of December 1, 1971, Minutes of the Medical Board, the Presbyterian Hospital in the City of New York.
105. Interview with Dick Webster, December 30, 1971, Folder "Dick Webster," Dean's Office Files, University of Southern California School of Medicine, Norris Medical Library, University of Southern California, Los Angeles, Calif.

CHAPTER 10

1. Kenneth M. Ludmerer, *Time to Heal: American Medical Education from the Turn of the Century to the Era of Managed Care* (New York: Oxford University Press, 1999), pp. 327–28.

2. Ludmerer, *Time to Heal*, pp. 214–18, 288–326, and 327–48.
3. Meeting of January 24, 1979, Minutes of the Staff Committee of the Medical Board, the Presbyterian Hospital in the City of New York, Archives and Special Collections, A. C. Long Health Sciences Library, Columbia University Medical Center, New York, N.Y.
4. The Structure of Graduate Medical Education and Its Financing, with agenda items for meeting of April 10, 1986, Executive Council Meetings and Agendas, Association of American Medical Colleges, Association of American Medical Colleges Archives, Washington, D.C.
5. From a sociological perspective, much more needs to be known about house officers' marriages, such as the precise number who married, the frequency and number of children, the occupations of spouses, and the degree to which spouses had to forego further professional education or work in jobs that were other than in their field in order to be the breadwinners of the family.
6. Herbert W. Nickens, Timothy P. Ready, and Robert G. Petersdorf, "Project 3000 by 2000—Racial and Ethnic Diversity in U.S. Medical Schools," *N Engl J Med*, 331 (1994): 473; Steven Shea and Mindy Thompson Fullilove, "The Entry of Black and Other Minority Students into U.S. Medical Schools: Historical Perspective and Recent Trends," *N Engl J Med*, 313 (1985): 936.
7. In the case of *Bakke v. the University of California* (1978), the US Supreme Court ruled that the use of specific quotas based solely on race was not permissible and thus ordered that Allen Bakke, a 34-year-old white engineer, should be admitted to the University of California, Davis, School of Medicine, which had rejected him twice. The decision did permit race to be used as one among many criteria and thus did not mark the end of affirmative action. Much has been written about this landmark judgment. See, for instance,Joel Dreyfus and Charles Lawrence, *The Bakke Case: The Politics of Inequality* (New York: Harcourt, Brace, Jovanovich, 1979); and Timothy J. O'Neill, *Bakke and the Politics of Equality* (Middletown, Conn.: Wesleyan University Press, 1985).
8. This number compared favorably with the percentage of women in other professions—for example, 2 percent in law and less than 1 percent in engineering. However, it was far less than the percentage of women physicians in European countries. For instance, in Germany 30 percent of doctors were women; in the Netherlands, 20 percent; in Great Britain, 25 percent; and in the Soviet Union, 75 percent. See Carol Lopate, *Women in Medicine* (Baltimore, Md.: Johns Hopkins University Press, 1968), p. 30.
9. Janet Bickel, Carolyn Galbraith, and Renee Quinnie, *Women in U.S. Academic Medicine Statistics* (Washington, D.C.: Association of American Medical Colleges, 1994), Table 1. Of course, the women's movement in its various guises encouraged women to enter many other nontraditional fields such as law, business, science, engineering, and academia.
10. Quoted in Ellen S. More, *Restoring the Balance: Women Physicians and the Profession of Medicine, 1850–1995* (Cambridge: Harvard University Press, 1999), p. 241. Unfortunately, race has continued to impact the experiences of African-American physicians. See, for instance, Marcella Nunez-Smith, Leslie A. Curry, JudyAnn Bigby, et al., "Impact of Race on the Professional Lives of Physicians of African Descent," *Ann Intern Med*, 146 (2007): 45–51; and Joseph R. Betancourt and Andrea E. Reid, "Black Physicians' Experience with Race: Should We Be Surprised?," *Ann Intern Med*, 146 (2007): 68–69.

11. Janet Bickel, "Scenarios for Success—Enhancing Women Physicians' Professional Advancement," *West J Med*, 162 (1995): 165–69; quotation, p. 166.
12. Notable studies of the history of women in medicine include Mary Roth Walsh, *"Doctors Wanted: No Women Need Apply": Sexual Barriers in the Medical Profession, 1835–1975* (New Haven: Yale University Press, 1977); Regina Markell Morantz-Sanchez, *Sympathy and Science: Women Physicians and American Medicine* (New York: Oxford University Press, 1985); Ellen S. More, *Restoring the Balance: Women Physicians and the Profession of Medicine, 1850–1995* (Cambridge: Harvard University Press, 1999); and Ann K. Boulis and Jerry A. Jacobs, *The Changing Face of Medicine: Women Doctors and the Evolution of Health Care in America* (Ithaca, N.Y.: Cornell University Press, 2008). For this study, the latter two works were especially helpful. From a sociological perspective, much more needs to be known about the demographics of residency, such as the distribution among the specialties by social class, ethnicity, religion, and race.
13. I was present at that meeting.
14. Alexander J. Walt, "The Challenge and a Vision for Reform of Graduate Medical Education," in Alexander J. Walt, Philip G. Bashook, J. Lee Dockery, and Barbara S. Schneidman, eds., *The Ecology of Graduate Medical Education* (Evanston, Ill.: American Board of Medical Specialties, 1993), pp. 2–3.
15. Recognition of Educational Activities at the Cleveland Clinic Foundation, May 12, 1987, Folder "Education Division," 3-PR20, Cleveland Clinic Archives, Cleveland, Ohio.
16. See, for instance, John N. Aucott, Julie Como, and David C. Aron, "Teaching Awards and Departmental Longevity: Is Award-Winning Teaching the 'Kiss of Death' in an Academic Department of Medicine?," *Perspect Biol Med*, 42 (1999): 280–87.
17. The absence of a strong reward system for teaching at academic medical centers is a major theme in Ludmerer, *Time to Heal*. This problem affected medical students as well as house officers.
18. Lewis Thomas, "What Doctors Don't Know," review of Melvin Konner's *Becoming a Doctor*, *New York Rev Books*, September 24, 1987, pp. 6–11.
19. Philip J. Snodgrass, *A Life in Academic Medicine* (New York: iUniverse, 2007), p. 142. This trend was the most pronounced in large "cognitive" specialties like internal medicine and pediatrics. It was less conspicuous in the surgical fields, where the smaller size of the programs and the need of all faculty—including the department chair—to maintain their operative skills continued to allow residents closer contact with the chairman.
20. David E. Rogers and Robert J. Blendon, "The Academic Medical Center: A Stressed American Institution," *N Engl J Med*, 298: 944, 1978.
21. See, for instance, Richard H. Saunders, "The University Hospital Internship in 1960: A Study of the Programs of 27 Major Teaching Hospitals," *J Med Educ*, 36 (1961): 597.
22. "The Experiences of Medical Students in Obtaining a Residency," a report of the Association of American Medical Colleges, 1986, with meeting of November 14, 1986, Minutes, Executive Staff Meetings, Georgetown University Hospital, Office of the Medical Director, Georgetown University Hospital, Washington, D.C.; August G. Swanson, "The 'Preresidency Syndrome': An Incipient Epidemic of Educational Disruption," *J Med Educ*, 60 (1985): 201–2.

23. Yasmine Iqbal, "Are Residents Applying Too Early for Fellowship Slots?," *Am Coll Physicians Obs*, March 2005, pp. 8–9. Many residents chose to take time off between residency and fellowship rather than run the risk of selecting a subspecialty too early and discovering once they had started that they had made a bad choice. They often spent this nonacademic year working in emergency rooms or intensive care units, which allowed them to pay down debts or accumulate savings. Beginning in the 2010–11 academic year, medical residents were permitted to apply for subspecialty fellowships during the third year of residency. The additional year of experience allowed many residents to be more confident about their choice of a subspecialty field.
24. The problem of faculty taking credit for others' work was one of a number of abuses of authorship, including plagiarism and fraud, that became widely publicized in the 1980s. See Ludmerer, *Time to Heal*, pp. 343–44.
25. "Commitment to an Educational Community," The Johns Hopkins Hospital House Staff Society Council Proposal, with meeting of October 29, 1991, Minutes of the Medical Board, the Johns Hopkins Hospital, the Alan Mason Chesney Medical Archives of the Johns Hopkins Medical Institutions, Baltimore, Md.
26. A splendid description of the contrasts between protest-era house officers and their predecessors is found in Fitzhugh Mullan, *White Coat, Clenched Fist: The Political Education of an American Physician* (New York: Macmillan, 1976). This book provides valuable historical insight into the political radicalization of house officers in the 1960s and 1970s; it has also achieved historical importance of its own as a valuable primary source documenting medical school and residency practices of that period.
27. B. Lamar Johnson Jr. to Sherman M. Mellinkoff, July 24, 1964, Folder "Medicine: Interns & Residents (House Staff) 1961–70," Box 11, Series 401, Administrative Subject Files of Franklin Murphy 1935–71 (Record Series 401), University Archives, Department of Special Collections, University Library, University of California, Los Angeles, Calif.
28. House Staff Petition to the Regents of the University of California, March 1964, Folder "Medicine: Interns & Residents (House Staff) 1961–70," Box 11, Series 401, Administrative Subject Files of Franklin Murphy 1935–71. As other letters in this folder reveal, the administration was sympathetic with the residents' demands, in no small part because they did not want to become noncompetitive with other Los Angeles teaching hospitals, which were paying house officers $1,200 per year more.
29. Rosemary Stevens, *In Sickness and in Wealth: American Hospitals in the Twentieth Century* (New York: Basic Books, 1989).
30. Meeting of October 3, 1967, Executive Faculty, Folder "Oct 1967-Feb 1968," Box 130, University of Michigan Medical School Records, Michigan Historical Collections, Bentley Historical Library, University of Michigan, Ann Arbor, Mich.
31. Meeting of October 3, 1967, Executive Faculty, Folder "Oct 1967-Feb 1968," Box 130, University of Michigan Medical School Records. In the late 1960s and early 1970s, medical students behaved in comparable ways in terms of appearance, demeanor, and activism. See Ludmerer, *Time to Heal*, pp. 238–43.
32. For instance, see meetings of April 12, 1974, and August 16, 1974, Executive Committee Meetings, the George Washington University Hospital, Office of

the Medical Director, the George Washington University Hospital, Washington, D.C.; executive committee meeting of September 14, 1983, Executive Board Minutes, University of Maryland School of Medicine, Dean's Office, University of Maryland School of Medicine, Baltimore, Md.

33. Joel H. Goldberg, "A New Look at House Officers' Incomes," *Hosp Physician*, March 1968, pp. 34–39.
34. House staff activism at Michigan illustrated the differing perspectives of house officers and administrators. In 1971, house staff stipends had increased by 16 percent, 36 percent, 21 percent, and 20 percent during the preceding four years. From the perspective of the faculty and administration, the house staff had clearly been an institutional priority. Yet the house staff, which considered the actual dollar amount the only meaningful figure, felt that they were not yet important to the hospital (Meeting of January 26, 1971, Executive Faculty, Folder "January-February 1971," Box 131, University of Michigan Medical School Records. Faculty at Michigan were also outraged that many house officers engaged in rampant moonlighting in local emergency rooms and intensive care units when not on duty at the university hospital—to the point that their performance at the university hospital was frequently slipshod because they were fatigued from the previous night's moonlighting (Robert A. Green to John A. Gronvall, August 1, 1975, Folder "House Officers Association 1973–6," Box 95, University of Michigan, Medical School Records).
35. Interns and Residents of the Boston City Hospital to the Honorable John F. Collins, May 25, 1965, Folder "Boston City Hospital—1965 Jan-June," Dean's Subject File, Harvard Medical School, Harvard Medical Archives, Rare Books and Special Collections, Francis A. Countway Library of Medicine, Harvard Medical School, Boston, Mass.
36. "Residents File Suit against California Medical Center Seeking to Limit Patient Load, Enjoin Overcrowding," news clipping dated January 16, 1970, with meeting of July 7, 1970, Minutes of the Meetings of the Joint Residency Program Committee, Folder "Joint Committee on Residencies Minutes/Gen Corres. 1968–1973," Box 468, Office of the Executive VP for Health Sciences/Dean of the Faculty of Medicine, Central Files, Archives and Special Collections, A. C. Long Health Sciences Library, Columbia University Medical Center, New York, N.Y.
37. Howard A. Nelson Jr. and Kirk Lipscomb to Louis Burroughs, June 17, 1969, Folder 8, Box 82, John Adriani Papers, National Library of Medicine, Bethesda, Md.
38. House Staff Requests, October 23, 1969, with meeting of November 3, 1969, Minutes of the Meetings of the Executive Committee of the Medical Staff, Howard University Hospital, Office of the Medical Director, Howard University Hospital, Washington, D.C.
39. Statement of Position of the House Staff Association of Columbia-Presbyterian Medical Center, with meeting of May 19, 1970, Minutes of the Medical Board, the Presbyterian Hospital in the City of New York, Archives and Special Collections, A. C. Long Health Sciences Library, Columbia University Medical Center, New York, N.Y.
40. Report of the House Staff Committee, with meeting of March 27, 1973, Minutes of the Medical Board, the Presbyterian Hospital in the City of New York.

41. Meeting of June 10, 1970, Board of Managers Minutes, the Presbyterian Hospital in the City of New York, Archives and Special Collections, A. C. Long Health Sciences Library, Columbia University Medical Center, New York, N.Y.
42. Joann S. Lublin, "Interns, Residents Turn to 'Unions' to Improve Wages, Patient Care," *Wall St J*, March 6, 1972, p. A1.
43. Lublin, "Interns, Residents," p. A14. The history of the unionization movement among house officers is much in need of study. For a fine introduction, seeRobert G. Harmon, "Intern and Resident Organizations in the United States: 1934–1977," *Milbank Quart*, 56 (1978): 500–30.
44. Ludmerer, *Time to Heal*, pp. 245–46.
45. A rich collection of clippings on the strike is found in House Staff Strike—Clippings File, Archives, the Mount Sinai Medical Center, New York, N.Y.
46. Quoted in David Bird, "The Sleepless Night Syndrome," *NY Times*, March 18, 1975. A fascinating window on the conservative attitudes of many physicians toward reducing the work hours of internship appeared in the pages of the *Journal of the American Medical Association*. In 1981, Norman Cousins, the editor of the *Saturday Review* and author of *Anatomy of an Illness as Perceived by the Patient* (New York: Bantam Books, 1981), wrote an essay for the journal in which he compared the internship with hazing (Norman Cousins, "Internship: Preparation or Hazing?," *JAMA*, 245 [1981]: 377). After receiving an avalanche of commentary, the journal subsequently published excerpts from many of the letters in "Internship: Physicians Respond to Norman Cousins," *JAMA*, 246 (1981): 2141–44. About 60 percent of the mail ran against the general thrust of the article. Much of the defense of the rigors of internship came from physicians who, having survived the experience, seemed determined not to permit others to escape. As interns, these doctors deplored the experience, but having survived, they changed their minds, claiming that it contributed to fortifying their moral character. As one wrote, "At the time I was an intern it seemed like a cruel price to pay to become a 'full-fledged physician.'... In retrospect I found it to be one of the most rewarding experiences that I have ever been through" (Letter of L. J. Turkewitz, p. 2141).
47. Quoted in Bird, "The Sleepless Night Syndrome."
48. Stevens, *In Sickness and in Wealth*, pp. 256–365.
49. Quoted in Stevens, *In Sickness and in Wealth*, p. 5.
50. Joel H. Goldberg, "Will House Staff Associations Become More Than Unions?," *Hosp Physician*, June 1971, p. 59.
51. Report of the House Staff Committee, with meeting of March 27, 1973, Minutes of the Medical Board, the Presbyterian Hospital in the City of New York.
52. Meeting of October 8, 1974, Small Committee, Folder "Small Committee," President/Dean's Papers (Chalmers Series), Mount Sinai School of Medicine, Archives, the Mount Sinai Medical Center, New York, N.Y.
53. Meeting of May 7, 1970, Transactions of the Medical Board of the New York Hospital, Archives, the New York Hospital-Cornell Medical Center, New York, N.Y.
54. Meeting of the House Staff of the Cleveland Clinic Foundation, February 21, 1970, Folder 2, Cleveland Clinic House Staff Committee Minutes 1972–1974, 11–TH, Cleveland Clinic Archives, Cleveland, Ohio.
55. Statement of Position of the House Staff Association of Columbia-Presbyterian Medical Center, with meeting of June 8, 1970, Minutes of the Meetings of the

Joint Residency Program Committee, Folder "Joint Committee on Residencies Minutes/Gen. Corres. 1968–1973," Box 468, Office of the Executive VP for Health Sciences/Dean of the Faculty of Medicine, Central Files.

56. Report of the House Staff Committee, with meeting of June 26, 1973, Minutes of the Medical Board, the Presbyterian Hospital in the City of New York.
57. Jay Greene, "Residents Are Employees, NLRB Rules," *Am Med News*, December 20, 1999, pp. 9–10.
58. Walt, Bashook, Dockery, and Schneidman, *The Ecology of Graduate Medical Education*.
59. Jordan J. Cohen, "Honoring the 'E' In Graduate Medical Education," *Acad Med*, 74 (1998): 108–13.
60. Waguih William Ishak, Sara Lederer, Carla Mandili et al., "Burnout during Residency Training: A Literature Review," *J Grad Med Educ*, 1 (2009): 237.
61. Herbert I. Freudenberger, "Staff Burnout," *J Soc Issues*, 30 (1974): 159–65.
62. Ishak, Lederer, Mandili et al., "Burnout during Residency Training," p. 237.
63. Samuel Shem, *The House of God* (New York: Richard Marek, 1978).
64. Shem, *The House of God*, p. 381. The term "gomer" had long been in use before its outing to the general public in *The House of God*. For more on the term, see Victoria George and Alan Bundes, "The Gomer: A Figure of American Hospital Folk Speech," *J Am Folklore*, 91 (1978): 568–81; and Deborah B. Leiderman and Jean-Anne Grisso, "The Gomer Phenomenon," *J Health Soc Behav*, 26 (1985): 222–32.
65. Information from Samuel Shem's website, www.samuelshem.com/v2/about/, visited December 4, 2012.
66. Samuel Shem and Stephen Bergman, "Resistance and Healing," in Martin Kohn and Carol Donley, eds., *Return to The House of God: Medical Resident Education 1978–2008* (Kent, Ohio: Kent State University Press, 2008), p. 222.
67. Shem and Bergman, "Resistance and Healing," p. 225.
68. Bergman provides his personal reflections on the novel in Shem and Bergman, "Resistance and Healing," pp. 221–36, and in the afterword to the 2003 Delta trade paperback edition of *The House of God*, pp. 391–97. A thoughtful analysis of the book is Howard Markel, "*The House of God* 30 Years Later," *JAMA*, 299 (2008): 237–39. Kohn and Donley, *Return to The House of God*, provides an outstanding account of the meaning of the book as well as a valuable discussion of graduate medical education during the ensuing four decades.
69. J. Pat Tokarz, William Bremer, and Ken Peters, *Beyond Survival* (Chicago: American Medical Association, 1979).
70. Stephanie Brown Clark, Neeta Jain, and Dagan Coppock, "Writing the Medical Training Experience in 1978 and 2006: Body Language in *The House of God*," in Kohn and Donley, *Return to The House of God*, pp. 117–20.
71. Suzanne Poirier, *Doctors in the Making: Memoirs and Medical Education* (Iowa City: University of Iowa Press, 2009), p. 66.
72. Poirier, *Doctors in the Making*, p. 26.
73. Poirier, *Doctors in the Making*, p. 156. As noted in the text, some memoirs were written by medical students, which leads to the larger observation that students as well as house officers developed burnout. For a discussion of this point, see Agnes G. Rezler, "Attitude Changes during Medical School: A Review of the Literature," *J Med Educ*, 49 (1974): 1023–30. That this problem has not abated with time is seen in Liselotte N. Dyrbye, Matthew R. Thomas, F. Stanford Massie et al., "Burnout and Suicidal Ideation among U.S. Medical Students,"

Ann Intern Med, 149 (2008): 334–41; and Julie M. Rosenthal and Susan Okie, "White Coat, Mood Indigo—Depression in Medical School," *N Engl J Med*, 353 (2005): 1085–88.

74. Conversation with David B. Hellmann, October 31, 2012.
75. Poirier, *Doctors in the Making*, pp. 2, 45, 77.
76. Carol Landau, Stephanie Hall, Steven A. Wartman, and Michael B. Macko, "Stress in Social and Family Relationships during the Medical Residency," *J Med Educ*, 61 (1986): 654–60.
77. Robert G. Petersdorf and James Bentley, "Residents' Hours and Supervision," *Acad Med*, 64 (1989): 181.
78. Clark, Jain, and Coppock, "Writing the Medical Training Experience in 1978 and 2006," p. 121.
79. Shem, *The House of God*, p. 364.
80. Shem, *The House of God*, p. 363.
81. Robert H. Moser, "Diseases of Medical Progress," *N Engl J Med*, 255 (1956): 606–14.
82. Ivan Illich, *Medical Nemesis: The Expropriation of Health* (New York: Pantheon, 1976). Among the notable histories of the bioethics movement are Renée C. Fox and Judith P. Swazey, *Observing Bioethics* (New York: Oxford University Press, 2008); John Hyde Evans, *The History and Future of Bioethics: A Sociological View* (New York: Oxford University Press, 2011); and Albert R. Jonsen, *The Birth of Bioethics* (New York: Oxford University Press, 2003).
83. Shem, *The House of God*, p. 86.
84. Shem, *The House of God*, p. 312.
85. Shem, *The House of God*, p. 193.
86. Shem, *The House of God*, p. 381.
87. Thomas McKeown, *The Modern Rise of Population* (New York: Academic Press, 1976);Thomas McKeown, *The Role of Medicine: Dream, Mirage, or Nemesis?* (Princeton: Princeton University Press, 1979).
88. Lewis Thomas, "The Technology of Medicine," in Lewis Thomas, *The Lives of a Cell: Notes of a Biology Watcher* (New York: Viking, 1974), pp. 35–42.
89. René Dubos, *Mirage of Health: Utopias, Progress, and Biological Change* (New York: Harper & Brothers, 1959).
90. Poirier, *Doctors in the Making*, p. 145.
91. Poirier, *Doctors in the Making*, p. 169.
92. See, for instance, Tait D. Shanafelt, Katherine A. Broadley, Joyce E. Wipf, and Anthony L. Back, "Burnout and Self-Reported Patient Care in an Internal Medicine Residency Program," *Ann Intern Med*, 136 (2002): 358–67.
93. Walt, "The Challenge and a Vision for the Reform of Graduate Medical Education," p. 4.

CHAPTER 11

1. Rick Mayes, "The Origins, Development, and Passage of Medicare's Revolutionary Prospective Payment System," *J Hist Med All Sci*, 62 (2006): 21–55. The intellectual leaders in the development of DRGs were John D. Thomson and Robert Fetter of Yale. Ironically, as Mayes points out (p. 34), the original purpose of DRGs was not cost control but the rationalization of medical practice to improve the quality of care and allow the better use of limited and expensive medical resources. Some have pointed out that not all patient conditions can be readily classified under the DRG system. For a discussion of this point, see Ganesh

G. Gupta, "Diagnosis-Related Groups: A Twentieth-Century Nosology," *Pharos*, Spring 1990, pp. 12–17.

2. Charles E. Rosenberg, *The Care of Strangers: The Rise of America's Hospital System* (New York: Basic Books, 1987).
3. Kenneth M. Ludmerer, *Time to Heal: American Medical Education from the Turn of the Century to the Era of Managed Care* (New York: Oxford University Press, 1999).
4. Though as noted in the last chapter, doctors sometimes erred by doing too much, and some patients survived an acute illness to experience years of progressive frailty or the ravages of multiple chronic diseases.
5. Ludmerer, *Time to Heal*, p. 358.
6. Meeting of May 3, 1989, Board of Governors Minutes, New England Medical Center Hospitals, Office of the President, New England Medical Center Hospitals, Boston, Mass. (quotation); Ludmerer, *Time to Heal*, pp. 349–69.
7. Of note, developments in medical practice also caused some specialties to disappear or be radically transformed. For instance, syphilology disappeared as a subspecialty after the discovery of penicillin, and polio, after the development of a vaccine. The virtual disappearance of patients requiring surgery for tuberculosis and other pulmonary infections—the beneficial consequence of new antibiotics—profoundly altered the content of thoracic surgery. Similarly, the introduction of the H_2-receptor antagonists, such as cimetidine, virtually eliminated the need for surgery in patients with peptic ulcer disease. This process continues today. New imaging techniques for studying the colon are replacing screening colonoscopies, and cardiac angioplasty for coronary artery disease is greatly reducing the need for cardiac bypass surgery, thereby forcing the fields of gastroenterology and cardiac surgery, respectively, to shift their focus.
8. Meeting of April 27, 1982, Minutes of the Medical Board, the Presbyterian Hospital in the City of New York, Archives and Special Collections, A. C. Long Health Sciences Library, Columbia University Medical Center, New York, N.Y.
9. Lara Goitein, "Market Forces and Graduate Medical Education," manuscript of presentation at Internal Medicine Resident Conference, Massachusetts General Hospital, January 11, 2001.
10. Even with the closure of these programs, the majority of residency programs remained in community-based teaching hospitals. Because of their much larger sizes, however, the university-based programs at tertiary care centers trained the majority of residents in the United States. See Molly Cooke, David M. Irby, and Bridget C. O'Brien, *Educating Physicians: A Call for Reform of Medical School and Residency* (San Francisco: Jossey-Bass, 2010), pp. 22, 165.
11. Letter of December 31, 1995, Chief Resident Letters, Massachusetts General Hospital, Massachusetts General Hospital Department of Medicine Archives, Boston, Mass.
12. Memorandum on Anesthesiology House Staff, April 13, 1982, Folder "Anesthesiology 1980–1986," Box 507746, the Johns Hopkins Hospital, House Staff Training Programs, the Alan Mason Chesney Medical Archives of the Johns Hopkins Medical Institutions, Baltimore, Md.
13. Paul T. Kefalides, "The Invisible Hand of Government in Medical Education," *Ann Intern Med*, 132 (2000): 686–88.
14. Ludmerer, *Time to Heal*, pp. 349–79.

15. Meeting of July 17, 1985, Minutes of the Medical Board, the Presbyterian Hospital in the City of New York, Archives and Special Collections, A. C. Long Health Sciences Library, Columbia University Medical Center, New York, N.Y.
16. Michael B. Edmond, “Taylorized Medicine,” *Ann Intern Med*, 153 (2010): 845–46.
17. See, for example, the focus on shortening the length of stay at the Massachusetts General Hospital described in Goitein, “Market Forces and Graduate Medical Education.”
18. To reduce expenses, many leading teaching hospitals laid off employees. Those losing jobs included not only janitors, food workers, and housekeepers but also those more directly involved with patient care, such as orderlies, technicians, and nurses. This frequently left important patient-related work undone, which sometimes fell to house officers. Layoffs represented an important financial tool for hospitals because two-thirds or more of their expenses went to employee salaries and benefits. The peak decade of nursing layoffs was the 1990s, but there was considerable pushback because the growing volume and acuity of patients required more, not fewer, nurses. In recent years many hospitals have once again been trying to hire more nurses. This has been difficult to do and significant shortages remain, largely because the availability of new nurses from nursing schools has diminished. Some hospitals have tried importing nurses from other countries, particularly the Philippines. Large shortages of nurses still exist, however. For more, see Peter I. Buerhaus, “Current and Future State of the US Nursing Workforce,” *JAMA*, 300 (2008): 2422–24.
19. Paul S. Russell, “Surgery in a Time of Change,” in John H. Knowles, ed., *The Teaching Hospital: Evolution and Contemporary Issues* (Cambridge: Harvard University Press, 1966), p. 58.
20. In 1978–79, as the chief resident in internal medicine at Barnes Hospital, I kept a log of every patient admitted to the internal medicine service during the year, which included the room and team to which the patient was assigned, the admitting complaint, initial findings, diagnostic and therapeutic plan, final results, and condition at discharge. The maximum number of patients a single team received on a “long call” day was four patients; this happened only a few times during the course of the year. The log is now in the possession of the Washington University School of Medicine Archives.
21. Letter of June 20, 1996, Chief Resident Letters, Massachusetts General Hospital.
22. It should not be presumed that support services became ideal. For instance, Lara Goitein, a medical intern at Massachusetts General Hospital in 1998–99, described the many system flaws that plagued her cohort of house officers, resulting from insufficient resources and personnel. “For example, cheap and overloaded computers which took 3 minutes to log on to, and often broke down so that you had to try logging on to three terminals before having success. Slow elevators, crowded with passengers, which took 8 minutes to arrive. Too few numbers of operators, so that calling labs or other ancillary services often meant 5 minutes on hold. Too few radiologists, especially at night, so that to review a film sometimes meant a wait of 45 minutes, all for a very cursory, and often erroneous, reading. Inadequate supplies, so that we couldn’t find paper for printing, or hemmocult [*sic*] solution, or hurricaine spray, or a central line. Overworked nurses, so that orders weren’t followed often until the very end of an eight hour shift. Overworked ancillary services, so that we had to beg and jump through hoops to get certain studies done” (Goitein, “Market Forces and Graduate Medical Education”).

23. See, for instance, Bruce C. Vladeck, "Hospital Prospective Payment and the Quality of Care," *N Engl J Med*, 319 (1988): 1411–14.
24. Conversation with David M. Kipnis, June 25, 2001.
25. John Laszlo and Francis A. Neelon, *The Doctors' Doctor: A Biography of Eugene A. Stead Jr., MD* (Durham, N.C.: Carolina Academic Press, 2006), p. 282.
26. Cooke, Irby, and O'Brien, *Educating Physicians*, p. 151.
27. A. McGehee Harvey, Victor A. McKusick, and John D. Stobo, *Osler's Legacy: The Department of Medicine at Johns Hopkins 1889–1989* (Baltimore, Md.: Department of Medicine of the Johns Hopkins University, 1990), p. 161.
28. Letter of December 21, 2001, Chief Resident Letters, Massachusetts General Hospital.
29. Letter of January 1, 2000, Chief Resident Letters, Massachusetts General Hospital.
30. Goitein, "Market Forces and Graduate Medical Education."
31. Goitein, "Market Forces and Graduate Medical Education."
32. Report of ACGME Task Force, with meeting of February 8–9, 1988, Minutes of the Meetings of the Accreditation Council for Graduate Medical Education, ACGME Archives, Chicago, Ill.
33. Meeting of December 8, 1990, Executive Committee Minutes, Accreditation Council for Graduate Medical Education, ACGME Archives, Chicago, Ill.
34. The document may be accessed at www.aamc.org/residentcompact.
35. Goitein, "Market Forces and Graduate Medical Education."
36. Deborah Villa, "A Chief Resident's Perspective," in Alexander J. Walt, Philip G. Bashook, J. Lee Dockery, and Barbara S. Schneidman, eds., *The Ecology of Graduate Medical Education* (Evanston, Ill.: American Board of Medical Specialties, 1993), p. 35.
37. Villa, "A Chief Resident's Perspective," p. 35.
38. Larry S. Schlesinger and Charles M. Helms, "Cost-Conscious Care, Housestaff Training, and the Academic Health Center," *Acad Med*, 70 (1995): 561–62.
39. Conversation with Dennis A. Ausiello, April 27, 2013.
40. Patrick A. McKee, "Is Scholarship Declining in Medical Education?," 24th John P. McGovern Award Lecture, American Osler Society, April 21, 2009 (American Osler Society, privately printed).
41. David A. Shaywitz and Dennis A. Ausiello, "The Demise of Reflective Doctoring," *NY Times*, May 9, 2000, p. D7.
42. David B. Hellmann, "Eurekapenia: A Disease of Medical Residency Training Programs?," *Pharos*, Spring 2003, pp. 24–26.
43. Sandeep Jauhar, "Teaching Hospitals Too Busy for Curiosity," *NY Times*, September 5, 2000, p. D8.
44. Lawrence K. Altman, "Socratic Dialogue Gives Way to PowerPoint," *NY Times*, December 12, 2006, p. D1. Lectures and conferences are an important part of graduate medical education, of course, but they should be intended as dessert, not a main course.
45. Cooke, Irby, and O'Brien, *Educating Physicians*, pp. 113–60; quotation, p. 150.
46. See, for instance, George M. Piersol, *Gateway to Honor: The American College of Physicians, 1915–1959* (Lancaster, Pa.: Lancaster Press, 1962), p. 31.
47. Christopher A. Feddock, "The Lost Art of Clinical Skills," *Am J Med*, 120 (2007): 374–78; Geoffrey McLennan, "Is the Master Clinician Dead?," *Acad Med*, 76 (2001): 617–19; Sandeep Jauhar, "The Demise of the Physical Exam," *N Engl J Med*, 354 (2006): 548–51; Abigail Zuger, "Are Doctors Losing Touch

with Hands-On Medicine?" *NY Times*, July 13, 1999, p. D1; Herbert L. Fred, "Hyposkillia: Deficiency of Clinical Skills," *Tex Heart J*, 32 (2005): 255–57.

48. See, for instance, Julia E. Connelly, "The Power of Touch in Clinical Medicine," *Pharos*, Spring 2004, pp. 11–13.
49. Fred, "Hyposkillia."
50. In recent years a few leading medical educators have championed the importance of the physical examination, pushing back against current trends. Particularly notable in this regard has been the work of the well-known internist, writer, and humanist Abraham Verghese. See, for instance, Abraham Verghese, "Culture Shock—Patient as Icon, Icon as Patient," *N Engl J Med*, 359 (2008): 2748–51; Abraham Verghese and Ralph I. Horwitz, "In Praise of the Physical Examination: It Provides Reason and Ritual," *Brit Med J*, 339 (2009): 1385–86; Abraham Verghese, Erika Brady, Cari Costanzo Kapur, and Ralph I. Horwitz, "The Bedside Evaluation: Ritual and Reason," *Ann Intern Med*, 155 (2011): 550–53.
51. Richard B. Gunderman, "Flexner after the Report," presentation at the Flexner Report Centennial Symposium, May 4, 2010, Louisville, Ky.
52. Jay Greene, "Residents Are Employees, NLRB Rules," *Am Med News*, December 20, 1999, pp. 9–11; Andrew C. Yacht, "Collective Bargaining Is the Right Step," *N Engl J Med*, 342 (2000): 429–31; Sujit Choudhry and Troyen Brennan, "Collective Bargaining by Physicians—Labor Law, Antitrust Law, and Organized Medicine," *N Engl J Med*, 345 (2001): 1141–44; Virginia U. Collier, Mohammadreza Hojat, Susan L. Ratner et al., "Correlates of Young Physicians' Support for Unionization to Maintain Professional Influence," *Acad Med*, 76 (2001): 1039–44.
53. Jordan J. Cohen, "White Coats Should Not Have Union Labels," *N Engl J Med*, 342 (2000): 431.
54. Lara Goitein to author, April 28, 2010. See also Goitein, "Market Forces and Graduate Medical Education."
55. Goitein, "Market Forces and Graduate Medical Education."
56. Lara Goitein to author, April 28, 2010.
57. William W. Parmley, "Reflections on Attending on the Cardiology Service," *J Am Coll Cardiol*, 37 (2001): 964.
58. N. R. Kleinfield, "For Three Interns, Fatigue and Healing at Top Speed," *NY Times*, November 15, 1999, p. A28.
59. Jordan J. Cohen and Robert M. Dickler, "Auditing the Medicare-Billing Practices of Teaching Physicians—Welcome Accountability, Unfair Approach," *N Engl J Med*, 336 (1997): 1317–20; Lisa I. Iezzoni, "The Demand for Documentation for Medicare Patients," *N Engl J Med*, 341 (1999): 365–67; Jon Schafer, "Department of Health and Human Services Moves to Rein in Medicare Audits of Teaching Hospitals," *J Investig Med*, 45 (1997): 319–23; Kefalides, "The Invisible Hand of Government," p. 688.
60. Allan H. Goroll, John D. Stoeckle, Stephen E. Goldfinger et al., "Residency Training in Primary Care Internal Medicine: Report of an Operational Program," *Ann Intern Med*, 83 (1975): 872–77.
61. Gerald T. Perkoff, "Teaching Clinical Medicine in the Ambulatory Setting: An Idea Whose Time May Have Finally Come," *N Engl J Med*, 314 (1986): 27–31.
62. John M. Eisenberg, "How Can We Pay for Graduate Medical Education in Ambulatory Care?," *N Engl J Med*, 320 (1989): 1525–31; Eugene C. Rich, Mark Liebow, Malethi Srinivasan et al., "Medicare Financing of Graduate Medical Education: Intractable Problems, Elusive Solutions," *J Gen Intern Med*, 17 (2002): 283–92; John Iglehart, "Medicare, Graduate Medical Education, and New Policy Directions," *N Engl J Med*, 359 (2008): 643–50.

63. Ludmerer, *Time to Heal*, pp. 359–62, 375–76.
64. Harold L. Lazar, Carmel A. Fitzgerald, Tazeen Ahmad et al., "Early Discharge after Coronary Artery Bypass Graft Surgery: Are Patients Really Going Home Earlier?," *J Thorac Cardiov Sur*, 121 (2001): 943–50. Similarly, a number of studies in the early 2000s on patients with broken hips showed that early hospital discharges to save money ultimately led to more complications and higher costs. See Ron Winslow, "Rush to Release Hip Patients Leads to Injury," *Wall St J*, January 14, 2003, p. D1.
65. Rosemary Gibson and Janardan Prasad Singh, *The Treatment Trap: How the Overuse of Medical Care Is Wrecking Your Health and What You Can Do to Prevent It* (Chicago: Ivan R. Dee, 2010); H. Gilbert Welch, Lisa M. Schwartz, and Steven Woloshin, *Over-Diagnosed: Making People Sick in the Pursuit of Health* (Boston: Beacon, 2011); Maggie Mahar, *Money-Driven Medicine: The Real Reason Health Care Costs So Much* (New York: Collins, 2006); Shannon Brownlee, *Overtreated: Why Too Much Medicine Is Making Us Sicker and Poorer* (New York: Bloomsbury, 2007).
66. Lara Goitein to author, April 25, 2010.
67. Cooke, Irby, and O'Brien, *Educating Physicians*, p. 152.
68. Kenneth I. Berns, "Preventing *Academic Medical Center* from Becoming an Oxymoron," *Acad Med*, 71 (1996): 117;David A. Blake, "Whither Academic Values during the Transition from Academic Medical Centers to Integrated Health Delivery Systems?," *Acad Med*, 71 (1996): 819.
69. Cheryl Ulmer, Dianne Miller, and Michael M. E. Johns, eds., *Resident Duty Hours: Enhancing Sleep, Supervision, and Safety* (Washington, D.C.: National Academies Press, 2009).
70. David Hellmann to author, June 6, 2013.
71. Ludmerer, *Time to Heal*, pp. 349–99.
72. Charles S. Bryan, "Medical Professionalism Meets Generation X: A Perfect Storm?," *Tex Heart I J*, 38 (2011): 468.
73. Conversation with Daniel M. Fox, November 12, 2010. Fox made this comment in the larger context of the contemporary attack on authoritarianism in medical education and practice. See Daniel M. Fox, "Systematic Reviews and Health Policy: The Influence of a Project on Perinatal Care since 1988," *Milbank Quart*, 89 (2011): 425–29, which documented the power of systematic reviews as opposed to individual experience across entire fields of medicine.
74. William B. Castle, "Historical Overview," in Maxwell Finland, ed., *The Harvard Medical Unit at Boston City Hospital*, vol. I (Boston: Harvard Medical School, 1982), p. 42.
75. *A Physician Charter: Medical Professionalism in the New Millennium* (Philadelphia: ABIM Foundation, 2007). The charter was originally simultaneously published in *Ann Intern Med*, 136 (2002): 243–46; and *Lancet*, 359 (2002): 520–22.
76. Conversation with Randall Burt, September 24, 2009.
77. Christopher L. Roy, Eric G. Poon, Andrew S. Karson et al., "Patient Safety Concerns Arising from Test Results That Return after Hospital Discharge," *Ann Intern Med*, 143 (2005): 121–28.
78. I was the attending physician.
79. Jonathan Epstein, "Lessons of Our Fathers," *J Clin Invest*, 120 (2010): 2243–47; "alive and grateful," p. 2244; "new appreciation," p. 2244; "pass the buck," p. 2244; "I was a cog," p. 2245.
80. Bradley Evanoff, Patricia Potter, Laurie Wolf et al., "Can We Talk? Priorities for Patient Care Different among Health Care Providers," in Kerm Henriksen,

James B. Battles, Eric S. Marks, and David I. Lewin, eds., *Advances in Patient Safety: From Research to Implementation*, vol. 1, Research Findings (Rockville, Md.: Agency for Healthcare Research and Quality, 2005), pp. 5–14. A major exception was intensive care units, where the ratio of nurses to patients was higher and where nurses typically worked much more closely with doctors.

81. Abigail Zuger, "For a Hospital Stay, Only a Select Few Qualify," *NY Times*, May 3, 2005, p. D6.
82. Danielle Ofri, "Sometimes, Doctors Find Answers Far Off the Charts," *NY Times*, December 7, 2004, p. D5.
83. Among these were introducing oneself, maintaining good eye contact, listening without unnecessarily interrupting, and sitting down beside the patient. In the early twenty-first century, most observers thought that medical education could and should do a better job of teaching these skills. Most medical educators recognized that for caring to be more than a manufactured product, however, physicians also needed genuine compassion, and the degree to which this quality was innate or could be taught was widely debated (Howard Spiro, "What Is Empathy and Can It Be Taught?," *Ann Intern Med*, 116 [1992]: 843–46; Laura Landro, "Teaching Doctors to Be Nicer," *Wall St J*, September 28, 2005, p. D1; Michael W. Kahn, "Etiquette-Based Medicine," *N Engl J Med*, 358 [2008]: 1988–89; "Can Caring for Patients Be Taught?," *Lancet*, 370 [2007]: 630).
84. However, even relatively simple or standardized procedures still needed to be performed carefully and thoroughly. For instance, the quality of colonoscopy examination was found to relate directly to the thoroughness with which the examination was performed. Doctors who spent more time examining the colon during the critical withdrawal phase of the procedure were much better at detecting abnormalities than those who worked more quickly (Robert L. Barclay, Joseph J. Vicari, Andrea S. Doughty, John F. Johanson, and Roger L. Greenlaw, "Colonoscopic Withdrawal Times and Adenoma Detection during Screening Colonoscopy," *N Engl J Med*, 355 [2006]: 2533–41).
85. Roberta Berrien, letter to the editor, *N Engl J Med*, 317 (1987): 456–57.
86. Leighton E. Cluff, "Reflections on the Lost Art of Caring," *Pharos*, Winter 2002; Leighton E. Cluff and Robert H. Binstock, eds., *The Lost Art of Caring: A Challenge to Health Professionals, Families, Communities, and Society* (Baltimore, Md.: Johns Hopkins University Press, 2001).
87. Daniel Munoz, "The Fast/Slow Paradox," *Hopkins Med*, Spring/Summer 2012, p. 47.
88. Munoz, "The Fast/Slow Paradox," p. 47.
89. Arnold S. Relman, "The New Medical-Industrial Complex," *N Engl J Med*, 303 (1980): 963–70.
90. Arnold S. Relman, "The Health Care Industry: Where Is It Taking Us?," *N Engl J Med*, 325 (1991): 856.
91. Lee S. Shulman, "Foreword," in Cooke, Irby, and O'Brien, *Educating Physicians*, p. ix.
92. I witnessed that episode.
93. John C. Duffy and Edward M. Litin, *The Emotional Health of Physicians* (Springfield, Ill.: Charles C. Thomas, 1967), p. vii.
94. Martha R. Fowlkes, *Behind Every Successful Man: Wives of Medicine and Academe* (New York: Columbia University Press, 1980).
95. Fowlkes, *Behind Every Successful Man*, pp. 42–43.

96. Fowlkes, *Behind Every Successful Man*, p. 200. See also Kristin Celello's study of the notion of marriage as women's work in *Making Marriage Work: A History of Marriage and Divorce in the Twentieth-Century United States* (Chapel Hill: University of North Carolina Press, 2009).
97. Quoted in Fowlkes, *Behind Every Successful Man*, pp. 192 ("loneliness"), 82 ("never came first").
98. Fowlkes, *Behind Every Successful Man*, p. 85.
99. Caution must be exercised in making judgments about the children. Systematic studies have not been performed, and there has always been a high degree of variability from one family to another. I do remember, however, attending a banquet where I sat next to a much older Harvard physician who regaled me with stories of 10 or 12 famous Harvard physicians of the 1940s, 1950s, and 1960s, all of whom were "heroes" of the profession with major discoveries or eponymous syndromes. Then he suddenly said to me, "Ken, it just occurred to me now—none of these individuals ever had children who amounted to anything in life or even were happy." Clearly, this is a subject rife for study.
100. Ellen S. More, *Restoring the Balance: Women Physicians and the Profession of Medicine* (Cambridge: Harvard University Press, 2001).
101. Wendy Levinson and Nicole Lurie, "When Most Doctors Are Women: What Lies Ahead?," *Ann Intern Med*, 141 (2004): 471–74.
102. Fowlkes, *Behind Every Successful Man*, pp. 193–201. In families with two working spouses, household duties usually were borne much more by the wife than the husband, which often led to considerable stress for working women. See Arlie Hochschild with Anne Machung, *The Second Shift* (New York: Avon, 1990).
103. Bryan, "Medical Professionalism Meets Generation X," 465–70; Emily Jovic, Jean E. Wallace, and Lane Lemaire, "The Generation and Gender Shifts in Medicine: An Exploratory Survey of Internal Medicine Physicians," *BMC Health Serv Res*, 6 (2006): 55; Jean M. Twenge, "Generational Changes and Their Impact in the Classroom: Teaching Generation Me," *Med Educ*, 43 (2009): 398–405; and Janet Bickel and Ann J. Brown, "Generation X: Implications for Faculty Recruitment and Development in Academic Health Centers," *Acad Med*, 80 (2005): 205–10. Different authorities use slightly different beginning and ending dates for the various generations.
104. Linell Smith, "Get a Life!?," *Hopkins Med*, Fall 2008, p. 22.
105. E. Ray Dorsey, David Jarjoura, and Gregory W. Rutecki, "Influence of Controllable Lifestyle on Recent Trends in Specialty Choice by US Medical Students," *JAMA*, 290 (2003): 1173–78.
106. N. R. Kleinfield, "New Doctors Step into a Turbulent World," *NY Times*, November 14, 1999, p. 30.
107. E. Ray Dorsey, David Jarjoura, and Gregory W. Rutecki, "The Influence of Controllable Lifestyle and Sex on the Specialty Choices of Graduating U.S. Medical Students, 1996–2003," *Acad Med*, 80 (2005): 791–96. In this study, 45 percent of male medical school seniors chose specialties with a controllable lifestyle, compared with 36 percent of women.
108. Michael J. Lepore, *Death of the Clinician: Requiem or Reveille?* (Springfield, Ill.: Charles C. Thomas, 1982), p. 301.
109. David E. Rogers, "On Iron Men in Wooden Ships: Some Thoughts on House Staff Training—1984," *Trans Am Clin Climatol Assoc*, 96 (1984): 212.

110. Fowlkes, *Behind Every Successful Man*; Daniel H. Funkenstein, *Medical Students, Medical Schools and Society during Five Eras: Factors Affecting the Career Choices of Physicians 1958–1976* (Cambridge, Mass.: Ballinger, 1978); Gardiner Harris, "Private Practices Are on Way Out," *St. Louis Post-Dispatch*, March 28, 2010, p. A4.
111. See, for instance, J. Paul Leigh, Richard L. Kravitz, Mike Schembri et al., "Physician Career Satisfaction across Specialties," *Arch Intern Med*, 162 (2002): 1577–84.
112. Jovic, Wallace, and Lemaire, "The Generation and Gender Shifts in Medicine."

CHAPTER 12

1. Arnold S. Relman, "Assessment and Accountability: The Third Revolution in Medical Care," *N Engl J Med*, 319 (1991): 1220–22.
2. John E. Wennberg and Alan Gittelsohn, "Variations in Medical Care among Small Areas," *Sci Am*, 246 (1982): 120–34. Wennberg's immense contributions to health services research arose from asking three basic questions: How much variation in medical practice occurs? How can we account for variation? How much variation is unwarranted?
3. C. M. Winslow, J. Kosecoff, R. H. Brook, M. R. Chassin, and D. E. Kanouse, "The Appropriateness of Use of Coronary Angiography and Coronary Artery Bypass Surgery," *Clin Res*, 34 (1986): 635A.
4. Marc A. Rodwin, *Medicine, Money, and Morals: Physicians' Conflicts of Interest* (New York: Oxford University Press, 1993).
5. Relman, "Assessment and Accountability," p. 1221.
6. As noted earlier, the story of consumerism in medicine remains to be told. Nancy Tomes is presently writing a book on the subject, which should prove to be a notable contribution.
7. Letter of June 30, 2004, Chief Resident Letters, Massachusetts General Hospital, Massachusetts General Hospital Department of Medicine Archives, Boston, Mass.
8. Quoted in Ramsey Flynn, "When Suitors Come Calling," *Hopkins Med*, Spring–Summer 2009, p. 33.
9. Quoted in Melissa Hendricks, "A Hard Day's Night," *Johns Hopkins Magazine*, February 2001, p. 43.
10. *Graduate Medical Education: Report of the Commission on Graduate Medical Education* (Chicago: University of Chicago Press, 1940).
11. Robert C. Friedman, J. Thomas Bigger, and Donald S. Kornfeld, "The Intern and Sleep Loss," *N Engl J Med*, 285 (1971): 201–3.
12. "Outline of Proposed House Staff Report," 1964–65, Folder "House Staff Council 1965–1970," the Johns Hopkins Hospital, House Staff Administrative Information, the Alan Mason Chesney Medical Archives of the Johns Hopkins Medical Institutions, Baltimore, Md.
13. James R. Boex and Peter J. Leahy, "Understanding Residents' Work: Moving beyond Counting Hours to Assessing Educational Value," *Acad Med*, 78 (2003): 939–44.
14. Gail Morrison, "Mortgaging Our Future—The Cost of Medical Education," *N Engl J Med*, 352 (2005): 117–19; S. Ryan Greysen, Candice Chen, and Fitzhugh Mullan, "A History of Medical Student Debt: Observations and Implications for the Future of Medical Education," *Acad Med*, 86 (2011): 840–45. In 2012, the median student debt rose to an all-time high of $170,000 (Darrell G. Kirch,

"Sequester or Not, Academic Medicine Must Transform," *AAMC Reporter*, October 2012, p. 2).

15. There was a paucity of data about moonlighting, though one observer believed the practice involved the "silent majority" of house officers, particularly those beyond the first two years of training. The activity was controversial and emotionally charged; house officers and faculty alike preferred to avoid discussing the subject. Among medical educators, it was politically correct to attribute moonlighting to the need of many residents to pay off their loans and support their families. This was undoubtedly true of many house officers. This explanation, however, did not take into account the fact that many debt-free residents also engaged extensively in moonlighting, a phenomenon that came to be called "my fellow resident's Porsche syndrome"—that is, my fellow resident drives a Porsche, I want one, too, so I'll moonlight to get one. Much more information is needed on this sensitive subject. For more on moonlighting, see Arthur J. Moss, "Moonlighting House Officers: The Silent Majority," *N Engl J Med*, 311 (1984): 1375–77.
16. John Z. Ayanian and Joel S. Weissman, "Teaching Hospitals and Quality of Care: A Review of the Literature," *Milbank Quart*, 80 (2002): 569–93; quotation, p. 589. See also Joel Kupersmith, "Quality of Care in Teaching Hospitals: A Literature Review," *Acad Med*, 80 (2005): 458–66.
17. Jerome P. Kassirer, the editor of the *New England Journal of Medicine*, pointed out that in this regard, teaching hospitals had much to learn from community hospitals. "Nonteaching hospitals have a substantial edge over teaching hospitals in many of the human dimensions of care" (Kassirer, "Hospitals, Heal Yourselves," *N Engl J Med*, 340 [1999]: 310).
18. On the Libby Zion case and its aftermath, see Natalie Robins, *The Girl Who Died Twice: The Libby Zion Case and the Hidden Hazards of Hospitals* (New York: Delacorte, 1995); David A. Asch and Ruth M. Parker, "The Libby Zion Case: One Step Forward or Two Steps Backward?," *N Engl J Med*, 318 (1988): 771–75; and Barron H. Lerner, *When Illness Goes Public: Celebrity Patients and How We Look at Medicine* (Baltimore, Md.: Johns Hopkins University Press, 2006), pp. 201–21.
19. Quotations in this paragraph are taken from Bertrand M. Bell, "Reconsideration of the New York State Laws Rationalizing the Supervision and the Working Conditions of Residents," *Einstein J Biol Med*, 20 (2003): 36.
20. New York State Committee on Emergency Services, *Final Report of the New York State Ad Hoc Advisory Committee on Emergency Services* (Albany: New York State Health Department, October 1987).
21. Bell, "Reconsideration of the New York State Laws," pp. 39–40.
22. Robert G. Petersdorf and James Bentley, "Residents' Hours and Supervision," *Acad Med*, 64 (1989): 179.
23. Bertrand M. Bell, "Supervision, Not Regulation of Hours, Is the Key to Improving the Quality of Patient Care," *JAMA*, 269 (1993): 403.
24. Bell, "Supervision, Not Regulation of Hours," p. 403.
25. Bell, "Reconsideration of the New York State Laws," pp. 36–40; Bertrand M. Bell, letter to the editor, *JAMA*, 298 (2007): 2865–66.
26. Robert G. Petersdorf, "Regulation of Residency Training," *B NY Acad Med*, 67 (1991): 331.
27. Associated Medical Schools of New York, "A View of the Proposed New York State Regulations Governing the Professional Activities of Residents," *NY State J Med*, 87 (1987): 587–89.

28. Analysis of Bell Committee Recommendations by GNYHA, Folder "New York State Commission on Graduate Medical Education," Graduate Medical Education Records, Dean's Office Files, College of Physicians and Surgeons of Columbia University, Archives and Special Collections, A. C. Long Health Sciences Library, Columbia University Medical Center, New York, N.Y.
29. See, for instance, Office of Planning to Dr. Katz/Participants/Members, January 20, 1986, Folder "Graduate Medical Education 1985–1987," Box 421, Office of the Executive VP for Health Sciences/Dean of the Faculty of Medicine, Central Files, Archives and Special Collections, A. C. Long Health Sciences Library, Columbia University Medical Center, New York, N.Y.
30. Bertrand M. Bell, "Greenhorns in White," *Wall St J*, February 9, 1995, p. A15.
31. Bell, "Reconsideration of the New York State Laws," p. 37.
32. Jordan J. Cohen, "It's about Time," *Assoc Am Med Coll Reporter*, May 2001, p. 2.
33. Linda T. Kohn, Janet M. Corrigan, and Molla S. Donaldson, eds., *To Err Is Human: Building a Safer Health System* (Washington, D.C.: National Academy Press, 2000). Some challenged the accuracy of those numbers. See, for instance, Rodney A. Hayward and Timothy P. Hofer, "Estimating Hospital Deaths Due to Medical Errors: Preventability Is in the Eye of the Reviewer," *JAMA*, 286 (2001): 415–20; Clement J. McDonald, Michael Weiner, and Siu L. Hui, "Deaths Due to Medical Errors Are Exaggerated in Institute of Medicine Report," *JAMA*, 284 (2000): 93–95. However, there was general agreement that the problem was serious.
34. Michael L. Millenson, "Pushing the Profession: How the News Media Turned Patient Safety into a Priority," *Qual Safety Health Care*, 11 (2002): 60.
35. Millenson, "Pushing the Profession," pp. 57–63.
36. Virginia U. Collier, Jack D. McCue, Allan Markus, and Lawrence Smith, "Stress in Medical Residency: Status Quo after a Decade of Reform?," *Ann Intern Med*, 136 (2002): 384–90.
37. DeWitt C. Baldwin Jr., Steven R. Daugherty, Ray Tsai, and Michael J. Scott Jr., "A National Survey of Residents' Self-Reported Work Hours: Thinking beyond Specialty," *Acad Med*, 78 (2003): 1154–63.
38. Also of interest, attitudes among residents toward the effects of sleep deprivation seemed to vary by specialty. For instance, one study of house officers at Johns Hopkins showed residents in pediatrics and psychiatry much more worried that sleep deprivation might lead to errors in patient management than residents in general surgery (Preliminary Report of the Survey on House Staff and Supervision, October 5, 1989, with meeting of November 29, 1989, Minutes of the Advisory Board of the Medical Faculty, the Johns Hopkins University School of Medicine, the Alan Mason Chesney Medical Archives of the Johns Hopkins Medical Institutions, Baltimore, Md.).
39. Baldwin, Daugherty, Tsai, and Scott, "A National Survey," pp. 1154–63; DeWitt C. Baldwin Jr., Steven R. Daugherty, Patrick M. Ryan, and Nicholas A. Yaghmour, "What Do Residents Do When Not Working or Sleeping? A Multispecialty Survey of 36 Residency Programs," *Acad Med*, 87 (2012): 395–402.
40. Jeffrey M. Drazen and Arnold M. Epstein, "Rethinking Medical Training—The Critical Work Ahead," *N Engl J Med*, 347 (2002): 1272.
41. Program Requirements for Residency Education in Thoracic Surgery, with meeting of September 10–11, 2001, Minutes of the Meetings of the Accreditation Council for Graduate Medical Education, ACGME Archives, Chicago, Ill.

42. Program Requirements for Residency Education in General Surgery, with meeting of February 12–13, 2001, Minutes of the Meetings of the Accreditation Council for Graduate Medical Education.
43. Cohen, "It's about Time," p. 2.
44. Meeting of February 14, 2000, Executive Committee Minutes, Accreditation Council for Graduate Medical Education, ACGME Archives, Chicago, Ill.
45. Meeting of June 9–10, 2002, Executive Committee Minutes, Accreditation Council for Graduate Medical Education.
46. Meeting of June 13–14, 1988, Minutes of the Meetings of the Accreditation Council for Graduate Medical Education.
47. The five original sponsoring organizations became "member organizations" of the independently incorporated ACGME, each with the power to appoint three individuals to the ACGME board. Those individuals, however, were responsible to the ACGME and not to the member organization that nominated them.
48. See the report of the executive committee retreat, December 1997, discussed at Leach's first meeting as executive director, meeting of February 16–17, 1998, and the ACGME's revised mission statement, with meeting of September 28–29, 1998, both in Minutes of the Meetings of the Accreditation Council for Graduate Medical Education.
49. Minutes of Council of Review Committee Residents, September 8, 2006, with meeting of September 12, 2006, Minutes of the Accreditation Council for Graduate Medical Education.
50. David C. Leach, letter to the editor, *Acad Med*, 76 (2001): 397.
51. Report of the ACGME Work Group on Resident Duty Hours, with meeting of September 9–10, 2002, Minutes of the Meetings of the Accreditation Council for Graduate Medical Education.
52. "Sleep-Deprived Doctors," *NY Times*, June 14, 2002, p. A34.
53. Rita Kwan and Robert Levy, *A Primer on Resident Work Hours*, 2nd ed. (Reston, Va.: American Medical Student Association, 2002), p. 14.
54. David M. Gaba and Steven K. Howard, "Fatigue among Clinicians and the Safety of Patients," *N Engl J Med*, 347 (2002): 1259.
55. Michael J. Green, "What (If Anything) Is Wrong with Residency Overwork?," *Ann Intern Med*, 123 (1995): 512. See also Linda Hawes Clever, "Who Is Sicker: Patients—or Residents? Residents' Distress and the Care of Patients," *Ann Intern Med*, 136 (2002): 391–93.
56. Ingrid Philibert, Paul Friedmann, and William T. Williams, "New Requirements for Resident Duty Hours," *JAMA*, 288 (2002): 1112–14.
57. Meeting of February 11–12, 2002, Minutes of the Meetings of the Accreditation Council for Graduate Medical Education.
58. Baldwin, Daugherty, Tsai, and Scott, "A National Survey," p. 1162.
59. Kenneth M. Ludmerer, *Time to Heal: American Medical Education from the Turn of the Century to the Era of Managed Care* (New York: Oxford University Press, 1999), p. 98.
60. "Improving the Safety of Health Care: The Leapfrog Initiative," *Eff Clin Pract*, 3 (2000): 313–16.
61. Kohn, Corrigan, and Donaldson, *To Err Is Human*; Committee on Quality of Health Care in America, *Crossing the Quality Chasm: A New Health System for the 21st Century* (Washington, D.C.: National Academy Press, 2001); Ann C. Greiner and Elisa Knebel, eds., *Health Professions Education: A Bridge to Quality* (Washington, D.C.: National Academies Press, 2003).

62. Meeting of September 22, 2004, Minutes of Meetings, American Board of Medical Specialties Executive Committee, American Board of Medical Specialties Archives, Chicago, Ill.
63. Meetings of September 23, 2004 ("visible external role"), and September 22, 2005 ("quest"), both Proceedings of the American Board for Medical Specialties, American Board of Medical Specialties Archives, Chicago, Ill.
64. ACGME Outcome Project Overview, with orientation materials for ACGME Review Committees, February 11, 2006, Accreditation Council for Graduate Medical Education Executive Committee Agendas, Accreditation Council for Graduate Medical Education Archives, Chicago, Ill. See also Paul Batalden, David Leach, Susan Swing, Hubert Dreyfus, and Stuart Dreyfus, "General Competencies and Accreditation in Graduate Medical Education," *Health Affairs*, 21, no. 5 (2002): 103–11; and David C. Leach, "Competence Is a Habit," *JAMA*, 287 (2002): 243–44. Many medical educators criticized the six core competencies because they were abstract and difficult to measure. For instance, one paper stated: "The difficulty is that core competencies attempt to distill a range of professional behaviors into arguable abstractions. As such, competencies can be difficult to grasp for trainees and faculty, who see them as unrelated to the intricacies of daily patient care" (M. Douglas Jones Jr., Adam A. Rosenberg, Joseph T. Gilhooly, and Carol L. Carraccio, "Competencies, Outcomes, and Controversy—Linking Professional Activities to Competencies to Improve Resident Education and Practice," *Acad Med*, 86 [2011]: 161).
65. Conversation with David Murray, a noted anesthesiologist and simulation expert, October 18, 2010; Rebecca Voelker, "Medical Simulation Gets Real," *JAMA*, 302 (2009): 2190–92. Of course, there were limits to simulation, and no one argued that it eliminated the need for involvement with patients. For instance, simulation offered surgical residents the opportunity to develop surgical technique but not surgical judgment.
66. Cheryl Ulmer, Dianne Miller Wolman, and Michael M. E. Johns, eds., *Resident Duty Hours: Enhancing Sleep, Supervision, and Safety* (Washington, D.C.: National Academies Press, 2009).
67. I served on the committee and suggested the title "Beyond Duty Hours."
68. I happened to be doing research for this book at the ACGME on that day and was informed of this by several of the officers.
69. Thomas J. Nasca, Susan H. Day, and E. Stephen Amis Jr., "The New Recommendations on Duty Hours from the ACGME Task Force," *N Engl J Med, 363* (2010): e3; John K. Iglehart, "The ACGME's Final Duty-Hour Standards—Special PGY-1 Limits and Strategic Napping," *N Engl J Med*, 367 (2010): 1589–91.
70. This was said to me by the chair of a prestigious department of internal medicine in June 2013.
71. Russell J. Nauta, "Residency Training Oversight(s) in Surgery: The History and Legacy of the Accreditation Council for Graduate Medical Education Reforms," *Surg Clin N A*, 92 (2012): 117–23; Russell J. Nauta, "The Surgical Residency and the Accreditation Council for Graduate Medical Education Reform: Steep Learning or Sleep Learning," *Am J Surg*, 201 (2011): 715–18.
72. Brian C. Drolet, Lucy B. Spalluto, and Staci A. Fischer, "Residents' Perspectives on ACGME Regulation of Supervision and Duty Hours—a National Survey," *N Engl J Med*, 363 (2010): e34.
73. Ryan M. Antiel, Scott M. Thompson, Darcy A. Reed et al., "ACGME Duty-Hour Recommendations—A National Survey of Residency Program Directors," *N Engl J Med*, 363 (2010): e12.

74. Quoted in Howard Markel, "A Book Doctors Can't Close," *NY Times*, August 18, 2009, p. D7.
75. Conversation with Thomas J. Nasca, June 11, 2010.
76. Joseph S. Alpert and William H. Frishman, "A Bridge Too Far: A Critique of the New ACGME Duty Hour Requirements," *Am J Med*, 125 (2012): 1.
77. Jay Greene, "GME Helps Community—and Bottom Line," *Am Med News*, 24 (April 2000): 12.
78. Lara Goitein and Kenneth M. Ludmerer, "Resident Workload—Let's Treat the Disease, Not Just the Symptom," *JAMA Intern Med*, 173 (2013): 655–56; Vineet M. Arora, Emily Georgitis, Juned Siddique et al., "Association of Workload of On-Call Medical Interns with On-Call Sleep Duration, Shift Duration, and Participation in Educational Activities," *JAMA, 300* (2008): 1146–53.
79. Jason Ryan, "Unintended Consequences: The Accreditation Council for Graduate Medical Education Work-Hour Rules in Practice," *Ann Intern Med*, 143 (2005): 82–83.
80. See, for instance, Laura A. Petersen, Troyen A. Brennan, Anne C. O'Neill et al., "Does Housestaff Discontinuity of Care Increase the Risk for Preventable Adverse Events?," *Ann Intern Med*, 121 (1994): 866–72; Christine Laine, Lee Goldman, Jane R. Soukup, and Joseph G. Hayes, "The Impact of a Regulation Restricting Medical House Staff Working Hours on the Quality of Patient Care," *JAMA*, 269 (1993): 374–78.
81. Damion Douglas, "Maintaining Duty-Hour Regulation through Improved Patient Handoff," *Resident Times*, Fall/Winter 2009, pp. 1–2; Erik G. Van Eaton, Karen McDonough, William B. Lober et al., "Safety of Using a Computerized Rounding and Sign-Out System to Reduce Resident Duty Hours," *Acad Med*, 85 (2010): 1189–95; Gautam Naik, "A Hospital Races to Learn Lessons of Ferrari Pit Stop," *Wall St J*, November 14, 2006, p. A1. Ironically, little was yet known about best practices in patient handoffs. See Lee Ann Riesenberg, Jessica Leitzsch, Jaime L. Massucci et al., "Residents' and Attending Physicians' Handoffs: A Systematic Review of the Literature," *Acad Med*, 84 (2009): 1175–87; and Max V. Wohlauer, Vineet M. Arora, Leora I. Horwitz et al., "The Patient Handoff: A Comprehensive Curricular Blueprint for Resident Education to Improve Continuity of Care," *Acad Med*, 87 (2012): 411–18.
82. See Abigail Zuger's observations in Susan Okie, "An Elusive Balance— Residents' Work Hours and the Continuity of Care," *N Engl J Med*, 356 (2007): 2667.
83. Holly Humphrey to David Hellmann, Daniel Goodenberger, and Kenneth Ludmerer, July 8, 2008.
84. George A. Sarosi, "Attending Rounds," *Ann Intern Med*, 153 (2010): 482.
85. I have in my possession a copy of this email exchange. One of the writers requested anonymity.
86. Ian Shapira, "Doctors Fear Work Caps for Residents May Be Bad Medicine," *Washington Post*, March 18, 2010.
87. Molly Cooke, David M. Irby, and Bridget C. O'Brien, *Educating Physicians: A Call for Reform of Medical School and Residency* (San Francisco: Jossey-Bass, 2010), pp. 141–42.
88. Ingrid Philibert, Thomas Nasca, Timothy Brigham, and Jane Shapiro, "Duty-Hour Limits and Patient Care and Resident Outcomes: Can High-Quality Studies Offer Insight into Complex Relationships?," *Ann Rev Med*, 64 (2013): 467–83.
89. A. Barnard, "Surgery Residents' Long Hours Draw Warning for Yale," *Boston Globe*, May 20, 2002, p. A1; David Kohn, "Hopkins Residency Program Loses Accreditation over Labor Rules," *Baltimore Sun*, August 27, 2003.

90. Christopher P. Landrigan, Laura K. Barger, Brian E. Cade, Najib T. Ayas, and Charles A. Czeisler, "Interns' Compliance with Accreditation Council for Graduate Medical Education Work-Hour Limits," *JAMA*, 296 (2006): 1063–70.
91. Meeting of September 12, 2006, Minutes of the Meetings of the Accreditation Council for Graduate Medical Education.
92. Philibert, Nasca, Brigham, and Shapiro, "Duty-Hour Limits," pp. 467–83. Of course, stress and depression among house officers hardly vanished, even though they were more rested. See Deborah Goebert, Diane Thompson, Junji Takeshita et al., "Depressive Symptoms in Medical Students and Residents: A Multischool Study," *Acad Med*, 84 (2009): 236–41; and Erin R. Stucky, Timothy R. Dresselhaus, Adrian Dollarhide et al., "Intern to Attending: Assessing Stress among Physicians," *Acad Med*, 84 (2009): 251–57.
93. Quoted in Liz Kowalczyk, "MGH Cited on Surgeons' Overload," *Boston Globe*, June 22, 2009.
94. Quoted in Janet Bickel and Ann J. Brown, "Generation X: Implications for Faculty Recruitment and Development in Academic Medical Centers," *Acad Med*, 80 (2005): 205.
95. Christopher P. Landrigan, Jeffrey M. Rothschild, John W. Cronin et al., "Effect of Reducing Interns' Work Hours on Serious Medical Errors in Intensive Care Units," *N Engl J Med*, 351 (2004): 1838–48.
96. See the letters to the editor on interns' work hours in *N Engl J Med*, 352 (2005): 726–28.
97. Amy K. Rosen, Susan A. Loveland, Patrick S. Romano et al., "Effects of Resident Duty Hour Reform on Surgical and Procedural Patient Safety Indicators among Hospitalized Veterans Health Administration and Medicare Patients," *Med Care:* 47 (2009): 723–31. See also Kevin G. Volpp, Amy K. Rosen, Paul R. Rosenbaum et al., "Mortality among Hospitalized Medicare Beneficiaries in the First 2 Years Following ACGME Resident Duty Hour Reform," *JAMA*, 298 (2007): 975–83.
98. Jennifer S. Myers, Lisa M. Bellini, Jon B. Morris et al., "Internal Medicine and General Surgery Residents' Attitudes about the ACGME Duty Hours Regulations: A Multicenter Study," *Acad Med*, 81 (2006): 1052–58; Sanjay V. Desai, Leonard Feldman, Lorrel Brown et al., "Effect of the 2011 vs. 2003 Duty Hour Regulation-Compliant Models on Sleep Duration, Trainee Education, and Continuity of Patient Care among Internal Medicine House Staff," *JAMA Intern Med*, 173 (2013): 649–55; Srijan Sen, Henry R. Kranzler, Aashish K. Didwania et al., "Effects of the 2011 Duty Hour Reforms on Interns and Their Patients," *JAMA Intern Med*, 173 (2013): 657–62.
99. Philibert, Nasca, Brigham, and Shapiro, "Duty-Hour Limits," p. 477.
100. Bell, "Reconsideration of the New York State Laws," p. 38.
101. Albert W. Wu, Susan Folkman, Stephen J. McPhee, and Bernard Lo, "Do House Officers Learn from their Mistakes?," *JAMA, 265* (1991): 2089–94; R. Jagsi, B. T. Titch, D. Weinstein et al., "Residents Report on Adverse Events and Their Causes," *Arch Intern Med*, 165 (2005): 2606–13; Arpana R. Vidyarthi, Andrew D. Auerback, Robert M. Wachter et al., "The Impact of Duty Hours on Resident Self Reports of Errors," *J Gen Intern Med*, 22 (2007): 205–9.
102. Hardeep Singh, Eric J. Thomas, Laura A. Petersen et al., "Medical Errors Involving Trainees: A Study of Closed Malpractice Claims from 5 Insurers," *Arch Intern Med*, 167 (2007): 2030–36.
103. Philibert, Nasca, Brigham, and Shapiro, "Duty-Hour Limits," pp. 473–74.

104. Philibert, Nasca, Brigham, and Shapiro, "Duty-Hour Limits," pp. 473–75, 478; Jay Jagannathan, G. Edward Vates, Nader Pouratian et al., "Impact of the Accreditation Council for Graduate Medical Education Work-Hour Regulations on Neurosurgical Resident Education and Productivity," *J Neurosurg*, 110 (2009): 820–27; meeting of June 8, 2013, Accreditation Council for Graduate Medical Education.
105. Adam A. Maruscak, Michael C. Ott, and Thomas L. Forbes, "Time to Refine Resident Duty Hour Guidelines," *J Grad Med Educ*, 4 (2012): 545–46.
106. See, for instance, Eugene Orientale Jr., "Length of Training Debate in Family Medicine: Idealism Versus Realism?," *J Grad Med Educ*, 5 (2013): 192–94; Cooke, Irby, and O'Brien, *Educating Physicians*, pp. 130, 158.
107. M. P. Schijven, R. K. Reznick, O. Th. J. ten Cate et al., "Transatlantic Comparison of the Competence of Surgeons at the Start of Their Professional Career," *Brit J Surg*, 97 (2010): 443–49; J. E. F. Fitzgerald and B. C. Caesar, "The European Working Time Directive: A Practical Review for Surgical Trainees," *Int J Surg*, 30 (2012): 1–5.
108. Lloyd Axelrod, Deep J. Shah, and Anupam B. Jena, "The European Working Time Directive: An Uncontrolled Experiment in Medical Care and Education," *JAMA*, 309 (2013): 447–48.
109. Axelrod, Shah, and Jena, "The European Working Time Directive," p. 448.
110. Kathlynn E. Fletcher, Sarah Nickoloff, Jeff Whittle et al., "Why Residents Consider Working beyond the Duty Hour Limits: Implications of the ACGME 2011 Duty Hour Standards," *J Grad Med Educ*, 3 (2011): 571–73. This study did not report how frequently residents broke the "+6" rule, only how frequently they considered it.
111. Julia E. Szymczak, Joanna Veazey Brooks, Kevin G. Volpp, and Charles L. Bosk, "To Leave or to Lie? Are Concerns about a Shift-Work Mentality and Eroding Professionalism as a Result of Duty-Hour Rules Justified?," *Milbank Quart*, 88 (2010): 350–81; quotation, p. 363.
112. *Unmet Needs: Teaching Physicians to Provide Safe Patient Care*, report of the Lucian Leape Institute Roundtable on Reforming Medical Education (Boston: National Patient Safety Foundation, 2010), p. 1.
113. John F. Christensen, Wendy Levinson, and Patrick M. Dunn, "The Heart of Darkness: The Impact of Perceived Mistakes on Physicians," *J Gen Intern Med*, 7 (1992): 424–31; Kirsten G. Engel, Marilynn Rosenthal, and Kathleen M. Sutcliffe, "Residents' Responses to Medical Error: Coping, Learning, and Change," *Acad Med*, 81 (2006): 86–93.
114. Meeting of February 13–14, 2005, Executive Committee Meetings, Accreditation Council for Graduate Medical Education.

CHAPTER 13

1. Sarah E. Brotherton and Sylvia I. Ertzel, "Graduate Medical Education, 2009–2010," *JAMA*, 304 (2010): 1255.
2. Molly Cooke, David M. Irby, and Bridget C. O'Brien, *Educating Physicians: A Call for Reform of Medical School and Residency* (San Francisco: Jossey-Bass, 2010), p. 8.
3. Brian David Hodges, "A *Tea-Steeping* or *i-Doc* Model for Medical Education?," *Acad Med*, 85, no. 9 (September Supplement, 2010), pp. S34–S44.
4. Hodges, "A *Tea-Steeping* or *i-Doc* Model."
5. Kelly J. Caverzagie, William F. Iobst, Eva M. Aagaard et al., "The Internal Medicine Reporting Milestones and the Next Accreditation System," *Ann Intern Med*, 158 (2013): 557–59.

6. Thomas J. Nasca, Ingrid Philibert, Timothy Brigham, and Timothy C. Flynn, "The Next GME Accreditation System—Rationale and Benefits," *N Engl J Med*, 366 (2012): 1051–56. The first seven specialties to employ milestones were emergency medicine, internal medicine, neurosurgery, orthopedic surgery, pediatrics, diagnostic radiology, and urology. A description of the milestones in each of these fields is found in the March 2013 supplement to the *Journal of Graduate Medical Education*.
7. Stuart E. Dreyfus, "The Five-Stage Model of Adult Skill Acquisition," *B Sci Technol Soc*, 24 (2004): 177–81.
8. Michael M. E. Johns, "The Time Has Come to Reform Graduate Medical Education," *JAMA*, 286 (2001): 1075–76. Not everyone endorsed the idea of shortening the length of residency for quick learners. For instance, the Alliance for Academic Internal Medicine argued that any time saved should be used to provide additional, enriching experiences (Steven E. Weinberger, Anne G. Pereira, William F. Iobst et al., "Competency-Based Education and Training in Internal Medicine," *Ann Intern Med*, 153 [2010]: 751–56). Traditionally, superior house officers had tended to seek longer training, either to more fully master a clinical specialty or to obtain research experience.
9. Nasca, Philibert, Brigham, and Flynn, "The Next GME Accreditation System," p. 1051. A description of the immense administrative burden of program directors is found in Jay Greene, "More Residency Directors Quitting," *Am Med News*, April 17, 2000, pp. 9–11. See also meeting of December 15, 2000, Executive Committee Minutes, Accreditation Council for Graduate Medical Education, Accreditation Council for Graduate Medical Education Archives, Chicago, Ill.
10. Sandra Jarvis-Selinger, Daniel D. Pratt, and Glenn Regehr, "Competency Is Not Enough: Integrating Identity Formation into the Medical Education Discourse," *Acad Med*, 87 (2012): 1185–90.
11. David Blumenthal, "New Steam from an Old Cauldron—The Physician-Supply Debate," *N Engl J Med*, 350 (2004): 1780–87; John K. Iglehart, "Grassroots Activism and the Pursuit of an Expanded Physician Supply," *N Engl J Med*, 358 (2008): 1741–49.
12. Quoted in Jennifer Proctor, "Addressing the Question of Physician Supply in America," *AAMC Reporter*, July 2001, p. 9.
13. John K. Iglehart, "The Residency Mismatch," *N Engl J Med*, 369 (2013): 297–99.
14. Iglehart, "The Residency Mismatch," p. 298.
15. Iglehart, "The Residency Mismatch," p. 298.
16. Many physicians remember the arduous effort it often took to obtain information before the 1990s. If on call, residents had to wait for a sufficient break in the workflow to run over to the medical library, often several buildings away. There, they did a literature search by hand using the *Index Medicus*, the standard guide to the medical literature. From there, they went to the library shelf to obtain the pertinent article—sometimes to find the volume not on the shelf or, if present, the article torn out.
17. Robert Wu, "Rise of the Cyborgs: Residents with Smart Phones, iPads, and Androids," *J Grad Med Educ*, 5 (2013): 161–62.
18. Emily Listfield, "Generation Wired," *Parade*, October 9, 2011, p. 9.
19. Listfield, "Generation Wired," p. 12.
20. Nicholas Carr, *The Shallows: What the Internet Is Doing to Our Brains* (New York: W. W. Norton, 2010); Sven Birkerts, "Reading in a Digital Age," *Am Scholar*, Spring 2010, pp. 32–44; Delese Wear, "A Perfect Storm: The Convergence of Bullet

Points, Competencies, and Screen Reading in Medical Education," *Acad Med*, 84 (2009): 1500–1504; and Matt Richtel, "Growing Up Digital, Wired for Distraction," *NY Times*, November 21, 2010, p. 1.

21. Sara H. Konrath, Edward H. O'Brien, and Courtney Hsing, "Changes in Dispositional Empathy in American College Students over Time: A Meta-Analysis," *Pers Soc Psychol Rev*, 15 (2011): 180–98.
22. Vineet M. Arora and Kevin G. M. Volpp, "Duty Hours: Time to Study?," *J Grad Med Educ*, 3 (2011): 281–84.
23. Conversation with David Hellmann, July 21, 2009.
24. Quoted in "Residency Rules," *Dome*, October 2003, p. 1.
25. David T. Stern and Maxine Papadakis, "The Developing Physician—Becoming a Professional," *N Engl J Med*, 355 (2006): 1796.
26. Jack Needleman, Peter Buerhaus, Soeren Mattke et al., "Nurse-Staffing Levels and the Quality of Care in Hospitals," *N Engl J Med*, 346 (2002): 1715–22; Ashish K. Jha, E. John Orav, Jie Zheng, and Arnold M. Epstein, "Patients' Perception of Hospital Care in the United Sates," *N Engl J Med*, 359 (2008): 1921–31; Jack Needleman, Peter Buerhaus, V. Shane Pankratz et al., "Nurse Staffing and Inpatient Hospital Mortality," *N Engl J Med*, 364 (2011): 1037–45.
27. David P. Sklar, "Faculty Supervision of Residents—Creating Important Moments of Magic," *Acad Med*, 88 (2013): 431–33.
28. Sklar, "Faculty Supervision of Residents"; S. M. Kilminster and B. C. Jolly, "Effective Supervision in Clinical Practice Settings: A Literature Review," *Med Educ*, 34 (2000): 827–40; Jeanne M. Farnan, Lindsey A. Petty, Emily Georgitis et al., "A Systematic Review: The Effect of Clinical Supervision on Patient and Residency Education Outcomes," *Acad Med*, 87 (2012): 428–42.
29. Tara J. T. Kennedy, Lorelei Lingard, G. Ross Baker et al., "Clinical Oversight: Conceptualizing the Relationship between Supervision and Safety," *J Gen Intern Med*, 22 (2007): 1080–85.
30. Steward Babbott, "Watching Closely at a Distance: Key Tensions in Supervising Resident Physicians," *Acad Med*, *85* (2010): 1399–1400; Anneke Sterkenburg, Paul Barach, Cor Kalkman et al., "When Do Supervising Physicians Decide to Entrust Residents with Unsupervised Tasks?," *Acad Med*, 85 (2010): 1408–17.
31. Dewitt C. Baldwin Jr., Steven R. Daugherty, and Patrick M. Ryan, "How Residents View Their Clinical Supervision: A Reanalysis of Classic National Survey Data," *J Grad Med Educ*, 2 (2010): 37–45.
32. Keith G. Shojania, Kathlyn E. Fletcher, and Sanjay Saint, "Graduate Medical Education and Patient Safety: A Busy—and Occasionally Hazardous—Intersection," *Ann Intern Med*, 145 (2006): 592–98.
33. Lawrence Loo, Nishant Puri, Daniel I. Kim et al., "'Page Me If You Need Me': The Hidden Curriculum of Attending-Resident Communication," *J Grad Med Educ*, 4 (2012): 340–45.
34. Kenneth M. Ludmerer, "Learner-Centered Medical Education," *N Engl J Med*, 351 (2004): 1163–64.
35. As always, there were disciplinary variations. Senior faculty tended to be the most visible to house officers in the surgical programs. They tended to be the least visible in large, nonprocedural fields such as internal medicine.
36. In internal medicine, this was the argument for replacing physician-scientists as teachers with "hospitalists"—internists, typically just out of an internal medicine residency, who specialized in the management of hospitalized internal medicine patients. Being exquisitely familiar with hospital routines and continually

present on the wards, hospitalists tended to care for comparable patients with slightly shorter lengths of stay than other faculty members. Having recently finished their residency, they often had more current facts immediately at their fingertips than many physician-scientists who taught on the wards only a few months a year. The point here is not to argue the relative merits of hospitalists and physician-scientists as clinical teachers. Some hospitalists made excellent teachers, while some eminent physician-scientists had become rusty in bedside skills. Rather, it is to suggest that graduate medical education was best served when faculty brought rigorous critical thinking to their teaching, regardless of their particular specialty or educational background. Studies of house officers confirmed this observation. Internal medicine residents considered "sharing of the attending physician's thought processes" the most important quality of good clinical teachers, followed by bedside teaching and role modeling—all of which trumped in importance the citing of literature, which residents felt they could do on their own. See Analia Castiglioni, Richard M. Shewchuk, Lisa L. Willett et al., "A Pilot Study Using Nominal Group Technique to Assess Residents' Perceptions of Successful Attending Rounds," *J Gen Intern Med*, 23 (2008): 1060–65; and Brita Roy, Analia Castiglioni, Ryan R. Kramer et al., "Using Cognitive Mapping to Define Key Domains for Successful Attending Rounds," *J Gen Intern Med*, 27 (2012): 1492–98.

37. Kevin B. Weiss, James P. Bagian, and Thomas J. Nasca, "The Clinical Learning Environment: The Foundation of Graduate Medical Education," *JAMA*, 309 (2013): 1687–88, quotation, p. 1688.
38. Eric S. Holmboe, Rebecca Lipner, and Ann Greiner, "Assessing Quality of Care: Knowledge Matters," *JAMA*, 299 (2008): 338–40.
39. Abigail Zuger, "When a False God Plays Tricks on the Faithful," *NY Times*, August 10, 2004, p. D5; Brendan Reilly, "Physical Examination in the Care of Medical Inpatients: An Observational Study," *Lancet*, 362 (2003): 1100–1105.
40. Kevin W. Eva, Carol L. Link, Karen E. Lutfey, and John B. McKinlay, "Swapping Horses Midstream: Factors Related to Physicians' Changing Their Minds about a Diagnosis," *Acad Med*, 85 (2010): 1112–17.
41. Mark L. Graber, Robert M. Wachter, and Christine K. Cassel, "Bringing Diagnosis into the Quality and Safety Equations," *JAMA*, 308 (2012): 1211. Jerome Groopman, in *How Doctors Think: Clinical Judgment and the Practice of Medicine* (New York: Oxford University Press, 2005), also emphasized that most diagnostic errors made by physicians resulted from cognitive mistakes.
42. Meeting of December 13, 2001, Proceedings of the American Board of Medical Specialties, American Board of Medical Specialties Archives, Chicago, Ill.
43. Victor R. Fuchs, "Current Challenges to Academic Health Centers," *JAMA*, 310 (2013): 1021–22.
44. Kenneth M. Ludmerer, *Learning to Heal: The Development of American Medical Education* (New York: Basic Books, 1985).
45. To Nasca, like Pellegrino, professionalism could not be "faked." A doctor's motivations and values were important, not simply outward behaviors. He believed that if true professional values had not been internalized, a doctor's moral compass and automatic choices might lead to nonprofessional behaviors if certain temptations presented themselves (conversation with Thomas J. Nasca, February 2, 2013).
46. Thomas J. Nasca to author, July 9, 2013.

47. Tricia Johnson, Mitul Shah, John Rechner, and Gerald King, "Evaluating the Effect of Resident Involvement on Physician Productivity in an Academic General Internal Medicine Practice," *Acad Med*, 83 (2008): 670–74.
48. Many medical educators also believed it would help if Medicare GME funding flowed to the clinical departments responsible for running the residency programs and not to the hospital itself, as was the existing policy. Many hospitals used this revenue stream for other worthwhile purposes not necessarily directly related to the educational mission. For an expression of this view, see Cooke, Irby, and O'Brien, *Educating Physicians*, pp. 117, 256.
49. John K. Iglehart, "Medicare, Graduate Medical Education, and New Policy Directions," *N Engl J Med*, 359 (2008): 643–50; John K. Iglehart, "The Uncertain Future of Medicare and Graduate Medical Education," *N Engl J Med*, 365 (2011): 1340–45.
50. Presentation of Kathleen Klink at board meeting of the Accreditation Council for Graduate Medical Education, September 29, 2013.
51. Conversation with Graham McMahon, October 17, 2013 (quotation); Graham T. McMahon, Joel T. Katz, Mary E. Thorndike, Bruce D. Levy, and Joseph Loscalzo, "Evaluation of a Redesign Initiative in an Internal-Medicine Residency," *N Engl J Med*, 362 (2010): 1304–11.
52. Nada Ratanawongsa, Cynthia S. Rand, Cathleen F. Magill et al., "Teaching Residents to Know Their Patients as Individuals: The Aliki Initiative at Johns Hopkins Bayview Medical Center," *Pharos*, Summer 2009, pp. 4–11; quotation, p. 8. In addition, I visited the Aliki program and have discussed it extensively with its leaders.
53. Quoted in Ratanawongsa, Rand, Magill et al., "Teaching Residents," p. 10.
54. Stanley Shi-Dan Liu, "An Oasis in Time," *Ann Intern Med*, 153 (2010): 614.
55. Ratanawongsa, Rand, Magill et al., "Teaching Residents," p. 6.
56. Liu, "An Oasis in Time," p. 615.
57. Liu, "An Oasis in Time," p. 615.
58. Ratanawongsa, Rand, Magill et al., "Teaching Residents," p. 10.
59. R. Neal Axon and Mark V. Williams, "Hospital Readmission as an Accountability Measure," *JAMA*, 305 (2011): 504–5; Alan J. Forster, Harvey J. Murff, Josh F. Peterson et al., "The Incidence and Severity of Adverse Events Affecting Patients after Discharge from the Hospital," *Ann Intern Med*, 138 (2003): 161–67; Scott Harris, "Discussion Grows over Hospital Readmissions," *AAMC Reporter*, June 2009, pp. 1, 4. Many factors influenced readmission rates, but a core problem was achieving adequate control of a patient's condition prior to discharge, as well as making certain that patients were educated about their problems before going home.
60. Sandeep Jauhar, "That Ounce of Prevention Grew Too Big," *NY Times*, December 2, 2003, p. D5.
61. Gardiner Harris, "Talk Doesn't Pay, So Psychiatry Turns Instead to Drug Therapy," *NY Times*, March 6, 2011, section 1, pp. 1, 21.
62. Innumerable physicians who have been allocated shorter and shorter amounts of time for each patient by their practice plans have complained of the shrinking duration of office visits. David Mechanic, studying administrative data, has argued that the average time of office visits has diminished much less than popularly perceived. He acknowledged, however, that the perception of time pressure was realistic because there is much more for doctors to do. See David

Mechanic, Donna D. McAlpine, and Marsha Rosenthal, "Are Patients' Office Visits with Physicians Getting Shorter?," *N Engl J Med*, 344 (2001): 198–204.

63. "The Future of Health Care," *Harvard Magazine*, March–April 1999, p. 51.
64. Randi Hutter Epstein, "Major Medical Mystery: Why People Avoid Doctors," *NY Times*, October 31, 2000, p. D7; Dwain Hanson, letter to the editor, *NY Times*, March 17, 2004, p. A17.
65. Hanson, letter to the editor, p. A17.
66. Abigail Zuger, "Dissatisfaction with Medical Practice," *N Engl J Med*, 350 (2004): 69–75; Linda Gundersen, "Physician Burnout," *Ann Intern Med*, 135 (2001): 145–48.
67. Andrea Sikon and David L. Bronson, "Shared Medical Appointments: Challenges and Opportunities," *Ann Intern Med*, 152 (2010): 745–46; Barbara Martinez, "Now It's Mass Medicine," *Wall St J*, August 21, 2000, p. B1.
68. See, for instance, Deborah Franklin, "Patient Power: Making Sure Your Doctor Really Hears You," *NY Times*, August 15, 2006, p. D5; Laura Landro, "Talking Points: Making the Most of Doctor Visits," *Wall St J*, October 31, 2007, p. D1.
69. William Hoffman, "Fed Up, Some Doctors Turn to 'Boutique Medicine,'" *ACP-ASIM Observer*, October 2001, pp. 1, 12–13; Troyen A. Brennan, "Luxury Primary Care—Market Innovation or Threat to Access?," *N Engl J Med*, 346 (2009): 1165–68; Michael Stillman, "Concierge Medicine: A 'Regular' Physician's Perspective," *Ann Intern Med*, 152 (2010): 391–92; Thomas S. Huddle and Robert M. Centor, "Retainer Medicine: An Ethically Legitimate Form of Practice That Can Improve Primary Care," *Ann Intern Med*, 155 (2011): 633–35.
70. Catherine Lucey and Wiley Souba, "The Problem with the Problem of Professionalism," *Acad Med*, 85 (2010): 1018; Jordan J. Cohen, "Lessons from Managed Care," *AAMC Reporter*, September 2001, p. 2.
71. Charles M. Kilo and Eric B. Larson, "Exploring the Harmful Effects of Health Care," *JAMA*, 301 (2009): 89–91.
72. Vijay M. Rao and David C. Levin, "The Overuse of Diagnostic Imaging and the Choosing Wisely Initiative," *Ann Intern Med*, 157 (2012): 874–76.
73. Herbert L. Fred, "Drawbacks and Limitations of Computed Tomography," *Tex Heart I J*, 31 (2004): 345–48; Reza Fazel, Harlan M. Krumholz, Yongfei Wang et al., "Exposure to Low-Dose Ionizing Radiation from Medical Imaging Procedures," *N Engl J Med*, 361 (2009): 849–57; Rebecca Smith-Bindman, "Is Computed Tomography Safe?," *N Engl J Med*, 363 (2010): 1–4; Bruce J. Hillman and Jeff C. Goldsmith, "The Uncritical Use of High-Tech Medical Imaging," *N Engl J Med*, 363 (2010): 4–6. Some suggested that the use of medical imaging be regulated. See David J. Brenner and Hedvig Hricak, "Radiation Exposure from Medical Imaging: Time to Regulate?," *JAMA*, 304 (2010): 208–9.
74. John H. Stone, "Incidentalomas—Clinical Correlation and Translational Science Required," *N Engl J Med*, 354 (2006): 2748–49.
75. Laura Landro, "Hospitals Set Blueprint for a Better 'Healing Environment,'" *Wall St J*, March 21, 2007, p. D9; Rhonda L. Rundle and Christina Binkley, "America's Most Luxurious Hospitals," *Wall St J*, August 27, 1999, p. W1; David W. Kennedy, Sarah H. Kagan, Kelly Breenen Abramson et al., "Academic Medicine Amenities Unit: Developing a Model to Integrate Academic Medical Care with Luxury Hotel Services," *Acad Med*, 84 (2009): 185–91.
76. Institute of Medicine, *Crossing the Quality Chasm: A New Health System for the 21st Century* (Washington, D.C.: National Academy Press, 2001).

77. Wendy Levinson and Philip A. Pizzo, "Patient-Physician Communication: It's about Time," *JAMA*, 305 (2011): 1802.
78. Rosemary Gibson and Janardan Prasad Singh, *The Treatment Trap: How the Overuse of Medical Care Is Wrecking Your Health and What You Can Do to Prevent It* (Chicago: Ivan R. Dee, 2010), p. 20.
79. Gibson and Singh, *The Treatment Trap*, p. 18.
80. Pamela F. Gallin, *How to Survive Your Doctor's Care: Get the Right Diagnosis, the Right Treatment, and the Right Experts for You* (Washington, D.C.: LifeLine Press, 2003); Thomasine Kushner, ed., *Surviving Health Care: A Manual for Patients and Their Families* (New York: Cambridge University Press, 2010); Thomas A. Sharon, *Protect Yourself in the Hospital: Insider Tips for Avoiding Hospital Mistakes for Yourself or Someone You Love* (Chicago: Contemporary Books, 2004); Kevin J. Soden and Christine Dumas, *Special Treatment: How to Get the Same High-Quality Health Care Your Doctor Gets* (New York: Berkley Books, 2003).
81. Consumer's Union, *When to Say "Whoa!" to Doctors: A Guide to Common Tests and Treatments You Probably Don't Need* (Yonkers, N.Y.: Consumer's Union, 2011).
82. Susan Morse, "How to Survive a Hospital Stay," *St. Louis Post-Dispatch*, January 8, 2007, p. H1;Tara Parker-Pope, "How to Get Treated Like a Doctor without Going to Medical School," *Wall St J*, February 3, 2004, p. D1; Thomas G. Donlan, "Does the Doctor Work for You?," *Barron's*, May 29, 2000, p. 50; Ranit Mishori, "The Danger of Too Many Tests," *Parade*, July 6, 2008, p. 6; Laura Landro, "Knowing When to Say 'No' to Tests," *Wall St J*, February 13, 2003, p. D3; Steven Findlay, "How to Improve Your Care," *USA Today*, March 23, 2011, p. 8A.
83. Regina E. Herzlinger, "Where Are the Innovators in Health Care?," *Wall St J*, July 19, 2007, p. A15.
84. Arthur Kleinman, "From Illness as Culture to Caregiving as Moral Experience," *N Engl J Med*, 368 (2013): 1377. See also Leighton E. Cluff and Robert H. Binstock, eds., *The Lost Art of Caring: A Challenge to Health Professionals, Families, Communities, and Society* (Baltimore, Md.: Johns Hopkins University Press, 2001). To philosophers, genuine caring represented compassion and moral commitment, not merely polite phrases that could be memorized and expressed without meaning. For instance, Brendan M. Reilly criticized physicians who, though "unfailingly polite," tended to "pretend kindness," thereby offering "a smarmy sham of the real thing" (Reilly, "Inconvenient Truths about Effective Clinical Teaching," *Lancet*, 370 [2007]: 705–10; quotations, p. 710).
85. Tait D. Shanafelt, Sonja Boone, Litjen Tan et al., "Burnout and Satisfaction with Work-Life Balance among US Physicians Relative to the General US Population," *Arch Intern Med*, 172 (2012): 1377–85; Bruce E. Landon, James Reschovsky, and David Blumenthal, "Changes in Career Satisfaction among Primary Care and Specialist Physicians, 1997–2001," *JAMA*, 289 (2003): 442–49; Abigail Zuger, "Dissatisfaction with Medical Practice," *N Engl J Med*, 350 (2004): 69–75.
86. Eric B. Larson and Robert Reid, "The Patient-Centered Medical Home Movement: Why Now?," *JAMA*, 203 (2010): 1644–45.
87. Tait D. Shanafelt, "Enhancing Meaning in Work: A Prescription for Preventing Physician Burnout and Promoting Patient-Centered Care," *JAMA*, 302 (2009): 1339.
88. Arnold S. Relman, *A Second Opinion: Rescuing America's Health Care* (New York: Public Affairs, 2007);Arnold S. Relman, "The Health of Nations: Medicine and the Free Market," *New Republic*, March 7, 2005, pp. 23–30.

89. David Brooks, "The Three Cheers for Irving," *NY Times*, September 22, 2009, p. A27. Another classic representation of the idea that many important dilemmas afford no technical solution is Garrett Hardin, "The Tragedy of the Commons," *Science*, 162 (1968): 1243–48.
90. David J. Rothman, "Medical Professionalism—Focusing on the Real Issues," *N Engl J Med*, 342 (2000): 1284–86; quotations, p. 1284.
91. Quoted in "A Better Way to Practice Medicine?," *Harvard Magazine*, May–June 2000, p. 60.
92. The Physician Charter was published in 2002 by the American Board of Internal Medicine Foundation, the American College of Physicians Foundation, and the European Federation of Internal Medicine. Within a decade the Charter was endorsed by more than 130 organizations and translated into 12 languages (Christine K. Cassel, Virginia Hood, and Werner Bauer, "*A Physician Charter*: The 10th Anniversary," *Ann Intern Med*, 157 [2012]: 290–91).
93. This, of course, was easier said than done, but it spoke to the contributions that enlightened medical leaders might make. Both managed care and fee-for-service contained perverse financial incentives for doctors and hospitals—the former, to do too little; the latter, to do too much. In responding to financial incentives, doctors showed they were human, not mean. However, it did lead many to hope that incentives for appropriate care could be developed.
94. Michael E. Porter and Elizabeth Olmsted Treisberg, "How Physicians Can Change the Future of Health Care," *JAMA*, 297 (2007): 1103–11; quotation, p. 1103.
95. Eliot Freidson, *Professionalism: The Third Logic* (Chicago: University of Chicago Press, 2001).
96. Arnold S. Relman, "Doctors as the Key to Health Care Reform," *N Engl J Med*, 361 (2009): 1225–27; Jordan J. Cohen, "Unions Are Bad Medicine for Doctors," *Acad Med*, 74 (1999): 905.
97. Mark Schlesinger, "A Loss of Faith: The Sources of Reduced Political Legitimacy for the American Medical Profession," *Milbank Quart*, 80 (2002): 185–235; quotation, p. 189.
98. Daniel M. Fox and Howard Markel, "Is History Relevant to Implementing Health Reform?," *JAMA*, 303 (2010): 1749–50; quotations, p. 1749 ("contingency"), p. 1750 ("self-interest").
99. Rajat K. Gupta, "Recovery and Reform," *B Am Acad* [of Arts and Sciences], Spring 2010, pp. 15–18.
100. Rosemary A. Stevens, "Public Roles for the Medical Profession in the United States: Beyond Theories of Decline and Fall," *Milbank Quart*, 79 (2001): 327–53; quotation, p. 337.
101. Presentation of Darrell G. Kirch, The Flexner Report Centennial Symposium, University of Louisville School of Medicine, May 4, 2010.
102. Michael E. Whitcomb, "Medical Education Reform: Is It Time for a Modern Flexner Report?," *Acad Med*, 82 (2007): 1.
103. Presentation of Darrell G. Kirch, The Flexner Report Centennial Symposium, University of Louisville School of Medicine, May 4, 2010.
104. Jordan J. Cohen, "Realizing Our Quest for Meaning," *Acad Med*, 79 (2004): 464–68; quotations, p. 464.
105. Of course, service and elevating the standards of medical care have always been the traditional mission of academic medical centers, not chasing dollars or pursuing growth. The well-known business author Jim Collins pointed out that the

optimum size of an organization is not necessarily the maximum size. In *How the Mighty Fall*, he found that corporate failure was much more likely to result from overreaching than from complacency. Companies put themselves on the road to ruin by confusing "big" with "great," thereby overdiversifying and abandoning core values and capacities. The analogy with academic medical centers was clear. See Collins, *How the Mighty Fall: And Why Some Companies Never Give In* (New York: HarperCollins, 2009).

106. Eryn Brown, "Poll: Most Doctors Deny 'Major Responsibility' for Cutting Costs," *St. Louis Post-Dispatch*, July 28, 2013, p. A16.
107. Gibson and Singh, *The Treatment Trap*, p. 105.
108. I am personally aware of these cases, which occurred in the emergency room of a major academic medical center.
109. Donald M. Berwick and Andrew D. Hackbarth, "Eliminating Waste in US Health Care," *JAMA*, 307 (2012): 1513–16; quotations, p. 1513. Waste could sometimes be surprisingly difficult to define. For a discussion, see Henry J. Aaron, "Waste, We Know You Are Out There," *N Engl J Med*, 359 (2008): 1865–67.
110. Steven E. Weinberger, "Providing High-Value, Cost Conscious Care: A Critical Seventh General Competency for Physicians," *Ann Intern Med*, 155 (2011): 386–88.
111. David B. Reuben and Christine K. Cassel, "Physician Stewardship of Health Care in an Era of Finite Resources," *JAMA*, 306 (2011): 430–32; Sean Palfrey, "Daring to Practice Low-Cost Medicine in a High-Tech Era," *N Engl J Med*, 364 (2011): e21.
112. Christine K. Cassel and James A. Guest, "Choosing Wisely: Helping Physicians and Patients Make Smart Decisions about Their Care," *JAMA*, 307 (2012): 1801–2.
113. Peter J. Greco and John M. Eisenberg, "Changing Physicians' Practices," *N Engl J Med*, 329 (1993): 1271–74; Lee Goldman, "Changing Physicians' Behavior: The Pot and the Kettle," *N Engl J Med*, 322 (1990): 1524–25.
114. John M. Eisenberg, *Doctors' Decisions and the Cost of Medical Care* (Ann Arbor, Mich.: Health Administration Press, 1986).
115. An important discussion of this subject is Deborah Korenstein, Minal Kale, and Wendy Levinson, "Teaching Value in Academic Environments: Shifting the Ivory Tower," *JAMA*, 310 (2013): 1671–72.
116. Janet D. Record, Cynthia Rand, Colleen Christmas et al., "Reducing Heart Failure Readmissions by Teaching Patient-Centered Care to Internal Medicine Residents," *Arch Intern Med*, 171 (2011): 838–39.
117. "Responsible Ordering: How a Small Group Got Big Results in Reducing Unnecessary Testing," *Breakthrough*, Holiday 2012, pp. 12–13, 19.
118. Victor R. Fuchs, "Eliminating 'Waste' in Health Care," *JAMA*, 302 (2009): 2481.
119. Stevens, "Public Roles for the Medical Profession," p. 348.
120. Richard M. Schwartzstein, Gary C. Rosenfeld, Robert Hilborn, Saundra Herndon Oyewole, and Karen Mitchell, "Redesigning the MCAT Exam: Balancing Multiple Perspectives," *Acad Med*, 88 (2013): 560–67. This was the first change in the MCAT examination since 1991. A comparison of the 1991 and 2015 examinations is found in "AM Last Page: The MCAT Exam: Comparing the 1991 and 2015 Exams," *Acad Med*, 88 (2013): 737.
121. Kenneth M. Ludmerer, *Time to Heal: American Medical Education from the Turn of the Century to the Era of Managed Care* (New York: Oxford University Press, 1999).

INDEX

Italicized page numbers indicate a table on the designated page. Page numbers followed by "n" and another number indicate a reference to an endnote on the designated page. For example, 400n90 points to endnote 90 on page 400.